With warm regards
Bill [illegible]

MEDICAL COMETS

Scholarly Contributions
by Medical Undergraduates

Dr. William C. Gibson

Medical Comets

Scholarly Contributions by Medical Undergraduates

UBC Alumni Association
University of British Columbia

Printed in Canada on acid-free paper

ISBN 0-88865-541-X

Canadian Cataloguing in Publication Data

Gibson, William Carleton, 1913-
Medical Comets

Includes bibliographical references and index
ISBN 0-88865-541-X

1. Medicine—Research—History—Anecdotes. 2. Medical students—Anecdotes. I. University of British Columbia. Alumni Association. II. Title.
R850.G52 1997 610'.72 C97-910564-1

UBC Alumni Association
6251 Cecil Green Park Road
University of British Columbia
Vancouver, BC V6T 1Z1

"A professor can never better distinguish himself in his work than by encouraging a clever pupil, for the true discoverers are among them, as comets amongst stars."

— *Carolus Linnaeus* (1707 – 1778)

This book is dedicated
to friends of medical students
and, in particular:

Cecil H. Green, MS (MIT), DSc Hon (Oxford)
Honorary Knight of the British Empire
Founder of Green Colleges in Oxford and Vancouver

Sir Richard Doll, DM (Oxford) FRS, FRCP
Her Majesty's Companion of Honour
Regius Professor Emeritus of Medicine, and
First Warden of Green College, Oxford

Paul B. Beeson, MD CM (McGill) KBE (Hon) FRCP, FACP
Professor Emeritus of Medicine, Yale
Nuffield Professor Emeritus of Clinical Medicine, Oxford

Robert J. Glaser, MD (Harvard) FACP
Teacher, clinician, editor of the medical student journal *The Pharos*
Dean, Vice-President and Acting President, Stanford

Contents

Foreword

Purnell W. Choppin, M.D.
President, Howard Hughes Medical Institute

A revolution in molecular biology over the past several decades has transformed our understanding of human health and disease. We have learned a great deal about how cells form the developing embryo and how our brains think and remember. We have identified the genes responsible for many inherited diseases, determined the three dimensional structure of the gene products, and correlated structure with function. We have a far better understanding of numerous medical problems, such as how certain viruses overcome the immune system and how genetic defects lead to the uncontrolled cell growth of cancer. This growing body of knowledge, in turn, has begun to yield important advances in clinical care, from new diagnostic procedures to the molecular design of pharmaceuticals.

One by-product of medical progress has been increasing specialization in biomedical research and clinical care. In the past, most research was carried out by physician-scientists, who moved easily between their laboratories and their patients' bedsides, searching for new ways to overcome problems they knew well from personal experience. Increasingly, however, it has become harder for physicians to achieve and retain expertise in both research and patient care. Many of those on the frontiers of medical research today are not physicians who deal with patients but scientists whose advanced training is biology and related disciplines. They are Ph.D.s or M.D./Ph.D.s and may work with fruit flies, worms or other model organisms rather than humans. Indeed, many researchers never see patients, although they rightly regard their efforts as essential to medical progress.

This increasing specialization within medical research has yielded a rich harvest of biological knowledge. Yet, for all its power and sophistication, medicine continues to be built on a foundation of patients and physicians. Far from being marginalized by the advent of molecular biology, physician scientists have become more important than ever before. They have a unique perspective on what is important in medical research, an expertise that exceeds the sum of their clinical and scientific skills. It is essential to the future of medicine that talented medical students be encouraged to undertake research. Indeed, this interest should be nurtured before they enter medical school, when they are undergraduates or even earlier.

The Howard Hughes Medical Institute has made a substantial commitment to the research training of medical students and physicians. One of these programs enables talented physicians with clinical experience to spend three years in full time basic research. Another program provides medical students with support to take a year off from their studies to receive training in research in their own institutions, and a third supports a program in which medical students spend a year carrying out research at the National Institutes of Health. These and other grants programs designed to enhance science education at every level from elementary school to graduate school. They complement the Institute's primary mission which is the support of biomedical research by approximately 300 outstanding scientists who are investigators located at over 60 medical school, universities and research institutes across the United States.

William Gibson has exemplified the best tradition of physician scientists throughout his own distinguished career. In *Medical Comets*, he reminds us in a remarkable way of the many contributions to medical progress that undergraduates and medical students have made over the centuries. With hundreds of examples, he shows how young scientists in college or medical school are capable of making important discoveries and clinical advances. His narrative covers not only familiar names such as Salvador Luria, Joshua Lederberg, Francois Jacob and other Nobel laureates of the past few decades, but others who also began making their mark at an early age. Also noted are physicians who gained fame in other arenas—writers such as Arthur Conan Doyle, poets such as John Keats and public health leaders such as Florence Sabin. In his conclusion, Gibson discusses why some medical students and undergraduates exhibit such proficiency at research, and what can be done to encourage the same interest in others.

If such encouragement is needed—and it is—it can be found here in *Medical Comets*. The stories told in the following pages make clear that research and clinical practice must coexist and are often guided into the future by our youngest scientists. Dr. Gibson gives us every reason to expect that today's students, like comets in the night sky, will be the next blazing lights to guide us beyond medicine's horizons.

Introduction

The appearance of *Young Endeavour*[1] some years ago caused a modest flurry of excitement among both medical students and their teachers. Professor John Fulton at Yale's Historical Library of the School of Medicine complained that it was the most frequently purloined book in an otherwise well-regulated storehouse of interesting works. As time went on the author received, from his contemporaries, emotional requests for a volume with the suggested title *Old Endeavour*. That must wait.

What follows in this new volume is a further account of the application of youthful "gray matter" to medical conundrums. Not all, or even many, of these triumphs have been earth-shaking, but they often foreshadowed great contributions later in life. Today it is a new climate that greets potential discoverers, as annual meetings of medical student investigators are held. This is especially so as the world's largest medical foundation, the Howard Hughes Medical Institute, under the enlightened presidency of Dr. Purnell Choppin, rallies to the support of a full year's research, or a Ph.D. acquisition by medical undergraduates who then return to their M.D. course. There is no limit to the benefits that await us.

The earth is degenerating these days. Bribery and corruption abound. Children no longer mind their parents. Every man wants to write a book and it is evident that the end of the world is fast approaching.
Assyrian tablet,
2800 B.C.

The truth is that the community is an aggregate of many members; and education is therefore the means of making it a community and giving it unity.
Aristotle,
384-322 B.C.

If no use were to be made of the labors of past ages the world must remain in the infancy of knowledge.
Cicero, 106-43 B.C.

The future for medical researchers becomes bright as, each year, trustees of foundations and other accumulations of capital realize the human potential that can be unlocked for the common good. An outstanding example is the Hannah Institute for the History of Medicine in Toronto, whose founder, Dr. Jason Hannah, once a neuropathologist at the Banting Institute at the University of Toronto, became the effective custodian of considerable Ontario Blue Cross funds when Canada's health system assumed the burden of hospitalization. With his enthusiastic directors, Hannah established one professorship in the history of medicine in each of Ontario's five medical schools, and has since provided fellowships for undergraduates seeking to devote part of their studies to medical historical research.

A generous bequest to the Medical Society of London by Sir John McNee is providing assistance to medical undergraduates in the London hospitals to pursue, during elective periods in their courses, important investigations. The best descriptions of such work are communicated to that ancient society and may be published in its *Transactions*. The bequest by a remarkable physician, Dr. Norah Schuster, to the Royal Society of Medicine in London continues to bring out the latent research and literary abilities of medical undergraduates anywhere in Britain.

A certain latitude has been exercised in this volume in describing some of our students as undergraduates, because some had their student careers interrupted by wars, illness, or misdirected efforts en route to their medical qualification.

We tend to meet any situation by re-organizing—and a wonderful method it may be for creating the illusion of progress, while producing confusion, inefficiency and demoralization.
Petronius Arbiter, First Century A.D.

The gods do not subtract from the allotted span of men's lives the hours spent in fishing.
Assyrian tablet, 2000 B.C.

The greatest liberation of thought achieved by the scientific revolution was to have given human beings a sense of a future in this world.
Sir Peter Medawar

Medical student societies have, over the centuries, provided to their members a forum for the presentation of new ideas backed up by their own research. The oldest medical society in the English-speaking world, the Royal Medical Society, inaugurated by the medical students at the University of Edinburgh in 1737, continues to this day to give medical students an audience for early descriptions of their investigations.

Slightly later, 1780, at Oxford, six medical students founded the Medical Society of Oxford, "a body for the promotion of medical knowledge in these walls." Oxford later fell upon such sad times that in some years only two students graduated from its "lost medical school." This, however, is in marked contrast to the flourishing medical school that has developed since the Lord Nuffield benefactions of 1936, and its postwar blossoming. It is today one of the world's top medical research and teaching establishments with 100 students graduating each year. The munificence of Dr. and Mrs. Cecil Green has produced a college at the Radcliffe Observatory (1772) which, among many other benefits, has offered housing to students completing their required 33 months of clinical work but whose undergraduate colleges can no longer accommodate them.

As medicine became more scientifically based, the work by undergraduates became less descriptive than it had been (in anatomy, for instance), and now tends to be concentrated on analytical work in the fields of biochemistry, physiology and pathology. From its inception, that talented group of pioneers at Johns Hopkins Hospital Medical School in Baltimore, openly encouraged their highly motivated students to research a problem during their four years of medical tuition. I say openly, for in some schools such practices were frowned on as being off track, frivolous, or designed to detract from the reputation of the professoriate.

The division of the contributions made by medical undergraduates into categories or principal subject fields is an ever-present problem, since some students made discoveries or at least advances in one field, only to be remembered for very different reasons in later years. To a degree it has been possible to describe their student work in rough chronological order, but nothing more.

It is hoped that the evidence adduced here will lead to more opportunities being opened to undergraduates in the health sciences to make contributions to knowledge and culture, from which our world can surely benefit.

Thus, as we begin a survey of further contributors we can be assured that history not only repeats itself, but that the recent and present student contributors are multiplied at an amazing and inspiring rate.

We can but agree with William Osler's view, expressed in his farewell address of 1905 as he left Johns Hopkins Medical School to become Regius Professor at Oxford: "Upon our heels a fresh perfection must tread, born of us, fated to excel us."

[1] William C. Gibson (Springfield, IL: Charles C. Thomas, 1959).

Medical Comets

Scholarly Contributions
by Medical Undergraduates

CHAPTER ONE

Anaesthetics

The history of surgical anaesthesia is the history of a discovery waiting to be made. From the experiments of the 19-year-old German medical student **Valerius Cordus** (1515-1544) using ether (which he synthesized from alcohol and sulphuric acid), to the 20th-century medical student work of J. Bailey Carter on ethylene, there are unrelated moments of hope. But until W.T.G. Morton's 1846 demonstration of ether as a reliable surgical anesthetic, there were more scattered shots at that target than there was hope. Information about ether, nitrous oxide, carbon dioxide and other agents was published sporadically, but in the three centuries from Cordus to Morton historians see the lack of application of these close calls—these brushes with the real world of unrelieved pain. The point was made in *Young Endeavour* that the role of medical students in the development of anaesthesia has been both key and exemplary.

As Sir Henry Dale, O.M., noted in his foreword to that volume, no one could "yet have found any reason for predicting the dimensions, still less the special direction, of the mature achievement that was yet to come" from early flashes of investigative genius, occasionally supplied with an excess of serendipity.[1]

Cordus' ether was noted by the peripatetic Swiss physician-alchemist, Paracelsus (Theophrastus Bombastus von Hohenheim, 1493?-1541), who found that chickens enjoyed its taste to such a degree that they would eat grain moistened with it until they were rendered unconscious. As the effect wore off, they would return unharmed to their former normal state. And yet no one then thought of surgical anaesthesia.

More than a century later ether was synthesized by two famous amateurs, Robert Boyle (1680) and Sir Isaac Newton (1704).

In 1718 medical student Johannes Bernard Quistorp (1692-1761), son of a Rostock pharmacist, wrote his graduation thesis at Leipzig, introducing the term "anaesthesia," and discussed its seven usages. The first was "*denegato sensationis per totum corporis*," in which there was no discernible effect on individual organs, respiration or pulse.

The name—aether—was contributed by the physician-chemist Frobenius in 1730. In 1743 its application on small pledgets of linen was recommended by Matthew Turner (a founder of the Warrington Academy) to treat headache, but no more general application was suggested.

Now the pendulum swings away from ether and towards nitrous oxide, the gas discovered by the Reverend Joseph Priestley in 1772, two years before he discovered oxygen. He was not long in promoting the idea that diseases of the lungs might be treated with various gases. By 1794 the physician and deposed professor of chemistry at Oxford, Thomas Beddoes, had an unusual pneumatic institution up and running at Bristol. With the help of James Watt of teakettle fame, Beddoes published a book on "factitious airs" and provided the setting for the discovery of nitrous oxide anaesthesia by the Cornish medical student Humphry Davy. Within six months of his arrival, Davy was manufacturing nitrous oxide and examining its cerebral effects on a remarkable group of volunteers such as Dr. Peter Mark Roget, of thesaurus fame, Tom Wedgwood, Richard Brinsley Sheridan, Robert Southey, the poet, Samuel Taylor Coleridge, Priestley's son and Watt's consumptive son. Davy was consuming nitrous oxide to relieve both his toothache and headache with repeated inhalations. (Beddoes acknowledged that as early as 1731 the Reverend Stephen Hales had an interest in this subject as well as in the measurement of blood pressure.)

Humphry Davy (1778-1829), the medical student, had little chance of continuing his indenture that he had begun with Dr. Borlase in Cornwall, nor of fulfilling his graduation requirements at Cambridge, so busy was he with his research. He published, in 1800, his soon-to-be-famous work on nitrous oxide and its respiration. He had no sooner completed this work, which clearly adumbrated nitrous oxide anaesthesia, than he prepared a paper read to the Royal Society of London on his development of a battery composed of 50 copper plates alternating with weak solutions of nitrous oxide and "sulphuret of potash." Davy commented that his device produced "pretty strong shocks," and "evolved gas from water."

Davy is best remembered for his farsighted remark in his classic *Researches, Chemical and Philosophical, Chiefly Concerning Nitrous Oxide*: "As nitrous oxide in its extensive operation appears capable of destroying physical pain, it may probably be used with advantage during surgical operations in which no great effusion of blood takes place."

Beddoes and Watt recalled the work of Richard Pearson (1765-1836) of Birmingham, in which ether was inhaled by tuberculous patients. Pearson's own observations were published when he was 30; in them, he described the use of "vapours of aether" in "consumptives."

In 1805 the ether story shifts to John Dalton, of atomic theory fame. He did not publish his work until 1820. By then the nitrous oxide pot was boiling, and a medical student at the University of Pennsylvania, **William P. C. Barton** (1786-1856), had written in 1808, "A Dissertation on the Chymical Properties and Exhilarating Effects of Nitrous Oxide Gas; and its Application to Pneumatick Medicine; Submitted as an Inaugural Thesis for the Degree of Medicine." At the age of 21 he repeated Davy's experiments with nitrous oxide and gave even more vivid descriptions of the results than those written by Coleridge or Southey. He speculated, but nothing more, on its possible use in medicine and surgery but did not grasp Davy's clearly stated notion of nitrous oxide as a general anesthetic. He mentioned that it had reduced the pain of his own head injury. Barton became the first chief of the Bureau of Medicine and Surgery of the U.S. Navy.

It were disgraceful, therefore, did we take the reports of others upon trust, and go on coining crude problems out of these, and on them hanging knotty and captious and petty disputations. Nature herself is to be addressed; the paths she shows us are to be boldly trodden; for thus, and whilst we consult our proper senses... shall we penetrate at length into the heart of her mystery.
William Harvey

For many reasons it is desirable that a medical student be conducted early in his career to the front line trenches of medical and physiological discovery. Let him realize that men as young as himself have made important contributions: that de Graaf at 23 years of age devised the first pancreatic fistula; that Helmholtz at 24 measured for the first time the heat production of frog muscle; that Johannes Müller at 25 had enunciated the principles of specific nerve energies. Let him discover that simple facts were once hidden in a fog of faulty observation and faulty reasoning, and that it was sometimes the enquiring minds of students like himself that made matters clear.
John Farquhar Fulton, 1930

Not long after he entered the U.S. Navy, Barton wrote: "A Treatise Containing a Plan for the Internal Organization and Government of the Marine Hospitals in the United States, Together with Observations on Military and Flying Hospitals and a Scheme for Amending and Systematizing the Medical Department of the Navy." The Secretary of the Navy was pleased with Barton's recommendations, but the Medical Department was not. Eighteen months later Barton wrote to the U.S. President of his "earnest wish... to retire from the scene of unavailing efforts."

His student years had seen the highly respected Benjamin Rush lecturing to medical students on ether. Rush asked his listeners concerning ether: "Might we not induce coma to a low degree of apoplexy in order to bear long operations and parturition well?" Rush's lectures for the 1815-1816 winter session have been preserved in a student's notebook.

No uniformity in life is found:—
In ev'ry scene varieties abound;
And inconsistency still marks the plan
Of that immortal noble being, Man,
As changeful as the April's morning skies,

His feeling and his sentiments arise;
And nature to his wond'rous frame has given
The mingled elements of earth and heaven.
In diff'rent climes and ages, still we find
The same events for diff'rent ends design'd;

And the same passion diff'rent minds can move
To thoughts of sadness or to acts of love,
Hence Genius draws his novel copious store;
And hence the new creations we adore:
And hence the scenic art's undying skill

Submits our feeling to its potent will;
From common accidents and common themes
Awakens rapture and poetic dreams;
And, in the trodden path of life, pursues
Some object cloth'd in Fancy's loveliest hues—

Humphry Davy,
from his prologue to *The Honey Moon* produced at Drury Lane,
January 30, 1805

The brilliant Philadelphia physician-chemist, James Woodhouse (1770-1809) was also lecturing at the university on nitrous oxide. One of his students, Benjamin Silliman, continued the interest in this gas on assuming the chair of chemistry at Yale University. The ether team was not silent either, as noted by George Bacon Wood, who graduated at Pennsylvania in 1818: "I remember well that it was quite the fashion among the boys in Philadelphia to inhale ether for its intoxicating effect." After the death of one subject the practice ceased, at least temporarily.

Back across the Atlantic in Britain, the ether devotees included Michael Faraday, who began life as a bookbinder's assistant; he read the volumes he was binding and went on to be Humphry Davy's right hand. He was familiar with the value of ether in alleviating pain, and is thought to have been the author of an unsigned note in 1818 in the *Quarterly Journal of Sciences and the Arts*, which stated: "A gentleman was thrown into a very lethargic state, which continued with occasional periods of intermission for more than thirty hours." Dale confirms that "Michael Faraday was later to observe the effects of ether and to recommend it as having advantages for such purposes over nitrous oxide ...some twenty-eight years before its practical application by Morton in Boston."

The county of Shropshire has long boasted of two medical innovators, **William Withering** (1775-1832), of digitalis fame, and **Henry Hill Hickman** (1800-1829), who introduced carbon dioxide as an anaesthetic agent. At the age of 24 Hickman published the results of his researches on its use in painless surgery on animals who had inhaled it in concentrated form. His pamphlet, "A Letter on Suspended Animation" received no attention from surgeons and in fact Sir Humphry Davy, President of the Royal Society of London, snubbed him completely.

As a result, Hickman appeared before the Académie de Médecine in Paris on October 21, 1828, to describe his work to an evaluating committee. Of that group only Baron Larrey, Napoleon's surgeon, took the matter seriously, so seriously that he offered to be Hickman's first human subject. Nothing came of his presentation in Paris. Hickman returned to Britain a broken man and reportedly died of tuberculosis within the year.

Crawford Long (1815-1878) had inhaled ether as a student at Pennsylvania and provided it for student revels in Jefferson, Georgia, where he set up his general practice. He administered this volatile agent to one of those former revellers, James Venable, in order to remove a small tumour from his neck on March 30, 1842. Unfortunately, Long did not publish this fact until 1848, but his account book clearly reflects the 1842 event. To return to the year 1842, a second tumour was removed from the patient later in that year and a toe was removed from a boy in the same year by Long.

However, two months prior to this, a student at the Berkshire College of Medicine, William Clarke, after experimenting on his classmates, used ether to successfully anaesthetize a Miss Hobbie while her dentist, Dr. Elijah Pope, painlessly removed a tooth.

Crawford Long has been handsomely remembered at the University of Pennsylvania, where in 1912 a memorial medallion by the Canadian physician-sculptor, R. Tait McKenzie, was unveiled. The inscription reads: "To Crawford Long. First to use ether as an anesthetic in surgery, March 30, 1842. From his alma mater."

The historic administration of ether anaesthesia by the Harvard student **William Thomas Green Morton** (1819-1868), on October 16, 1846, changed the way surgery was to be done around the globe. In the five years previously there had been only 184 operations at the Massachusetts General Hospital, possibly because of the pain involved for patients, but Professor John Collins Warren, age 68 in the fateful year of 1846, was open-minded enough to permit the dentist-turned-medical student to show what ether could do. The successful anaesthesia that Morton provided, before a packed surgical theatre, was soon communicated to the world by the orthopaedist Henry Jacob Bigelow, who as a student had produced a different agent—nitrous oxide—at Harvard College. Before sending his eyewitness account of "Ether Day" to the *Boston Medical and Surgical Journal*, he carefully checked it with Dr. Oliver Wendell Holmes, who like Bigelow had been a winner of the Boylston Essay Prize on graduation from Harvard Medical School. Bigelow's paper on the October 16 revolution was published on November 18, 1846.

Morton was no flash-in-the-pan student. He had investigated beforehand the effect of ether on fish, insects, his spaniel dog and himself. He was a skilled dentist who had studied dentistry with Horace Wells in Hartford, Connecticut (the luckless pioneer in nitrous oxide anaesthesia). Morton, though, was so bogged down with litigation and notoriety after "Ether Day" that he never completed medical school.

The news quickly flew to London where the surgeon Robert Liston employed ether given by Mr. Squire, a medical student, to anaesthetize a patient whose leg had to be amputated. Students at University College, including Joseph Lister and his classmate Joseph Clover (of later anesthetic fame) must have been astounded by the highly successful outcome. Their report describing the proceedings said of the patient: "Presently he awoke, and when the cloth was removed from his stump, and he saw that his leg was gone, the unbounded wonder and delight of the patient was scarcely greater than that of the spectators." Liston, schooled in pre-anaesthetic days, had amputated the leg in 30 seconds!

There is one ghost that continues to haunt this whole subject of medical students' role in anaesthesia and it concerns Caleb Bentley Matthews. He graduated from the University of Pennsylvania Medical Faculty in 1824 having presented his thesis, "On Inhalation of Ether" in that year. Sadly, this thesis, bound with others of the same date, cannot be found by the university authorities. It predated Morton's demonstra-

Like the tumultuous billows of the sea
Succeed the generations of mankind;
Some in oblivious silence pass away,
And leave no vestige of their lives behind.

Others, like those proud waves which beat the shore,
A loud and momentary murmur raise;
But soon their transient glories are no more.
No future ages echo with their praise.

Like you proud rock, amidst the sea of time,
Superior, scorning all the billows' rage,
The living Sons of Genius stand sublime,
The immortal children of another age.

For those exist whose pure ethereal minds,
Imbibing portions of celestial day,
Scorn all terrestrial cares, all mean designs,
As bright-eyed eagles scorn the lunar ray.

Theirs is the glory of a lasting name,
The meed of Genius, and her living fire;
Theirs is the laurel of eternal fame,
And theirs the sweetness of the muse's lyre.
Humphry Davy,
from *The Sons of Genius*

tion by 22 years. A.C.R. Callisen's *Medical Bibliography*, published in Copenhagen in 1832, specifically refers to Matthews' work. Not only did his thesis disappear, but Matthews himself disappeared into the Homeopathic Medical College of Pennsylvania, where he taught materia medica and therapeutics, dying at age 50, strangely unsung.

In the succeeding century, modifications in the technique of administering anaesthetics abounded and gradually new chemical agents were developed. A medical student at the University of Chicago, J. Bailey Carter, working with Professor A.B. Luckhardt in physiology, did yeoman service in establishing a new gas and anaesthetic, ethylene.

It all began with the reported losses suffered by flower growers whose carnations, shipped into Chicago and placed in greenhouses heated with illuminating gas, "went to sleep." It was found that four per cent of the gas was ethylene and that this was the culprit.

Over the years ethylene was shown to be a non-toxic anaesthetic agent when administered to frogs, white rats, dogs, guinea pigs, white mice and rabbits. It was compared in its effects with other well-known agents. Eventually a medical student, J.B. Carter, inhaled ethylene briefly, with no untoward effects. Professor Luckhardt was next, to be followed by the distinguished surgeon Dallas B. Phemister and his colleague Eugene Cary.

Next, this anaesthetic was repeated on the professor six times spread over three weeks. Bailey's anaesthesia was compressed into seven sessions in the same period, Sunday being the preferred day for these trials. Appropriately, their conclusion was: "No late or evil effects were in evidence." Carter must have been relieved to graduate in 1924!

Local anaesthesia became the subject of later research, such as that carried out at the Karolinska Hospital in Stockholm by two young chemists. In his inaugural dissertation in 1948, Nils Löfgren described the new synthetic drug "Xylocaine," which he and his colleague Bengt Lundquist had perfected with the help of the Wallenberg Foundation. Löfgren praised Lundquist for carrying out the first human trials "in heroic experiments on himself." They described the effectiveness of Xylocaine on body surfaces, and noted its great stability in water as well as its use without the necessity of epinephrine, especially in hand surgery.

Dental surgery, which started so much research into anaesthesia, had come full circle, more than a century later, with a new synthetic agent.

Youthful contributors range all the way from Valerius Cordus in 1540 to Wells, who wrote a book on the teeth at age 23 and recorded the use of nitrous oxide on himself at age 29, to Faraday, who was 26 when he published "On Ether," to Henry Hickman, who experimented on carbon dioxide anaesthesia at age 24, and to Marguerite-Louise Baur, the Zurich medical student, who under the supervision of Professor Henry Sigerist wrote her 1927 graduation dissertation on her research in the laboratory on the soporifics of the past, now tested by her on frogs.

Not to be outdone, Yale medical undergraduates were also stirring in the field of anaesthesia, and in 1910 a paper by **Herbert Thoms** (1885-1972), an undergraduate, was published under the title "A New Apparatus for the Administration of Rectal and Pharyngeal Anesthesia." His teacher, Dr. J.M. Flint, who had been an undergraduate researcher at

Johns Hopkins under Osler, suggested that Thoms investigate the problem facing the anaesthetist in certain types of regional surgery. Thoms designed and built his own apparatus, which is very well illustrated in his undergraduate paper.

Two Harvard medical students who became concerned with the lax manner in which ether was being administered, **Harvey Cushing** (1869-1939) and **Amory Codman** (1869-1940), devised an "Ether Chart." Medical students had been used to monitor patients under anaesthesia and there were some fatal consequences. Cushing and Codman introduced a chart for each surgical patient on which respiration, pulse and temperature were regularly recorded during the operation. Together they prepared a paper sharply critical of the methods then in use and the hospital authorities were greatly upset. In fact, they persuaded Cushing and Codman that they had better not publish the paper. However, what they did in its preparation had a successful outcome and after their endeavour the unconscious patient received far more attention. Harvey Cushing persisted and six years later brought back to the United States from Italy a modification of Riva-Rocci's pressure-measuring apparatus so that systolic and diastolic pressures could be recorded on the anaesthetic charts in addition to the other data that they had already prescribed.

[1] Attributed to Horace Walpole, 1754, to describe the three Princes of Serendip (Ceylon) "making discoveries by accident or sagacity, of things they were not in quest of."

When I was a boy I wanted to know about the clouds and the grasses, and why the leaves changed colour in the autumn; I watched the ants, bees, birds, tadpoles and cadis worms; I pestered people with questions about what nobody knew or cared anything about.
John Hunter

CHAPTER TWO

Anatomy

The *Fabrica* of 1543 is the first modern work of a creator. Not that Vesalius created the science of human anatomy—that was done by the Alexandrians--but he remade it. Here and there are original observations and keen comments but all are the work of transmuters or transmitters. To appreciate what he did, compare the beggarly treatises of his predecessors in the sixteenth century and others, with the royal volume of the 'Fabrica.' We enter a new world. To have completed before his twenty-ninth year a task of this magnitude, at such a period when dissections were difficult to make and authority difficult to resist, is a feat to which the literary history of the profession offers no parallel. In itself, for what it contains, but still more for what it did, the 'Humani corporis fabrica' is one of the great books of the world with which in the literature of Medicine only the 'De motu cordis' of Harvey is to be compared. The one revolutionized anatomy the other created modern physiology. This work of Vesalius is the first modern treatise on anatomy based upon dissections of the human body. To appreciate the extraordinary character of the descriptions and of the plates they must be compared with contemporary works. Vesalius really described the body as we know it, for the first time fully and for the first time accurately. It is difficult to say whether in text or figure the departure from the anatomy of the day is the more striking. There are grave mistakes of omission and of commission but they appear insignificant in a volume full of such

Andreas Vesalius (1514-1564)

Modern medicine owes much to Andreas Vesalius who published the first great text on human anatomy since the Christian era began. His contribution stands with that of William Harvey in the magnitude of its influence on science.

Vesalius was born in 1514 in Brussels. His father was court pharmacist to King Charles V, whom he accompanied on journeys throughout his vast kingdom. His grandfather was a court physician who wrote a commentary on Rhazes, the great Arab clinician (860-962). His great-grandfather was physician to Emperor Maximilian's wife. His great-great-grandfather was also a physician and wrote a discourse on the works of Avicenna (980-1036), the physician-geologist of Bagdad. Vesalius wrote a book of commentaries himself, also on the "Ninth Book of Rhazes," as his baccalaureate dissertation. Vesalius was still in the medieval tradition of Arabic medicine, but he was to make his mark as a humanist, a student of Galen, before he became the first modern anatomist himself. He thus represents all three stages in his own course of development.

As a comparatively young boy Andreas showed an interest in anatomy, dissecting rats, cats and dogs and in studying a skeleton retrieved from gallows not far from his home. His preliminary studies in the classics were made at Louvain under Johann Guenther of Andernach, later to be his teacher of anatomy in Paris.

When a medical student in Paris, Vesalius relied on the Cemetery of the Innocents at Montfaucon for a supply of bones. At times he had to compete for those bones with vicious dogs. His other outstanding teacher in Paris was Jacobus Sylvius, later to be his severest critic. It is known that Vesalius was an extremely hard worker in his student days in Paris. Guinterius Andernacus wrote of Vesalius, "a young man, by Jove, of great promise, possessing a singular knowledge of medicine, erudite in both languages [Latin and Greek] and most skilled in dissecting bodies."[1]

Vesalius came to Paris already knowing human anatomy. His knowledge was superimposed upon the emotional background of a potential rebel—and it was not long before he was in full revolt against what he saw in Paris, as his words suggest:

> The lecturers are perched up in a pulpit like jackdaws, and arrogantly prate about things they have never tried, but have committed to memory from the books of others, or placed in written form before their eyes. The dissectors are so ignorant of language that they are unable to explain their dissections to the onlookers and merely botch what they are supposed to exhibit in accordance with the instructions of the physician, who never applies his hand to the dissection, but contemptuously steers the ship out of the manual, as the saying goes. Thus everything is wrongly taught, days are wasted in absurd questions, and in the confusion less is offered to the onlooker than a butcher in his stall could teach a doctor.
>
> Except for eight muscles of the abdomen, disgracefully mangled and in the wrong order, no one... ever demonstrated to me any single muscle, or any single bone, much less the network of nerves, veins and arteries.

After witnessing two incompetent dissections, Vesalius jumped into the third one—done on a dog—to show his fellow students the true and beautiful "fabric of the body," to be followed by many more such demonstrations.

In 1536 a war with France was brewing, so he returned to his home in Louvain to serve in the army. He carried on further anatomizing and during 1537 published his dissertation on Rhazes, "*De singulum corporis partium affectuum curatione*," printed in Louvain by his friend of Paris days, Rutger Resch, and reprinted in Basel by Robert Winter. This he dedicated to his friend and patron Nicolaus Florenas, physician to the Emperor. With the same spiritual broom used on Galen he began his re-editing of Rhazes, then "cleansed of errors and clothed in elegant Latin style." One is reminded of the service performed somewhat earlier by another purgative spirit, Lorenzo Valla, in his "Elegant Latin Language" (1476).[2]

In the same year (1537) Vesalius sought the liberal atmosphere of Padua, near the free-trading and free-thinking city of Venice. He graduated as Doctor of Medicine at Padua on December 5 and was made professor of anatomy and surgery the next day. Within four months, and with the help of his friend Calcar, a Belgian pupil of Titian, he raised some eyebrows as he published six *Tabulae Anatomicae* for his students. He did the dissections himself and this fact brought large numbers of students to see and hear him. Three of the studies were drawn by him of dissections of the blood vessels, and the other three were by the artist Stefen van Calcar. Only six months after taking up his Chair, and in order to provide his students with an interim text, he personally re-edited his teacher Guinterius' *Institutiones Anatomicae* (a commentary on Galen), published in May 1538.

Vesalius' publications now began to pyramid in a truly amazing manner. In 1539, at the age of 25, he published his *Epistola Docens* on venesection, which was a commentary on the feud between those in favour of blood-letting on the side of the body torn with disease, as against those holding the opposite view.

He then turned to Galen's texts, three volumes of which he edited for the Venetian publishers Giunta.[3] However, in 1540, convinced that he must put down a record of his own findings in human dissections, he

important contributions. To the middle of the sixteenth century anatomy was taught from the writings of Galen, not from what was seen in the public dissections. From what the great Master had written there was no appeal and the veneration with which his works were regarded were as for a gospel, like the feeling men have towards the sacred Scriptures. Imagine the surprise of the easy-going old professors who held the chairs of anatomy to have a huge volume thrust into their hands filled from cover to cover with descriptions and figures with which they were unfamiliar. And written by a young man of twenty-eight! Headed by his old teacher Sylvius a storm of opposition soon raged, and a vindication of Galen was attempted, but it was soon found that the old anatomy, correct enough in places, was largely that of swine, dogs and monkeys, while the 'Fabrica' contained descriptions and figures from human dissections. To understand the phenomenon, almost unique in the history of science, of a revolution of this character effected by so young a man, we must remember that from boyhood Vesalius had a perfect passion for dissecting. After devoting his energies to the anatomy of the domestic animals, he robbed graveyards and gallows for human skeletons, while as early as 1534-36 as prosector to Sylvius and Guinterius in Paris he had opportunities to dissect the human body. His reputation must have been remarkable, as at the age of twenty-three he was appointed Professor at Padua, one of the leading schools of Europe. The 'Fabrica' remains a monument of human effort, one of the greatest in the history of our profession.

William Osler, written in the *Fabrica*, which he sent to McGill University from Rome in 1909.

started to write his 700-page *De Fabrica Humani Corporis*, which he completed in August 1542. His publishing, though overpowering, did not prevent his continuing to teach anatomy from human dissections. What Vesalius was doing for students at the dissecting table, his Paduan pupil Montanus was to do eventually for medical student-teaching at the bedside. The virulent criticism that descended upon Vesalius caused him to burn his manuscripts and leave Padua, where he had made such a great contribution. He went to the Spanish court of the marauding Charles V and his son Phillip II. After an absence of 17 years Vesalius wrote a letter to his successor Fallopius at Padua regretting his remove from the academic life—"that most delightful life, which, teaching anatomy, I passed in Italy, the true nurse of intellect.... I look forward to see the ornaments of our science continue to bud forth in the school from which I was, while yet a youngster, dragged away to the dull routine of medical practice and to the worries of continual journeys." No more complete isolation from his old subject can be imagined than that behind the Pyrenees, where he complained he could not even obtain a skull to anatomize. At age 50, Vesalius died on the island of Zante in Greece while returning from a pilgrimage to Jerusalem.

"Furthermore, these pernicious men are not above speaking slander, if they notice any one who knows things of which they are ignorant, they admit that he is well versed in those subjects but deny that he is a physician .... Just as if a man should be considered a physician only when he is nothing else, or as if unlimited diligence in any of the branches of study subservient to medicine would impair one's knowledge of the art itself .... The physicians who advance this opinion are those with no knowledge of medicine except for some drugs that cleanse the bowels, and syrups that cause the evacuation of humours."
Vesalius, *Epistola Chynae*, 1546

Vesalius was also a physiologist. He removed the spleen in an animal, with no ill-effects (as Christopher Wren was to do a century later). Vesalius cut the recurrent laryngeal nerve producing aphonia or loss of voice as Galen had done before him. He sliced living muscle tissue in the long axis of the fibres and found little or no disability. He pierced the thoracic wall of animals and kept them alive by artificial respiration through a bellows.

Vesalius' pupil and successor, Fallopius, taught Fabricius, who, in turn, taught William Harvey at Padua. Thus passed on the spirit of enquiry from an anatomist interested in physiology, to a physiologist who finally made sense of the anatomy of the heart and circulation. One is reminded of the words of Jean Fernel (1497-1557): "Anatomy is to physiology as geography is to history—it gives the setting of the events."

There are those who speak lightly of the pen changing the world more effectually than the sword, and yet when scholars contemplate the year 1543 they cannot but believe that it is so. In that year the writings of two physicians shook the world of thought. These were the posthumous astronomical work of Copernicus, *De Revolutionibus Orbium Coelestium*, and *De Humani Corporis Fabrica* of Vesalius.

Lorenzo Bellini (1643-1704)

Galileo, during his time at Pisa, numbered among his associates such men as the histologist Malpighi and the physicist Borelli. The latter was one of the first to attempt purely physical explanations for the microscopic workings of the body organs. Associated with him in this was a medical student, Lorenzo Bellini, whose name is still applied to the "straight tubules" of the kidney that conduct the newly formed urine to the apex of the "pyramids of Malpighi," on its way to the ureter and bladder.

In 1662, the 19-year-old Bellini was anatomizing a deer, sent to Borelli by the Duke of Tuscany, when he discovered the "straight tubules." Although the great anatomist, Eustachius, after whom is named the Eustachian tube of the ear, had mentioned minute tubules in the kidney, it remained for the alert Bellini to clearly grasp their nature and meaning. It is likely, moreover, that a pupil of the physicist Borelli should propose a purely physical theory to account for the separation of the urine from the large amount of blood which coursed through the kidneys—a volume of blood now known to be as much as 1000 litres per day.

Bellini pictured the "serous" or fluid part of the blood giving rise to the urine by some sort of separation within the peripheral tissue of the kidney, and then continuing through the channels, already mentioned, to the bladder. The blood corpuscles, on the other hand, remained in the blood vessels and left the kidney by the renal veins. The degree of separation of these elements depended upon the comparative sizes of the urine-bearing tubules and the veins leaving the kidney.

Bellini could see no cause to introduce any chemical theory into the discussion and wrote: "Inside the body changes of mechanical pressure suffice to explain all that takes place. A gland is simply a closed vessel with extremely small perforations of different shape and size.... There is not the slightest necessity for complicating the matter with ferments."

This eminent pupil of Borelli became professor of anatomy at Pisa and eventually physician to Cosimo III at Florence. He wrote "*De Urinis et pulsibus, de missione sanguinis, de febribus, de morbis capitis, et pectoris*," published in Frankfurt and Leipzig in 1695, and described calcification of the coronary arteries. Bellini's name is associated in physicians' minds today, however, with his undergraduate contribution on the kidney tubules, "*Exercitatio anatomica de structura* Et *usu rerum*," published in Florence in 1662.

Johann Conrad Peyer (1653-1712) and **Jean Conrad Brunner** (1653-1727)

These two Swiss medical students were distinguished for their discoveries each made at the age of 24. Peyer first published, at Schaffhausen, his work on what is still referred to as "Peyer's patches" in his dissertation, "*Exercitatio anitomico-medica de Glandulis Intestinorum.*" These were associated at that time with typhoid fever. Brunner, on the other hand, discovered the glands still known by his name in the submucosa of the duodenum, though he did not publish his work until 15 years later when he became professor of medicine at Heidelberg. His student work had actually been done at Strasbourg and will be discussed later under endocrinology.

Johann Hamm (Hamen) (1650-1723)

Next in the chronology comes Johann Hamm (Hamen) from Arnheim in Holland. He was, as a medical student, working with Anthony van Leeuwenhoek in Leyden when in 1674 he discovered the structure of human spermatozoa under his microscope. Leeuwenhoek confirmed the discovery, extended the observation to other animals, and then sent the work to the Royal Society of London in one of his 375 communications to that body. In Leeuwenhoek's quaint phraseology the sperms became "little men" and "little women." Leeuwenhoek did not begin publishing until the age of 41, but he continued to work and to write till the end of his life.

OXFORD ANATOMY

News from the dead; Or a true and exact Narration of the miraculous deliverance of Anne Greene, who being Executed at Oxford, December 14, 1650, afterwards revived; and by the care of certain Physitians there, is now perfectly recovered. Together with the manner of her Suffering and the particular meanes used for her Recovery.
Written by a Scholler in Oxford [Richard Watkins], Whereunto are prefixed certain Poems. Lichfield, Oxford, 1651.

Ann Green was a slippery quean,
In vain did the jury detect her;
She cheated Jack Ketch, and then the vile wretch
'Scap'd the knife of the learned dissector.

William Petty (1621-1675) in that year "achieved considerable notoriety by reviving with [Thomas] Willis, a murderess, Ann Green, who had been hanged in the Oxford Parks by the executioner, Jack Ketch, and declared dead by the Sheriff. She was bled, put to bed to a warm woman and revived with spirits. According to Evelyn [the diarist] 'The young scholars joined and made a little portion, and married her to a man who had several children by her, she living fifteen years after.'
Alastair Robb-Smith & H.M. Sinclair, A *History of the Teaching of Anatomy in Oxford*, 1950

Osler adds: "Anne Greene a servant born in 1628 was unjustly and unsuccessfully hanged for nearly half an hour, while her friends 'thumped' her and jerked with all their weight on her legs, 'the sooner to dispatch her out of her paine'. Even so, when Petty and [Thomas] Willis came to anatomize her they found her breathing."

Johann Friedrich Meckel (1724-1774)

In the year after Hamm's death Johann Friedrich Meckel was born in Wetzlar. This birth began a distinguished line of Prussian anatomists that was to number his son Phillip (1756-1803), professor of anatomy at Halle, two grandsons, Johann Friedrich (1781-1833), called the Younger, and known as "the German Cuvier," and August Albrecht (1790-1829), professor of anatomy at Berne.

Johann Friedrich Meckel, the Elder, wrote his graduation thesis "*De quinto pare nervorum cerebri*" at the age of 24, describing the ganglion which still bears his name. Phillip graduated in Strasbourg in 1777 with a dissertation of great merit on the internal ear, "*De labyrinthi auris contentis*."

The younger Meckel is known for his work on "Meckel's diverticulum" but he was also to bring to public notice the classical texts of embryology by Caspar Friedrich Wolff (1733-1794), by translating them into German. Wolff, known to every student for the "Wolffian body" or primitive kidney, wrote the first of his revolutionary doctrines in his graduation thesis "*Theoria Generationis*" in 1759. His view, like Harvey's, was that the embryo develops gradually, and is not a mere prefabricated creature in miniature awaiting release from the ovary. Few have rivalled the originality of thought displayed by this master observer and "father of embryology."

The more complete you make your book, Lyell, the fewer I shall sell of it.
John Murray, Publisher,
to Darwin's Cambridge teacher.

Charles Darwin (1758-1778), son of Erasmus Darwin

This promising youth died of a dissecting wound at the age of 20. He was a great favourite among the students and professors at the University of Edinburgh and reported his research as an undergraduate to the Aesculapian Society on his "Experiments Establishing a Criterion between Mucaginous and Purulent Matter, and an Account of the Retrograde Motions of the Absorbent Vessels of Animal Bodies in Some Diseases." This was published in 1780 at Lichfield, where his distinguished father Erasmus Darwin and his family resided. For his research he was given the gold medal of the student society.

Antonio Scarpa (1752-1832)

Scarpa was one of those fireballs whose precocity was legendary. A pupil of Morgagni, Scarpa was made professor of anatomy at Modena at the age of 22. Two years earlier his student research had led to the publication of an historic treatise on "The Round Window of the Ear." Then followed his work on the secondary membrane of the tympanum, the naso-palatine innervation, the nerves of the heart, the cremasteric fascia, Scarpa's triangle of the thigh, and intimal changes in arteriosclerosis.

At the age of 31 Scarpa became professor of anatomy and clinical surgery at the University of Pavia, and left that famous school in his debt as he pioneered in the clinical treatment of aneurysms, inguinal hernia and cataract. From his earliest student days Scarpa added lustre to the Pivia of Spallanzani and Volta.

Johannes Müller (1801-1858)

Müller was one of the greatest physiological teachers of all time and numbered among his students Helmholtz, Remak, Gruby, du Bois Reymond, Brucke, Henle and Rudolf Virchow. Müller established a dynasty or several dynasties, such as Henle who taught Koch, who taught William Welch at Johns Hopkins and Paul Ehrlich. At the age of 22 Müller published in Leipzig his work "*De Respiratione Foetus commentario physiologica.*" He graduated from Bonn University in 1825; his thesis described his discovery of the Müllerian duct. He will be discussed more fully in the chapter on the nervous system.

Jacob Henle (1809-1885)

Another precocious contributor to the science of anatomy was Jacob Henle. At age 18 he entered the University of Bonn, where he encountered the great teacher and physiologist Johannes Müller, who invited him, in his second semester, to illustrate the structure of glands in the body. In accord with that excellent custom in German medical schools, Henle transferred to Heidelberg, where some of Europe's greatest clinicians were teaching.

An hypothesis that becomes dispossessed by new facts dies an honourable death; and if it has already called up for examination those truths by which it was annihilated it deserves a moment of gratitude.
Jacob Henle

It was an amazed professorate that received Henle's highly original thesis on "The Optic Membranes in Man and Animals," founded upon his own anatomical investigation. Müller was so impressed with Henle that he took him with him to visit Paris laboratories. Eventually Henle visited Berlin, where he met Felix Mendelssohn. Müller became professor in Berlin upon the death of the anatomist Rudolphi, the father-in-law of one of the greatest of all medical discoverers, Johannes Evangelista Purkinje.

As a child Henle suffered from periostitis and unfortunately this recurred throughout his life. His time in Bonn as an undergraduate was spent in the bosom of Müller's family. Henle loved to converse with Müller and to play duets on the piano with Müller's wife. For his student activities at Bonn University, Henle was imprisoned for four weeks and then sentenced to six years in a fortress prison. However, the great biologist and statesman von Humboldt interceded and had Henle freed. Henle's graduation thesis of 1832 occasionally surfaces in the catalogues of rare book dealers today, where it demands a great price.

Gabriel Gustav Valentin (1810-1883)

This talented pupil of Purkinje graduated from the gymnasium in Breslau in 1828 and thereafter entered the medical faculty of Breslau. His graduation thesis of 1832 concentrated on the embryonic development of muscle tissue. In 1836 he discovered the nucleolus of cells. One of his greatest accomplishments was his work with Purkinje in which they described the ciliary motion in epithelial tissue. By the year 1884 he was writing on the action of pancreatic juice on starch.

John Goodsir (1814-1867)

The development of bone and of teeth occupied a number of medical student investigators. John Goodsir came to his work in medical school with a rich background of microscopical observations on the marine forms dredged up from the Firth of Forth, Scotland, where he lived. His study of sponges provided many clues when he came to investigate bone growth. While an undergraduate at Edinburgh he embarked upon a study of the embryonic development of teeth, and charted the stages through which the teeth passed until eruption was complete. This formed the basis of his later work carried on as curator of the Museum of the College of Surgeons, Edinburgh, where he produced his monumental treatise on the development of bone in general. Even at that early date he clearly understood the concept of bone builders versus bone absorbers, and of the balance that had to be struck between these two activities. He eventually succeeded Monro Tertius in the chair of anatomy at Edinburgh, thus bringing to an end a reign by three members of the same family for 128 years. It was to Goodsir that Virchow dedicated his milestone "Cellular Pathology" in 1858, "as one of the earliest and most acute observers of cell-life, both physiological and pathological." In 1845 Goodsir's published work contained the germinal idea of the theory eventually announced by Virchow, omnis cellula e cellula.

William Bowman (1816-1892)

One of the fathers of histology or microscopic anatomy was William Bowman. With an artist mother and a botanically-and geologically-oriented father, Bowman grew up with "intense longings to penetrate the secrets of nature," as he put it. William attended an unusually enlightened school in Birmingham, founded by the father of Sir Rowland Hill, the author of the British system of penny post. After an explosion that affected one of his hands, this nascent investigator was cared for by an excellent surgeon, Joseph Hodgson, who influenced the boy to study medicine.

Hence at age 16, Bowman became apprenticed to Mr. Hodgson, the founder of the Birmingham Eye Hospital, a fellow of the Royal Society of London, and president of the Royal College of Surgeons. Fellow apprentices, or "pupil dressers" to Hodgson included Francis Galton, whose description of the life of medical students of the third decade of the 19th century includes, among other things, a student tour of Europe with Bowman.

Few students can have surpassed the high standards set by Bowman, during the years he spent at the Birmingham General Hospital. His notes are preserved in a group of case books, wherein he sketched, in colour, what he was seeing—undoubtedly due to his mother's artistic influence. His first publication was a shared work, with Frederick Ryland, in 1837, "A Treatise of the Diseases and Injuries of the Larynx and Trachea."

As a student, Bowman was a founder of the Birmingham University Medical Society and read a paper one month after its inception, on "*Spinal Paraplegia*." He followed this with papers on influenza, haemorrhage from external injury and emphysema. In his student post-mortem work he measured the size of the orifices in the heart. The physician for whom he carried out this exercise, Peyton Blakiston, rewarded Bowman with a fine microscope that he prized throughout his life. Bowman has been referred to by the well-known Birmingham medical historian, Dr. Ben Davis, as "the father of histology in the United Kingdom as well as the founder of British ophthalmology."

In 1837 Bowman transferred to King's College, London, and studied under that pioneer physiologist, Robert Bentley Todd. As a medical undergraduate Bowman was made joint editor with Todd of *The Cyclopaedia of Anatomy and Physiology*, and had responsibility for researching and reporting on the histology of the skin, mucous membranes, nerves, organs of sense, lungs, liver, testes, kidneys, bone, muscle and cartilage.[4]

In the midst of all this, Bowman was admitted in 1837 to the Royal College of Surgeons in the member category—a qualification to practice then in general use. Eight years after entering King's, his enormous task on the *Cyclopaedia* was completed. The great anatomist of a later era, Sir Arthur Keith, is said to have hailed this joint effort as without parallel: "No one has ever discovered so many new anatomical facts in so short a period."

Four years after his London degree Bowman was made a fellow of that most prestigious company of scientists, the Royal Society of London, having read to them at the age of 23 his landmark paper, "On the Minute Structure and Movements of Voluntary Muscles." Well into the 20th-century histology (from the Greek *histos* meaning tissue) was to be found within most British departments of physiology. Bowman was well placed, then, to correlate structure and function in his discoveries, notably in the kidney. As John Fulton commented, "When he first entered King's College, London, he was already well launched on a research career." Fulton adds that "Bowman described the capsule surrounding the Malpighian body and showed that the cavity of this capsule is continuous with the uriniferous tubule."

When another student discoverer, Helmholtz, invented the ophthalmoscope in 1851, Bowman was the first to use it in Britain. Ophthalmic surgery gradually gained Bowman's attention and he founded the Association for the Advancement of Medicine by Research. He became the first president of the Ophthalmological Society of the United Kingdom. His book on ophthalmic surgery was dedicated to his early teacher in the Birmingham General Hospital, "in grateful recognition of early kindness and encouragement during five years spent within the walls of that noble institution." Addressing the students at King's College in 1851, Bowman paid a great tribute to an educational institution too often overlooked as a teaching treasure: "The one thing more than another in the circumstances of my own education, which I am now inclined to look back upon with a special thankfulness, it is that for several years a large hospital was my home."

Frederick Oldfield Ward (1818-1877)

Frederick Ward was educated at Dr. Knox's School in Tonbridge up to the age of 15 when he entered the medical school of King's College Hospital, London. There he distinguished himself, winning a medal in chemistry in 1835 and one in botany in 1837. At the age of 20, and while still a medical student he published his *Human Osteology*, one of the most unusual books in the long history of anatomy.

The volume was the size and shape of a small prayer book, but what it lacked in size it made up in substance. The simplicity of its prose and illustrations is something rarely found in expensive medical texts today.

In the preface Ward says that his little volume was the product "partly of researches in the museum and dissecting room, prosecuted at intervals during the last five years: partly of a careful perusal and comparison of the best English and foreign works on the subject." His aim, he said, was brevity. "But holding that true brevity consists not in expressing ideas in a small space but in conveying them in a short time, I have not thought it inconsistent with this design to dilate freely upon some obscure and difficult points which have been passed over in a few lines by previous writers .... Whatever contradictory statements came under my notice in the course of this comparison were noted down, and made the subject of careful research in several extensive anatomical collections .... which afforded me the opportunity of comparing nearly two hundred specimens of each bone."

This Vesalian spirit went further. Ward tested the oft-reported elasticity of the clavicle by hammering it longitudinally against a stone wall and observing its spring. He tested too the strength of the lateral condyle of the femur and found that each cubic inch could support "four hundred weight without sensible alteration." A second edition of his book appeared in 1856 and a third in 1875. Ward died in 1877.

The initial hostile reception of the *Origin of Species* and especially the ignorant and contemptuous attack by Bishop Samuel Wilberforce has become proverbial. But contempt rapidly gave way to acclaim.... When even the ill-tempered Bishop Wilberforce reluctantly confessed his error, Darwin's champion, Thomas Henry Huxley, remained unsatisfied. "Confession unaccompanied by penitence ... affords no ground for mitigation of judgement; and the kindliness with which Mr. Darwin speaks of his assailant, Bishop Wilberforce, is so striking an exemplification of his singular gentleness and modesty, that it rather increases one's indignation against the presumption of his critic." Huxley called Darwin's book "the most potent instrument for the extension of the realm of natural knowledge which has come into men's hands since the publication of Newton's *Principia*.... It was badly received by the generation to which it was first addressed, and the outpouring of angry nonsense to which it gave rise is sad to think upon. But the present generation will probably behave just as badly if another Darwin should arise, and inflict upon them what the generality of mankind most hate—the necessity of revising their convictions."
Daniel J. Boorstin,
The Discoverers (1983)

Thomas Huxley (1825-1895)

The calm of the Victorian era was shattered by two medical students and their theory of evolution. Charles Robert Darwin (1809-1882) and his "bulldog," Thomas Huxley, were to hold the stage in England for almost 60 years as they indoctrinated and divided the country.

Darwin entered upon medicine at Edinburgh but gave it up after two terms because some of the lectures were "incredibly dull." He then decided to study for the church but gave that up, ending by taking his B.A. at Cambridge. He sailed on the H.M.S. *Beagle* as naturalist to the expedition that lasted from 1831 to 1836. It was in that year, as he sought to classify the specimens brought back, that he made journal notes of his theory of evolution.

In the same year Thomas Huxley was moving from the school at Ealing where his father taught, in order to support his seven children, to Coventry where self-education became the order of the day. At the age of 12, Thomas was lighting his candle early in the morning in order to read Hutton's *Geology*. His brother-in-law, Dr. Cooke of Coventry, early stimulated Thomas' interest in anatomy, and it is recorded that the young student contracted an infection while attending an autopsy. He read Sir William Hamilton's *Logic* and taught himself German.

Huxley at the age of 15 was keeping a journal and speculated on "what would become of things if their qualities were taken away." He noted down quotations from Goethe, and speculated on the origin of the colours in the sunset. His social conscience was rapidly maturing and he wrote: "I think now that it is against all the laws of justice to force men to support a church with whose opinions they cannot conscientiously agree. I wonder what will be my opinion ten years hence?" At least one bishop was to find out clearly what Huxley's views were to be, as will be outlined presently.

Huxley spent some time in making a galvanic battery that would deposit carbon. He was forever experimenting with things electrical and wrote in his journal on January 30, 1842: "I have for some time been pondering over a classification of knowledge"—at age 16. By then he was apprenticed to Dr. Chandler at Rotherhithe near the East London docks, and he never forgot the mixture of poverty and ignorance that he saw there. He was too young to be admitted to the University of London, and so studied in the Library of the College of Surgeons whenever he could. (This glorious library has been the sanctuary of the serious student of medicine for generations. Its rebuilding after direct bomb hits in World War II has been a godsend to a new generation of students.)

Through Sydenham College, Huxley was able to prepare for the matriculation examinations of the University of London, in which he won the Medal of the Apothecaries Society for his paper in botany. With his brother, J.E. Huxley, he entered Charing Cross Hospital Medical College in October 1842.

This is how Huxley described the essence of his student discovery: "The only instruction from which I obtained the proper effect of education was that which I received from Mr. Wharton Jones, who was the lecturer on physiology. ... The extent and precision of his knowledge impressed me greatly, and the severe exactness of his method of lecturing was quite to my taste. I do not know that I have ever felt so much respect for a teacher before or since.... It was he who suggested the publication of my first scientific paper—a very little one—in the *Medical Gazette* of 1845, and most kindly corrected the literary faults which abounded in it."

It is possible that Huxley's attendance at post mortem examinations sharpened his interest in microscopic structures. He spent so much time over the microscope that his classmates, seeing him from the courtyard outside, dubbed him "The Sign of the Head and the Microscope." At the age of 19 he wrote his first paper, "On a Hitherto Undescribed Structure in the Human Hair Sheath," still known as "Huxley's layer." He continued his brilliant record by winning the prize in chemistry, and at graduation in 1845 won the gold medal for anatomy and physiology.

He immediately joined the Naval Medical Service and under the kindly eye of Sir John Richardson, the explorer and naturalist, was posted as Assistant Surgeon to H.M.S. *Rattlesnake* about to set off for Australia. Delays were noted in his diary: "December 10, 1846. In Plymouth Sound. Thank God! Fitting out is at last over. We have no more caprices to fear but those of the wind—a small matter after having been exposed to those of the Admiralty."

For all his success at university he was commendably cautious as he wrote: "I must keep two points in view, 1st that I am simply a student; 2nd from the peculiar circumstances in which I am placed, care and caution in observation may help me to become a teacher with regard to particular points."

In the period of more than seven months that it required to reach Australia Huxley had time to ruminate further: "Naturalizing for systematic purposes is not *à mon gré*. My memory is not sufficiently selective of these facts to give me any hope of attaining profound systematic knowledge—and furthermore all the naming and determining of place is far better done by those who sit in museums at home .... But what I *can* do and they *cannot* and where therefore the chief value of my position is: I can observe 1. the 'habits' of living bodies, 2. their mode of development and generation, 3. their anatomy by dissection of the fresh specimens, 4. their histology by microscopic observation." Obviously he was still Wharton Jones' disciple, now in action. It speaks well, too, for the value of a medical training when a man sets out to observe even the lowest forms of life clinically, in their habitat, and before they reach a museum.

Huxley's years with the H.M.S *Rattlesnake* were varied and interesting. Ashore he was observant too, and noted that even in 1847 he wit-

If all the books in the world except the *Philosophical Transactions* [of the Royal Society of London] were destroyed, it is safe to say that the foundations of physical science would remain unshaken and that the vast intellectual progress of the last two centuries would be largely, though incompletely, recorded.
Thomas Henry Huxley (1866)

It is a peculiarity of the physical sciences that they are independent in proportion as they are imperfect; and it is only as they advance that the bonds which unite them become apparent.
Thomas Huxley,
Science and Culture

nessed an operation in Hobart, Tasmania, done under ether anaesthesia, which had been introduced less than a year previously by a Boston medical student.

In Sydney Huxley became engaged to Henrietta Heathorn. They were married in England eight years later and lived to raise eight children.

On his return with H.M.S. *Rattlesnake* to England in 1850 Huxley tried to find a publisher for his scientific papers. The Admiralty was not interested. Huxley therefore resigned his commission and appealed to the Royal Society, which responded nobly, thanks to a grant from H.M. Government; today, such Peter-versus-Paul methods of financing research are still occasionally practiced.

At the age of 25 Huxley was made Fellow of the Royal Society and a year later was awarded its gold medal and elevated to its Council. Despite this, he was turned down for posts he sought at the Universities of Toronto, Cork, Aberdeen and King's College, London. His mother died, his father took ill and Huxley was on the point of settling in Australia as a general practitioner when the School of Mines in London appointed him lecturer in palaeontology.

With this appointment began 40 years of ceaseless work, turning out scientific papers, sitting on Royal Commissions, on the London School Authority, and as a Governor of Eton. The publication of Darwin's *Origin of Species* in 1859 was Huxley's great opportunity to become a teacher to a whole generation. His speeches and writings soon attracted universal attention. His subjects were not confined to evolution but ranged over the whole field of knowledge. He was a pioneer in adult education, and always the poor man's friend. He excoriated injustice, prejudice and privilege. His lay sermons in the modern vernacular may be said to have "comforted the afflicted and afflicted the comfortable." Amidst all his crusading he found time to establish in 1871 the first true laboratory of biology. He founded two scientific journals, which may be considered the forerunners of the modern *Nature*. He was best-known in America for his appearance at the opening of the Johns Hopkins University in 1876 where he spoke "On University Education." There was no music, no prayer and no benediction. President D.C. Gilman described the reaction of the Board: "Huxley was bad enough; Huxley without prayer was intolerable."

From the age of 15 Huxley felt keenly the injustice of a state-supported church. In 1860 Oxford heard even stronger views when he debated the subject of evolution with Bishop Samuel Wilberforce. The bishop asked if it was through his grandfather or his grandmother that Huxley claimed descent from a monkey. Huxley's classic reply was this: "I asserted—and I repeat—that a man has no reason to be ashamed of having an ape for his grandfather. If there were an ancestor whom I should feel shame in recalling it would rather be a man—a man of restless and versatile intellect—who, not content with equivocal success in his own sphere of activity, plunges into scientific questions with which he has no real acquaintance, only to obscure them by aimless rhetoric, and distract the attention of his hearers from the real point at issue by eloquent digressions and skilled appeals to religious prejudice."

Huxley died at the age of 70. Without his talents Darwin's theory would never have been so widely spread, and education in Britain would have been the poorer. From a medical student uncertain of his first published reports, but supported in them by one superb teacher, Huxley became one of the greatest teachers of the last century, a contributor and editor of the top rank, and a scientist-statesman with few equals. Huxley died in 1895, predeceased by Darwin in 1882. Huxley's fellow student discoverers, Helmholtz and Oliver Wendell Holmes, died a few months ahead of Huxley.

Henry Gray (1827-1861)

Gray's *Anatomy* is still known to medical students the world over, though it was first published in 1858 when Henry Gray was 31 years old. The author had won prizes for his undergraduate publications 10 years earlier, but too little credit is sometimes given to his classmate, Henry Van Dyke Carter (1831-1897). The preface of the *Anatomy* notes: "In the majority of cases the illustrations have been copied or corrected by recent dissections, made jointly by the author and Dr. Carter." Carter's life is outlined below.

Gray's *Anatomy* is said to have been the first textbook in which surgical anatomy was discussed along with general morphology. The clarity of the text owed much to Timothy Holmes, the editor, who, after Gray's death from smallpox, became the guiding spirit in future editions. As Dr. Noel Poynter, Director of the Wellcome Institute for the History of Medicine in London, has pointed out, there were 32 British editions of the *Anatomy* in its first century. There have been many since. The centennial edition comprised 1500 pages containing 1300 illustrations. In that special edition a relative of Gray provided the electron micrographs. The first two editions in Britain, containing 750 pages with 363 illustrations, were published by John W. Parker, printer to Cambridge University. He is famous for having introduced steam-driven presses against great opposition. He also used this press for the printing of Bibles.

Mr. Gray has published a book that is not wanted. It is low and unscientific in tone; and it has been compiled for the most part, in a manner inconsistent with the profession of honesty which we find in the Preface. Mr. Gray has worked without fairly appreciating the intellectual condition and requirements of the present race of Medical Students.
Medical Times and Gazette, March 5,1859

It was while preparing the second edition of his classic that Gray was stricken with small pox, which he contracted from a nephew whom he was nursing at the time. One might have thought that a new type of *Anatomy*, such as Gray presented to the world, would have received unqualified acclaim. However, the *Medical Times* reviewed the first edition with what has been referred to as "slashing criticism." *The Lancet*, however, thought well of the volume. It should be remembered that Gray's *magnum opus* had to compete with well-established texts such as those by Quain, Sharpey, Winslow and Bichat. Perhaps Gray's apprenticeship as the surgical curator of his hospital's pathology museum developed in him a perspective not always found in academic anatomists. Sadly, his manuscript for a volume on tumours, on which he was working at the time of his death, has never been found.

The writing of Gray's *Anatomy* has been characterized by Bishop as a "stupendous achievement." The combined efforts of Gray and Carter produced 183 illustrations from their original dissections together, done while they were demonstrators in anatomy at St. George's Medical School in London.

Carter, in the year of the appearance of the first edition, joined the Indian Medical Service and retired with the rank of Surgeon General in 1888 after 30 years of service. He became Professor of Anatomy and Physiology and Principal of Grant Medical College in Bombay. During his extensive experience he published descriptions of "Madura Foot," or

"Carter's Mycetoma." Among his other areas of study were leprosy, and spirillum fever with which he won the Stewart Prize of £500 sterling offered by the British Medical Association. He carried on the microscopic anatomical work which he had begun with Henry Gray.

Gray's student work included a 341-page essay that won for him the Triennial Prize of the Royal College of Surgeons in 1848. His subject was "The Origin, Connection and Distribution of the Nerves of the Human Eye and its Appendages," illustrated by comparative dissections of the eye of other vertebrate animals. The Recorder of the Royal College of Surgeons, an able historian, wrote that "the whole thing gives evidence of his enthusiastic and painstaking industry." This student dissertation is probably without parallel as a comprehensive survey of the phylogeny of the nervous structures associated with vision and eye movements. After dealing with the visual apparatus of the cuttlefish and octopus, he details the arrangements in fish, reptiles and birds. He then starts on the mammals and includes the stag, horse and porpoise. The anatomy of the trigeminal and facial nerves is covered, together with the distribution of the sympathetic nerves. Finally, he writes a 257-page treatise on the structures associated with vision in the human.

As a student Gray reported his studies of both the gross and microscopic structures involved in vision, rotating the eyeball, closing the eyelids, regulating the nutrition of the eye, controlling the secretion of tears and regulating the size of the pupil and the curvature of the lens. He pursued the orbital nerves back to their origin. Upon graduation he carried his earlier work further and wrote a paper on the development of the retina and optic nerve and of the membranous labyrinth of the ear and the auditory nerve. In 1852 he published a paper on the development of the ductless or inwardly secreting glands of the chick and a year later described a remarkable ovarian cyst that contained brain tissue. At the age of only 25 he was made a Fellow of the Royal Society. In the same year he was awarded the Astley Cooper Prize of 300 guineas for his dissertation, "On the Structure and Use of the Spleen." Another gifted young investigator, Christopher Wren, had also described the spleen and its surgical removal.

Gray's undergraduate labours fitted him to produce the book that still bears his name and is still in daily use. Although a gifted dissector and illustrator, Gray repeatedly said that his book was but an extension of his teaching arm, and that he had written it for students who wanted to learn rather than for anatomists alone.

As Conan Doyle wrote: "For him who has mastered Gray's *Anatomy*, life has no further terrors."

Joseph Lister (1827-1912)

Illustrated earlier was the determinative influence of Wharton Jones on the student life of Thomas Huxley in 1845. In 1852 Jones was influencing another student investigator, Joseph Lister, at University College, London. Having come to the medical school with a B.A. degree, and being skilled in microscopy through association with his father's researches on achromatic lenses, Lister was attracted to the physiological laboratory of Professor William Sharpey. Wharton Jones was still closely associated with physiology though immersed in clinical work.

Lister's excellent microscopy was the key with which he unlocked the secrets of the muscle of the iris, and that of the skin, in two undergraduate studies. He wrote in his first paper, "Observations on the Contractile Tissue of the Iris": "Our knowledge of the cause of the movements of the iris was, till within the last few years, in a very unsatisfactory condition .... An operation for artificial pupil, by excision, performed by Mr. Wharton Jones at University College Hospital, on the eleventh of August of the present year (1852), placed in my possession a perfectly fresh portion of a human iris.... I proceeded to avail myself of this somewhat rare opportunity of investigating the muscular tissue of the human iris. On placing under the microscope, four hours after the operation, portions of the tissue carefully teased out in water with needles, I found that some of the muscular fibre-cells had become isolated, and presented very characteristic appearances."

This paper was published in the first volume of the *Quarterly Journal of Microscopic Science* in 1853, as was his second paper, "Observations on the Muscular Tissue of the Skin." Lister showed the minute muscles that elevate the hairs on the skin surface during fright or other suitable stimulation.

It may seem to some that Lister's excursion into muscle structure and function had no connection with his later work. The common denominator was his superb microscopy. If ever Pasteur's dictum, "Fortune favours the prepared mind" was applicable, it was to Lister. He saw everything he investigated in physiological terms. In this he was ahead of his time, though in tune with his teachers, Sharpey, Wharton Jones and Robert Liston the surgeon. Undoubtedly his boyhood interest in botany had stimulated the inquisitive part of his nature.

Consequently, an outbreak of "hospital gangrene" in London caused Lister to ask its basic causes. At Edinburgh, where he became an extramural lecturer in surgery in 1853, Lister began his researches on coagulation of the blood and inflammation in the web of the frog's foot.

Lister had learned and practiced the essentials of physiological observation as an undergraduate and these he now brought to his clinical problems of what he called "sepsis" and "putrefaction" in wounds. He reasoned from Pasteur's experiments on putrefaction in organic matter that micro-organisms could be at the root of putrefaction in his patients' tissues.

In May 1866, in Glasgow, Lister first treated suppurating wounds with crude German creosote. Soon carbolic acid was isolated and came to be used. Lister was not satisfied with this fierce chemical treatment of human tissues, as noted in Sir Howard Florey's "Lister Oration," presented to the Canadian Medical Association in Vancouver in 1954. Florey reproduced Lister's notes of 100 years ago, from which it was clear that Lister was in search of a tissue-friendly antibiotic to curb infection.

Lister's pre-eminence as a surgeon has tended to obscure the fundamental apprenticeship that he served in physiology. He always urged upon his students his view that it is "by collateral knowledge that healing is most frequently advanced."

William Turner (1832-1916)

William Turner was the son of an upholsterer and cabinetmaker. In 1850 he entered St. Bartholomew's Hospital Medical School where he studied with Sir James Paget, who had himself been a student contributor to science. At the end of his first year Turner won the prize in chemistry and botany. In 1853 he was awarded the coveted scholarship in anatomy and physiology and in his graduation year of 1857 Turner won the gold medal offered by the Society of Apothecaries, a very great honour. This was awarded for his researches in materia medica.

Turner's ability was recognized early in his student career and he was invited to present his paper "An Examination of the Cerebrospinal Fluid" by the Royal Society of London. To fill a vacancy caused by illness at the University of Edinburgh Medical School, Professor Goodsir (1814-1870), also a medical student contributor, asked Sir James Paget to provide an interim senior demonstrator in anatomy. Paget suggested Henry Gray, but of course by that time Gray was heavily engaged in producing his great *Anatomy*.

Professor Goodsir was happy to have the highly recommended Turner help with the teaching in Edinburgh even before Turner had received his Bachelor of Medicine degree in London in 1857. John Goodsir was keen on student investigators because he himself had established a great reputation for his own undergraduate work on the embryology of the teeth and bone and later in life produced a monumental work on the building up and tearing down of bone as an everyday process. Goodsir's interests were broad and together with his colleague, Joseph Lister the surgeon, he published a paper on the structure of nerve fibres soon after the pair had gone north to Scotland to teach and do research. William Turner succeeded Professor Goodsir in the chair of anatomy at Edinburgh.

With Sir George Humphry, the Cambridge anatomist, Turner founded the *Journal of Anatomy and Physiology*, which had a profound influence on British science.

Munk's Roll of the Royal College of Physicians concludes: "Sir William Turner takes a foremost place in English medicine during the Victorian age. Coming to London poor and friendless, he made his way by sheer force of character, first as a good teacher and as an original investigator in anatomy." Turner eventually became the Principal of the University of Edinburgh.

Student contributors to the science of osteology seem to have been legion in the early 19th century. The famous **Jonathan Hutchinson** (1829-1913), as a student, was studying the notched teeth in infantile syphilis. In the year of his qualification in medicine he began his observations on inflammation of the eye in infants and young persons suffering from the congenital form of the disease. Meantime his contemporary, Julius Wolff, in Germany, was just graduating with a thesis written on the experimental reproduction of bone. Wolff thought of bone as being in a continual state of flux and like another student investigator, Oldfield Ward, he studied the neck of the femur to show how the details of structure met the problem of function. With the help of his engineering friend Culmann, Wolff made a design analysis of the neck of the femur that led him to his law of bone formation that stated that the amount of growth in a bone depends on the need for that growth.

Another contemporary in this field was Joseph Samson Gamgee, who was born in Leghorn in 1828 and took up the study of medicine at University College Hospital, London. As an undergraduate he won the Liston Clinical Medal for his essays on the treatment of fractures. A year before he graduated, his paper, "On the Advantages of the Starched Apparatus in the Treatment of Fractures and Diseases of the Joints" was published. This 89-page volume, printed by H.K. Lewis in London, contained Gamgee's revolutionary idea of getting the fractured bone into proper alignment as soon as possible, with anesthetic if necessary, rather than waiting for the soft-tissue swelling to subside, which was then the usual procedure. Gamgee applied the porous pasteboard splints and starched bandages even to sprains and to diseased joints to bring them rest. He sought to provide the patient with a light and therefore portable strong splint in the form of a cast that could be easily cut open. He wrote that he was weary of "multifarious and inefficient contrivances rich in wood and leather, splints, straps and buckles, hooks and screws, bolts and hinges, which have been prolifically devised for the treatment of fractures." During Gamgee's residency in surgery at University College Hospital, London, he was depended upon, to a great extent, by the famous surgeon John Erichson, who himself had been a student contributor (on the coronary circulation). Gamgee was meticulous in the fitting of casts and wrote of the need to respect the soft parts; he said: "There must be no squeezing like that of an old college friend's hand when seen after a long absence.... The soothing surgical pressure is like that which you interchange with the hand of a lady."

Georges Benjamin Clemenceau (1841-1929)

Not many great political leaders can claim to have had a medical training. Not only did Clemenceau strike a blow for anatomy in his thesis of May 13, 1865, "*Notions d'Anatomie et de Physiologie générales*," he was the famous political leader of France 1906-1909, and in World War I, 1917-1920. He reminds us of such prime ministers as Dr. Sun Yat Sen and Dr. Juan Negrín.

William Osler (1849-1919)

Sir William Osler is identified in the public mind with McGill University in Montreal (1870-1884), the University of Pennsylvania in Philadelphia (1884-1889), Johns Hopkins Hospital Medical School in Baltimore (1889-1905), and with Oxford University (1905-1919). However, as a budding microscopist he owed his early training to his home province, Ontario. He had the good fortune to learn his craft under the tutelage of the Reverend W.E. Johnson at Trinity College School in Weston, Ontario, from grinding stones and fossils to the microscopic world of fresh water polyzoa.

On ascending to Trinity College at the University of Toronto (a university started by an Anglican bishop "to counteract the seditious influence of Harvard"), Osler pursued further microscopic studies culminating, in 1869, in his first publication, "Christmas and the Microscope." He wrote: "Upon putting a slide under the microscope before I had properly focused, I saw the dim outline of some little creature kicking and struggling as though it were in a net." It turned out to be one of the *tardigrada*, or little water bears, that had become entangled in the gelatinous tube of *encyonema prostratum*.

While still a medical undergraduate at Toronto, Osler published a paper on "Canadian Diatomaceae," describing in detail their reproduction and development. Additionally, he gave a description of the microscopic features of the trachea of the mouse, followed by a demonstration of live nematodes *trichinella spirallis* in a cadaver being dissected, presumably that of someone who had eaten undercooked pork.

The great pathologist Maude Abbott commented on Osler's undergraduate propensity: "His interest in the post-mortem room and his free use of the microscope are among the most conspicuous acts in his history, revealing as they do, the quick grasp of essentials which was the outstanding feature of his genius." In 1872, while still a student, Osler assisted his chief at the Medico-chirurgical Society by the demonstration of pathological material and published his first classic case reports with autopsy findings. His M.D. thesis was awarded a special prize for its originality. An excellent study of Osler's early years as a microscopist has been recently published by Alvin E. Rodin and J.D. Key. Osler the pathologist will be discussed in a later chapter.

A contemporary of Osler, **Paul Ehrlich** (1854-1915), while still a student developed a triacid stain that permitted the clear definition of the nucleus, the cytoplasm, and other details of the interior of cells in thin dried films of blood. Ehrlich's major discoveries will be dealt with in another chapter.

At the age of 22, **Giulio Bizzozero** (1846-1901) described the formation of the blood elements in the bone marrow, especially the white blood corpuscles. He is best-known for giving the blood-platelets their name and showing that they have a role in the coagulation of blood (1882).

By the Advice of that excellent Man, Dr. Wilkins, I first set upon this Enterprize [*Micrographia, or Physiological Descriptions of Minute Bodies made by the Help of magnifying Glasses*] yet still came to it with much Reluctancy, because I was to follow the Footsteps of so eminent of Person as Dr. Wren, who was the first that attempted anything of this Nature; whose original Draughts do now make one of the Ornaments of that great Collection of Rarities in the King's Closet. This Honour which his first Beginnings of this kind have received, to be admitted into the most famous Place of the World, did not so much incourage, as the Hazard of coming after Dr. Wren.
Robert Hooke, *Micrographia* (1665)

Santiago Ramón y Cajal (1852-1934)

No story of student contributions to anatomy would be complete without a reference to the colourful Spaniard, Don Santiago Ramón y Cajal. His rise from the lowliest teaching post to the Nobel Prize in Medicine is a romance in itself. What he did for science in Spain is a record of one man's triumph against poverty, ignorance and prejudice.

Cajal, to use his mother's name, was born in the villa of Petilla de Aragon,[5] the son of a "barber surgeon second class." The most mischievous boy for miles around, Santiago became a legendary figure when he hollowed out a tree trunk and, making an unusually successful cannon of it, blew down the wall of a grandee's palace. Time spent in jail failed to temper his high spirits, but his father's hunting activities were soon shared with him. Together they tramped the hills in search of game, and eventually Santiago developed his flair for drawing and sketching. By judicious visits to cemeteries he built up a fine collection of human bones that he drew to perfection. By the age of 18 he had completed a creditable atlas of osteology. It was never published, since in Spain foreign medical volumes were the rule. However, the sheets, later displayed at the Instituto Cajal in Madrid, were both beautiful and faithful.

By dint of great sacrifice Santiago and his brother graduated with the degree Bachelor of Medicine from the University of Zaragoza. Santiago became lecturer in microscopic anatomy in Valencia while his brother went off to South America where for some 30 years he was private secretary to a king of the Pampas, and returned to Zaragoza to become professor of gynaecology.

In Valencia Cajal wrote a set of notes for his students in histology, as Osler did in Montreal at about the same time, and came to the conclusion that there was little to write about on the microscopic structure of the nervous system. The knowledge of this important part of the body was hidden in an impossible thicket of ignorance and speculation.

At this stage Cajal went to Madrid to take his higher degree of Doctor of Medicine. He saw there for the first time the capillary circulation in the web of the frog's foot—the preparation which was to serve Lister so well. He found a psychiatrist in Madrid named Simarro, who had beautiful silver-stained preparations of nervous tissue. Some he had stained by his own method, and some after the method of Camillo Golgi, the Italian anatomist of Pavia.

On Cajal's return to Valencia he began to stain, with silver, the nervous system of insects and mice. He had so little money that he had to put many sections on one microscope slide. What he saw excited him. He wrote his first paper and sent it to *The Catholic Daily* in Zaragoza. He sent reprints of it to the crowned heads of Europe but received no glowing acknowledgements. Undeterred, he stained more minute structures and wrote more papers. He was made professor at Barcelona and eventually at Madrid. Here the voice of scorn came repeatedly to his ears—who did this Cajal think he was, writing papers for journals beyond the Pyrenees?

Cajal had come out of his laboratory in 1885 to give help in a serious cholera epidemic that swept Spain—and for this help he was given a beautiful microscope by the people of Zaragoza. In the same epidemic there appeared on an English team of researchers sent out by St. Thomas' Hospital, London, a man who was to make Cajal's name famous. He was Charles Sherrington, also destined to receive the Nobel Prize in Medicine—and in the same branch of medicine, the study of the nervous system. They did not meet in Spain, but Sherrington learned enough Spanish to read Cajal's papers, which came to him later when he was foreign secretary of the Royal Society in London.

Sherrington, whose research on the physiology of the nervous system began while he was a student, found in Cajal's early papers the structural facts that his physiological experiments made him surmise. Before long he had Cajal invited to London to give the Croonian Lectures at the Royal Society. From that day Cajal never looked back, and the sceptics in Spain were silenced. Sherrington had some fine lantern slides made of Cajal's microscopic specimens, but Cajal refused to show them. He wanted his audience to look into real microscopes to see real structures, and his strategy worked. There was nothing aloof about the reception of his work in Britain. Cambridge accorded him an honourary degree, and Oxford colleges dipped into their archives to find that they had ancient connections with Spanish universities, such as Salamanca.

This was all very well, but Cajal's curiosity overcame him, and at times when he should have been getting an honour he would be found in a botanical garden. He arose early and every morning took up his place before 8 a.m. at one of the bridges over the Thames, to watch the millions come to work in the city.

Cajal became recognized abroad, and finally in Spain. He was made a life Senator and a great Instituto Cajal was built to honour him. He preferred to work at home, however, writing and editing, and, like a picador, sharpening his lances for the endless polemics which he carried on with opponents of his neurone theory. His speech on receiving the Nobel

The ideal of science is to elucidate the dark mysteries and unknown forces which invest us, for the benefit of our descendants, and to make the world more agreeable and intelligible, while we ourselves are forgotten like the seed in the furrow.
The emotion lights the cerebral machine which acquires by it necessary heat, the forge where fortunate intuitions and hypotheses will be wrought.
No one ignores the fact that the one who knows and does is valuable compared to the one who knows and goes to sleep.
Ramón y Cajal,
Rules and Counsels for the Scientific Investigator, 1923

Grey matter abounds in countries with grey skies.
Genius, like the inhabitants of the depths of the sea, moves by its own light.
Only the doctor and the dramatist enjoy the rare privilege of charging us for the annoyance they give us.
As long as our brain is a mystery, the universe, the reflection of the structure of the brain, will also be a mystery.
Ramón y Cajal,
Charlas de Cafe, 1932

Prize in 1906—a prize shared with his caustic opponent Golgi—was a masterpiece of scientific prose. Golgi's was, unhappily, a bitter denunciation of his rival.

Cajal did for the finer anatomy of the nervous system what Vesalius did for gross anatomy. He described what was there to be seen, rather than what authorities decreed to be there. Both began as student contributors, dependent upon the dry bones of gallows and cemeteries. Both left scientists in their debt.

Frederick Augustus Dixey (1855-1935)

While Dixey is widely known as a pioneer of osteogeny, his fame as a collector of butterflies is worldwide. He was born in London in 1855 where his grandfather was optician to Queen Victoria and his father took up the same profession. Strangely, Frederick Dixey arrived at Wadham College, Oxford, with a scholarship in classics. However, he went on to University College, London, and became a demonstrator in physiology to Sir Edward Sharpey-Schafer. He qualified to practice medicine through his Oxford degree in 1884 and from then on his life rotated around Wadham, Christopher Wren's college.

Dixey was the first to demonstrate that although the shaft of bone making up the terminal phalanx of a digit was laid down in cartilage, its tip and ungual tuberosity are laid down in membrane. He saw that the thimble-like cap of membrane bone developing at the terminal part of a digit is distinct from the cartilaginous bone of the proximal part of the phalanx. His undergraduate work was communicated to the Royal Society of London in 1879 by Sharpey-Schafer. However, Dixey was not made a Fellow of the Royal Society until 1910, thanks to his fame then as an entomologist. In fact, his scientific interests were varied. He wrote on vital statistics, the epidemiology of influenza and the natural history of diphtheria. He was a confirmed Darwinian. Dixey was killed by a motorcar in 1935 as he was crossing Park Lane on his way to a meeting of the Entomological Society, and his son said, "He died with his mind full of the work he hoped to do." The *Lancet* noted: "Both in the subjects which he chose for investigation and in the manner of their treatment we can see the value of his previous work in medical fields."

Willem Einthoven (1860-1927)

While Einthoven is known as "the father of electrocardiography" as well as the Nobel Prize winner in 1924, he actually began his life as a medical student at Utrecht as an anatomist. He was well-known for his athletic activities there, which brought him great acclaim as a rower, gymnast and fencer. They also brought him a broken arm, the mechanics of which intrigued him. With the anatomist Koster he wrote his first paper, "Some Remarks on the Elbow Joint," which was an engineering and anatomical analysis of the problem that he had encountered. His doctoral thesis (1886) was produced under the supervision of the eminent scholar Franz Cornelius Donders and was entitled "Stereoscopic Vision Through Colour Variation." Remarkably, at the age of 25 Einthoven achieved the professorship of physiology of the great university of Leyden. He is encountered later, under the cardio-vascular system.

A lesser-known medical student, this time in Berlin, was Leonor Michaelis (1875-1949), a pupil of Emil Fischer and Du Bois Reymond.

From the laboratory of Professor Oskar Hertwig he produced a paper on the histology of milk secretion, which won him a faculty prize. A further student paper described the fertilizing of the ovum in amphibians. His M.D. thesis described the first cleavage of the frog's egg. Within a year he produced, for medical students, a short textbook on embryology which, under his eye, went through nine editions. His abilities led to a position as Paul Ehrlich's private assistant at the state institution for serological research, where his vital staining of mitochondria with Janus green brought him great renown. This technique was taken to the United States by Professor Cowdry. The multilingual Michaelis became a Fellow of the Rockefeller Institute in 1929.

Joseph Hugo Vincent Disse (1852-1912)

Disse has been rescued from oblivion by Professor Rudi Schmid, the liver specialist of the University of California at San Francisco. He writes, "The name Disse is familiar to most hepatologists because it graces the narrow space separating the liver's fenestrated sinusoidal membrane from the plasma membrane of the hepatocyte plates." Born in 1852 in Westphalia, where his father was the district physician, Disse studied medicine under the happy German custom of moving from the University of Würzburg, to Göttingen, München and Erlangen. At the University of Erlangen he produced his thesis, "Contributions to the Anatomy of the Human Larynx," in 1875 and was granted his Doctor of Medicine degree for it. As Schmid has written: "Disse was an experimental pathologist of unusually wide scope whose scientific interests ranged from human and animal anatomy, histology and embryology to anatomical pathology, often with an emphasis on functional or evolutionary aspects. His published works comprise treatises on the origin of blood cells and vascular structures in incubated hens' eggs (1879); the expansion of the paranasal sinuses after birth (1889); the early evolution of the olfactory nerve (1897); the growth of the eye's anterior chamber in the field mouse (1906); and various articles on the evolution or fine structure of the gastric mucosa, the kidneys and the urinary tract and the matrix of bones and teeth . . . . In this panoply of scientific contributions, his description of the mammalian liver's perisinusoidal space seems to have received only scant attention."

His important work on the lymphatics of the liver depended on subcutaneously injected India ink. "Disse's interpretation of these remarkable findings was that the liver cell not only produces bile draining into the biliary system but also is the fountainhead of the hepatic lymph system that eventually abuts the venous system. He clearly recognized the anatomical separation of the lobular blood and lymph tracks and detected what is now known as the hepatocyte's plasma membrane and the collagen fibres beneath the sinusoidal endothelium."

John Charles Grant Ledingham (1875-1944)

The distinguished bacteriologist and pathologist, John Charles Grant Ledingham, began his medical career at Aberdeen, Scotland, in 1897 by dissecting out and describing the entire musculature of the chimpanzee. In need of a medium for its publication, he, with a fellow student, founded the *Proceedings of the Society of Anatomy and Anthropology of Aberdeen University*. This came to the notice of Francis Galton, the geneticist, and thereafter they engaged in considerable correspondence. Ledingham confirmed Galton's discovery of the strange numerical relationships between the finger print patterns on the various digits. In later life Ledingham rose to be director of the bacteriological department of the famous Lister Institute in London and was eventually made director of the institute itself. His best-known studies were those on variola, vaccinia and avian molluscum published in 1926.

Frederic Wood Jones (1879-1954)

Wood Jones entered the London Hospital Medical School in 1897 and had a distinguished student career there. He won prizes and scholarships, and graduated in 1904. As a student he contributed to the *Journal of Anatomy and Physiology* many notes on the musculature of the bladder and urethra, the development of the fundus of the stomach and a method of "reconstruction" of a human embryo by placing together photographic reproductions of serial sections cut through the fixed and preserved embryo. The originality of his approach impressed his fellow students and his professors.

Like his biographer, W.E. Le Gros Clark, the professor of anatomy at Oxford, Wood Jones was greatly attracted to the tropical areas of the world. On graduation from the London Hospital he went straight to Singapore and thence to the Cocos Islands as the medical officer to a telegraph company that was making extensions of its cable to the islands of Malaysia, New Zealand, Australia and the Great Barrier Reef. Wood Jones' colourful personality was well summed up by John Fulton's friendly bookseller Eric Bligh in London, who in the 1930s supplied Fulton, the American at Oxford with some superb and inexpensive volumes.

In writing to Fulton, who was then at Magdalen College, Bligh said, "I think, on the whole, Wood Jones is the most magnificent man I've ever known. An absolutely glorious figure: such enthusiasm, such avidity for experience (that's why he's let the London world of professors and jobs go to the devil), such sincerity, such enormous humour, such trueness and magnetic geniality of manner. His marriage of course was a vast romance. Mrs. Wood Jones was the daughter of George Clunies Ross... If you do not happen to be familiar with the extraordinary story of the Clunies Ross family and the Cocos Islands, do get Wood Jones, 'Coral and Atolls.'"

Wood Jones did not spend too long in any one place. He returned to England in 1907 as assistant to Elliot Smith, who was interested in the archaeology of Nubia. Then Wood Jones reported on the burial and treatment of the body in the pre-dynastic period in Egypt up to the Ptolemaic period. He paused long enough to publish his volume *Coral and Atolls*. From being a lecturer in anatomy at the University of Manchester he became a demonstrator at St. Thomas' Medical School, London, and from 1912 to 1914 was the professor of anatomy at the London Medical School for Women.

With the outbreak of war in 1914 he became captain in the Royal Army Medical Corps and served in the orthopaedic wards of the special military hospital at Shepherd's Bush in London. By the end of the war he was made Registrar of Neurology under the Pensions Board. His study, "The Principles of Anatomy as Seen in the Hand," was published in 1920 after he had taken the chair of anatomy at Adelaide University in Australia, where he spent eight years. After professorships at Melbourne in Australia and at the University of Manchester, he settled down as professor of human anatomy at the Royal College of Surgeons in London and conservator of its great museum. Professor Le Gros Clark wrote of Wood Jones' "originality of approach," and his "restless curiosity." It is a fascinating story of a hyperactive medical student who remained productive until he died at age 75.

George Washington Corner (1889-1981)

This long-lived ornament of the medical profession was born in Baltimore. His grandfather was one of the original trustees of Johns Hopkins, his university and hospital.

At the age of 16 George Corner entered the Johns Hopkins University and after his freshman year became interested in biology and veterinary medicine. In some way he gained access to the U.S. Department of Agriculture publications on Texas cattle fever and the wonderful research in that field by Theobald Smith. Corner was not to be fenced in by the official curriculum and managed to substitute biology for second-year Latin. He learned in the laboratory to cut tissues for microscopic slides while at the same time writing a term paper for J.B. Watson in psychology, "A Personal Study of Mental Imagery." He finished off three years of college entrance before entering the Hopkins medical faculty by spending the summer at the U.S. Fisheries Laboratory at Beaufort, North Carolina, working on the translucent eggs of southern sea urchins. Entering Johns Hopkins Medical School with 70 other students of Yale, Harvard, Princeton and a few Californians, he was taught anatomy by Professor Mall and the scholarly Florence Sabin. He formed a small journal club that had Dr. Sabin as its mentor. The restless Corner sought research time from Professor Mall who agreed to the proposal, subject to Corner immediately writing the normal anatomy examination. Corner did that successfully. Thereafter he spent four years as a research student with Mall in the interstices of the Hopkins timetable. His research problem concerned the pancreas, where Eugene Opie in pathology was already making inroads. Corner joined a flourishing history of medicine club that was fired up by Harvey Cushing.

Before his medical graduation Corner produced a paper on "Mithridatium and Theriac," and at the same time took classes from the medical artist Max Broedel.

Graduating tenth in his class Corner went off for the summer to Freiburg to hear the lectures of the great pathologist Ludwig Aschoff. After two summers with the Grenfell Mission in Labrador, Corner sought an internship with Howard Kelly, the young professor of obstetrics and gynaecology, but Professor Mall offered him an assistantship that started him on his long and fruitful life in endocrinology. From Mall's laboratory he then went off to the University of California in Berkeley with the Hopkins graduate Herbert Evans.

In a productive life of 92 years, Corner added to medical knowledge of everything from infusoria to the endocrine control of reproduction, on which he became a world authority. He agreed with Thomas Huxley that in this life it was wise to "spin the gossamers as well as forge the anchors of the mind." His finest student contribution was on the structural unit of the pancreas. That was undoubtedly his springboard into the realm of endocrinology, in which he became a renowned leader.

Louis Gross (1895-1937)

Killed in an aircraft crash en route to his new research post at the University of Southern California, this remarkable student has been eulogized by his teacher, Dr. Maude Abbott:

> Louis Gross was born in Montreal on 5th May, 1895 and entered the Faculty of Medicine of McGill University with a scholarship from the Montreal High School in 1916. During his undergraduate period, he won various prizes for extracurricular work and led his class on the aggregate during the five years of the course, graduating in 1921 with the Holmes gold medal, the highest award in the gift of the Faculty. Immediately thereafter he was appointed Douglas fellow in pathology and spent the next five years teaching and working in the department of pathology under the guidance of Prof. Horst Oertel, who directed him to the study of the vascular architecture of the various organs and the effect thereon of advancing age and various pathological changes. In the injection method with subsequent roentgenological examination, he developed a very successful personal technique and published in rapid succession four papers on the structure and functions of the circulation in the kidney, spleen, liver, placenta and lung. Finally, as the climax of these preliminary studies, there appeared in 1921 his classic monograph, "The blood supply to the heart in its clinical and anatomical aspects," (1921) which, published at the age of 26, immediately won international recognition as an authoritative contribution of great scientific value, and remains his masterpiece.

Histology is an exotic meal... Taken compulsorily in large doses it is impossible to digest, but after repeated tastings in small draughts it becomes completely agreeable and even addictive... Those who teach it ... content themselves with small earnings, and hence have few enemies.
Pio del Rio-Hortega,
Madrid, 1933

Salvador Edward Luria (1912-1991)

Luria won the Nobel Prize in 1969. Forty years earlier he had entered the medical faculty of the University of Turin. While an undergraduate he began his illustrious career by work in tissue culture research under the distinguished Professor Giuseppe Levi. Luria graduated in 1935 with the M.D. degree, summa cum laude. After three years in the army his life concentrated on the problem of avoiding the Nazis. He fled to Paris in 1940 and emigrated to the United States, where he became a very productive researcher.

George Emil Palade

George Emil Palade won the Nobel Prize in Medicine in 1974. He was born in 1912 in Moldavia, Romania, and at age 18 began his medical studies at the University of Bucharest. He started research as a medical student in the anatomy laboratory, graduating in 1940. During World War II he served in the medical corps of the Romanian Army. Postwar, in 1946 he an opportunity to work in the laboratory of Professor Robert Chambers at New York University. Palade was offered a post at Rockefeller University where he successfully combined the techniques of cell fractionation and electron microscopy, and later autoradiography. Both there and at Yale University he was joined in research by Dr. James Jamieson, an outstanding graduate of the University of British Columbia. Palade shared the 1940 Nobel Prize with Albert Claude and Christian R. de Duve for their work on the microscopic structure and functions within a cell that laid the foundations for modern cell biology.

One of Palade's great contributions was his insistence that cellular protein factories and their malfunction lead to diseases, especially degenerative diseases. Like other medical student researchers he succumbed to the temptation to found a periodical, in this case *The Journal of Cell Biology*.

Renato Dulbecco (1914)

Born at Catanzaro, Italy, Dulbecco entered the University of Turin at the age of 16. His brilliant work in his first year of medicine propelled him into research within the anatomy department under Professor Giuseppe Levi on tissue cultures, neurology and experimental biology. That laboratory also contained such scholars as Salvador Luria and Rita Levi-Montalcini. In 1936 he did his military service in medical work. He returned to pathology in 1938 and during World War II was posted first to the French front and later to Russia, where he was seriously wounded. After several months of hospitalization he joined the Italian underground as the German occupation of Italy unfolded. Dulbecco was a physician for the partisans and joined the Committee for National Liberation in Turin. He served in the first post-war government there.

Dulbecco returned to his former laboratory but was offered a post at the University of Indiana where he shared a laboratory with James Watson, of helical DNA fame. Dulbecco's work took him to the California Institute of Technology, the Rockefeller University in New York, Glasgow and the Salk Institute, as well as to the Imperial Cancer Research Foundation in London, England. Eventually he settled at the University of California at San Diego.

[1] Guinterius, a liberal Catholic taught another great contributor, Michael Servetus, who discovered the lesser circulation from the right to the left heart through the lungs, which he first described in *Restitutio Christianismi* (1553). Servetus, at the age of 20, began publishing his supposedly heretical works for which he was burned at the stake by John Calvin at Geneva in 1553. Guinterius described Servetus as "a man who would be an ornament of any branch of letters, and one who is second to none in the Galenical doctrine." (William Tyndale of Oxford had been similarly burned in 1536 for translating into English the New Testament.)

[2] The frauds in translation uncovered by Valla in his beautifully printed *Elegantia* (as seen in the Sherrington copy in the University of British Columbia's Woodward Library) were of the magnitude of the half-truths in Galen uncovered by Vesalius.

[3] Vesalius generously referred to Galen later as "after Hippocrates the prince of medicine," and "easily the foremost among the teachers of anatomy."

[4] Carl F.W. Ludwig (1816-1895) published in 1842 his Marburg M.D. thesis summarizing his student work on a purely physical theory of the formation of urine. He was not cognizant of Bowman's contemporary paper.

[5] His schooling, in part, was in the region of Huesca, where Michael Servetus was born, in 1511. From the village, Villanueva, he derived his alternate name Villanovanus, under which he practised medicine until hunted down by the Inquisition for John Calvin, who burned him at the stake in 1553.

CHAPTER THREE

Bibliography

> *"There is no better float through posterity than to be the author of a good bibliography."* -Osler

Progress in medicine has depended more upon the written word than it has in any other branch of science. The scholars, who because of their own trials in self-education were determined to simplify the use of the world's literature, form a unique group. Each was a profound student of nature as well as an innovator in the field of bibliography. They are considered here because they began their work as bibliographers while undergraduate students—when their own personal struggle to codify knowledge was their daily occupation.

Conrad Gesner (1516-1565)

Conrad Gesner is the first of these great men. Osler said that he did not know if Gesner should be placed in his *Bibliotheca Prima*, where the greatest scientific contributors were arrayed, and added, "But I love him so much I must put him there. Besides he is the father of bibliography." Gesner, the son of a poor furrier in Zurich, graduated in medicine in Basel in 1541 after enduring many privations. Gesner's education was undertaken by his great-uncle, Hans Frick, a man with an interest in botany that was soon communicated to his student. In addition, a dedicated teacher by the name of J.J. Amman took this promising lad into his own home and tutored him for three years in Latin and Greek.

Gesner's father was killed as he fought beside Zwingli in the War of the Protestant Reformation, so that Conrad, aged 15, had again to seek help, which he found in the home of the Strasbourg scholar, Wolfgang Capito, where he learned Hebrew. At age 16, with a small bursary from Zurich, he set off for France and unfortunately encountered nothing but closed minds at the University of Paris. Returning to Switzerland to teach classics, Gesner began to prepare for his study of medicine. In time, he went to Montpellier, and in 1541 completed his medical doctorate in Basel. It was in the course of his undergraduate studies that he became convinced, as Billings was to be convinced 300 years later—of the need for the orderly recording and description of all books which would assist scholars in pursuing knowledge.

He had already begun to gather material for his *Bibliotheca Universalis*, an attempt to list and annotate the titles of all books in Greek, Latin and Hebrew ever published. Only youth can start such projects. Even the erudite Gesner little dreamed that his catalogue would reach 20 volumes. Ironically his volume on medical books (Volume XX) was never completed.

Gesner was at once a great botanist, zoologist and scholar, editing the works of the brilliant Valerius Cordus, who, in his teens, revolutionized botany, and first synthesized ether. Gesner's bibliographic methods have long been applied in all fields of knowledge, not merely in the medical.

Gesner died of pleurisy at the age of 49, worn out by 20 years of incessant work—his practice by day and his writing by night on his bibliography, his Greek dictionary, his volumes of botany, his five-volume *Historia Animalium*, and his book of selected readings from contemporary surgeons. He was ennobled in the year before his death. For a man who was dogged by poor health and poor eyesight he set a record for creative activity.

Although Otto Brunfels (d. 1534) wrote his graduation thesis in his native town of Basel in 1530 on a botanical subject, and is discussed in that chapter, he also published in that same year a 78-page catalogue of illustrious physicians.

Gabriel Naudé (1600-1653

Gabriel Naudé, while a medical student in Paris, was given charge of Henri de Mesme's library. His graduation in medicine took place at Padua. Soon thereafter he published his great work *Aduis pour dresser une Bibliotheque* (1627).

Having graduated at Padua, he devoted his life to books, being librarian successively to Cardinal Bagni and Cardinal Barbarine in Italy and to Richelieu in 1642 and Mazarin in 1643 in France. Finally his labours took him to Sweden, where he was librarian to the Queen. His major work was the collecting of Mazarin's first library, which was cruelly dispersed in 1652 during the Fronde Rebellion. Naudé died while on the way home to help Cardinal Mazarin to begin afresh. That would have been a tall order, since Mazarin's library contained 6000 volumes, for which he had paid 20,000 livres to Cordesius, Canon of Limoges.

Albrecht von Haller (1708-1777)

Albrecht von Haller, also a Swiss scholar, was a child prodigy, born in Berne into an aristocratic family. His immense bibliographical papers began with his compilation of 2000 short biographies from his own pen at eight years of age, and with the writing of a Greek dictionary with Chaldee and Hebrew editions at age 10. Throughout his professional life at Göttingen and after his nostalgic return to Berne at the age of 45, he continued this scale of literary production. He is memorialized in Berne in the Hallerianum as the greatest physiologist of his time. His discoveries on the irritability of muscle and the sensibility of nerve were masterpieces. He lives also in his poems and in his country's literature.

Of Haller, Osler writes, "He is the greatest bibliographer in our ranks.

To learning and judgment he added that indispensable quality in a bibliographer, accuracy." His *Bibliotheca medicinae practicae* of four volumes contained an analysis of 52,000 publications.

Robert Watt (1774-1819)

There is perhaps no stranger story in the history of medicine than that of Dr. Robert Watt's *Bibliotheca Britannica*, the "brain child" of his early student days of 1793, the manuscripts of which were discovered in 1864 bound up in two sacks in the possession of his youngest daughter who died insane in the poorhouse.

Watt was born in 1774 on a poor farm in Ayrshire, 18 miles from Glasgow. After all manner of hardships he reached the University of Glasgow, where from 1793 to 1795 he studied arts. Here he began his monumental bibliographic research. He transferred to Edinburgh, seeking to do divinity but eventually settled on medicine. His medical studies were interrupted by financial stringency that forced him into school-teaching for a time. He finally graduated at Glasgow in 1799 and set out for the slate-roofed town of Paisley. There he lived the life of a general practitioner until 1810, when he was granted his M.D. degree from the "University and King's College of Aberdeen," and moved to Glasgow to begin teaching in the theory and practice of medicine. He was a pioneer in social medicine and in the study of the views of superstitious people on the causes of central nervous system disease.

If we think of the Eighteenth Century merely as an age of incisive thinking of materialism and anthropolatry, an age of conscientious clearness, of polish, of self-conceit, as well as scepticism, then Carlyle is right and Voltaire is its chief exponent and representative. But while the conflict with authority was carried on outwardly by the polemics of Voltaire and the literary industry of the encyclopedists, the predominant features, the essential facts of the movement, were the peremptory spirit of free enquiry, together with laborious research and broad systemization. The results of these efforts were utilized by Voltaire and his associates as sturdy weapons of offence. The best minds were inflamed by an inexhaustible and universal curiosity. It was not sometimes in politics and sometimes in religion, as formerly, but in religion, politics, philosophy, man and society, moral and physical sciences, all, everything, became at once the object of study, doubt, and system. In all this it was Haller who was the High Priest; he not only attended the altar, but developed the ceremonials. He was the paragon and epitome of the period. He lived his religion and exemplified it. Voltaire only preached.

C. B. Reed, 1916

Shortly after settling in Glasgow, Watt opened his extensive and discerning library to his medical students. He published in 1812 a *Catalogue of Medical Books for the Use of Students Attending Lectures*. This rare document has been made available to present generations through the researches and scholarly pursuits of Dr. Francesco Cordasco of Long Island University (republished by William F. Kelleher, New York, 1950). Watt opened his "Address to Medical Students on the Best Method of Prosecuting Their Studies" thus:

> It is not from having spent a certain number of years at schools of medicine, it is not from having repeatedly paid fees to the most eminent teachers, nor from the charm of degrees, diplomas and other academical honours, that diseases are to be cured. No, it requires real medical skill, and that can only be acquired from diligent and unwearied exertion.
>
> The reading of the student is too often confined to systems and to compilations, which are generally the works of men of no experience, or of men writing under the influence of preconceived opinions. By the first, materials of little value are as readily selected as those of real importance; while, by the last, only such facts are recorded as go to support a particular theory. To obtain correct views in medicine it is necessary to have recourse to original writers, to such as write from actual observation, who have seen and treated the diseases they describe.
>
> Many students, however, are neither possessed of such works or have access to them. To remedy this defect, the present plan of establishing a Library is undertaken and it is hoped that it will meet the approbation of those for whose benefit it is intended.

He was clearly not speaking to those to whom James Atkinson (1759-1839) addressed his *Medical Bibliography*—"To all idle medical students in Great Britain, sit," with a picture of the human sacrum.

Watt's reputation rests largely upon his monumental *Bibliotheca Britannica*. This was developed gradually by the addition, to the medical titles, of works in law, divinity and other subjects. At the age of 43, Watt had a premonition of his early death and wrote that he saw himself "verging towards the afternoon of life in an impaired state of health." Accordingly he retired to Campvale and there worked until his death two years later on his *Bibliotheca Britannica* or a "General Index to the Literature of Great Britain and Ireland Ancient and Modern, including such foreign works as have been translated into English or printed in the British Dominions, as also a copious selection of the writings of the most distinguished authors of all ages and nations." From his sick-bed he supervised the work of his two literary sons and just before his death a few sheets of this first section came to his sick-bed from the printers. Four hundred subscribers are listed as having contributed to the support of the publication. The sons died of tuberculosis and Watt's widow received nothing from the publisher, who failed. The 50,000 titles dealt with were found on slips of paper among the possessions of Watt's daughter. Today they fill 15 volumes on authors and 54 volumes on subjects in the Paisley Free Library. Watt's undergraduate dream of someday preparing a great bibliography of published works in English was finally realized.

During the period of my early physiological researches, it often happened to me to make a discovery, and when, according to a custom which I still follow, I consulted the authors after I had finished the work, I found the whole discovery in Haller. I was greatly provoked, I cursed more than once this wretched book where everything was to be found; but I drew this conclusion which will console many young doctors who have similar back luck, even if I found things which others had discovered before me, I could, if I continued working, find facts still undiscovered.
F. Magendie,
translated by Olmsted

John Shaw Billings (1838-1913)

Billings, as an undergraduate, made a discovery that influenced the lives of more potential medical discoverers than any other single development in medical literature.

He was born in Cotton Township in Switzerland County, Indiana, on April 12, 1838. His father ran a country cross-roads store at Allensville. The family moved to Rhode Island to farm but later returned to Indiana. They were originally descended from John Howland who came to America on the *Mayflower*, and through every vicissitude and tribulation in the west maintained one thing that is central to this chapter's theme—the New Englanders' love of literature.

The seal of [the Hopkins] degree should be a guarantee that its possessor is not only a well educated physician in the fullest sense of the word but that he has learned to think and investigate for himself, and is therefore prepared to undertake, without danger of failure from not knowing how to begin, the study of some of the many problems still awaiting solution.
John Shaw Billings

At an early age John Shaw Billings became saturated with the printed word, and by the age of eight he had read the Bible through completely. At the age of 10 he embarked on the study of Latin, with a grammar, a copy of Caesar and a dictionary. Fortunately he found a ready and sympathetic tutor in the local cleric. He taught himself Greek and geometry and on the strength of these entered Miami University at Oxford, Ohio, at the age of 14.

Having already learned to study by himself, he was able to carry his college work with ease. This gave him the time to browse in the university's 8000-volume library. This collection was remarkable chiefly for the fact that it could be consulted only on Saturday mornings, at which time each student could borrow two books.

While not "exophthalmic with bibliomania," as Harvey Cushing used to say of some of his book-collecting colleagues, Billings definitely became an addict in his early years. Later, of course, he was characterized by Dr. Oliver Wendell Holmes as "a bibliophile of such eminence" that he regarded him "as a positive danger to the owner of a library if he is ever let loose in it alone."

Living on 75 cents a week—mostly on milk and eggs, according to Weir Mitchell—Billings had no money for entertainment. He was of a practical turn of mind, however, and quickly found a method of climbing into the university library on six days of the week, so that he had, in effect, a private library of 8000 volumes. He sampled a wide variety of them, shelf by shelf, and the broad knowledge gained there enabled him to tutor other students, as a means of supporting himself.

In 1857 Billings graduated near the top of his class and became a lecturer with a touring magic lantern show. By 1858 he had earned enough money to enable him to enter the Medical College of Ohio, founded by Daniel Drake (now the University of Cincinnati).[1] He graduated in 1860 after a concentrated course, made doubly so by his simultaneous employment as caretaker of the dissecting rooms. In addition, he "lived in" at one of the hospitals.

Billings' undergraduate discovery was made in the performance of that melancholy duty of writing a graduation thesis, in 1860. What he found greatly influenced his life, as he relates it:

> This has happened in this wise: In the thesis just referred to, it was desirable to give the statistics of the results obtained from certain surgical operations as applied in the treatment of epilepsy. To find these data in their original and authentic form required the consulting of many books, and to get at these books I not only ransacked all the libraries, public and private, to which I could get access in Cincinnati, but for those volumes not found here (and these were the greater proportion), search was made in Philadelphia, New York and elsewhere, to ascertain if they were in any accessible libraries in this country.
>
> After about six months of this sort of work, and correspondence, I became convinced of three things. The first was, that it involves a vast amount of time and labour to search through a thousand volumes of medical books and journals for items on a particular subject, and that the indexes of such books and journals cannot always be relied on as a guide to their contents. The second is, that there are in existence somewhere, over one hundred thousand volumes of such medical books and journals, not counting pamphlets and reprints. And the third was, that while there was nowhere in the world a library which contained all medical literature, there was not in the United States any fairly good medical library, one in which a student might hope to find a large part of the literature relating to any medical subject, and that if one wished to do good bibliographical work to verify the references given by European medical writers, or to make reasonably sure that one had before him all that had been seen or done by previous observers or experimenters on a given subject, he must go to Europe and visit, not merely one, but several of the great capital cities in order to accomplish his desire.
>
> It was this experience which led me, when a favourable opportunity offered at the close of the war [1865] to try to establish, for the use of American physicians, a fairly complete medical library,

and in connection with this to prepare a comprehensive catalogue and index which should spare medical teachers and writers the drudgery of consulting ten thousand or more different texts, or of turning over the leaves of as many volumes to find the dozen or so references of which they might be in search.

Following graduation, Billings acted as demonstrator in anatomy at his alma mater and was about to enter surgical practice when the Civil War supervened. Passing at the top of a list of applicants he was appointed first lieutenant and assistant surgeon in April 1862, and sent to Cliffburne General Hospital, Washington, D.C. This institution he found to be "in an extremely filthy and dilapidated condition—no drainage whatever, no sinks, no water within half a mile." How it had served formerly as the barracks of the Fifth United States Cavalry is hard to imagine. However, Billings plunged in, and his career as designer and builder of hospitals began.

Billings' army career was demanding and varied. In 1863 he was sent to work under Surgeon General of the army of the Potomac, Jonathan Letterman. In the Battle of Chancellorsville he had the experience "of handling wounded without an ambulance corps, and getting them off when the troops were falling back. . . . We lost altogether between ten and fifteen thousand men." At the Battle of Gettysburg he operated on casualties for seven days continuously—yet found time to keep up his case notes and statistics on the number of gunshot wounds, cases of tetanus and secondary haemorrhages.

These details of Billings' career are cited as proof of the man's sheer ability and physical endurance. In 1862, with his successful excision of the ankle joint, he was the forerunner of Lister—another student discoverer—whose oft-quoted case of excision of the wrist was to be published in 1865.

In August 1864 Billings' field service came to an end, and on the last day of the year he was assigned to the Surgeon General's office in the War Department at Washington. There he was to spend 31 productive years, leaving as his memorial, the great Surgeon General's Llibrary and its invaluable *Index Catalogue*.

Billings' great opportunity to follow up his student discovery came in 1868, when Surgeon General Barnes—to his eternal credit—gave him a sum of $80,000, remaining unspent in Civil War hospital funds, to establish a medical library worthy of the name. At the time of Billings' arrival in the Surgeon General's office, the library comprised 2,253 volumes, indexed in a 31-page catalogue. By 1872, the catalogue was 454 pages long. By the time Billings retired from the army (1895) the first series of 16 volumes of the *Index Catalogue* was completed and the next series was about to commence.

Billings achieved his ambition because he knew how to state his case clearly—something he may have learned in his magic-lantern show days—something that he certainly developed in his Civil War service. He was able to establish the *Index Medicus* in 1879 and get an appropriation from Congress in 1880 to start printing his *Index Catalogue*. Hume has given a most scholarly account of Billings' development of this unique bibliographic enterprise, and also gives some indication of his satisfaction as it developed: "Billings once said that a librarian is in one respect only a sort of hod carrier, who brings together the bricks made by one set of men in order that another set of men may build therewith—but he is apt to take quite as much pride and satisfaction in the resulting structure, provided it be a good one, as if he built it himself."

An undergraduate who had enjoyed a collection of 8000 volumes, and who recognized too that a real medical bibliographical service was needed in the world, was unlikely to be backward in producing arguments for his project. He simply told the incredulous that, "Books are properly compared to tools of which the index is the handle." He bluntly told Congress that the cost of printing his *Index Catalogue* would compare with the cost of an "expedition to the North Pole, five miles of subsidized railroad, one company of cavalry, or a small post office building." In terms of the cost of modern military aircraft, Billings today would undoubtedly have some astronomical but sound demands to make of Congress.

The Washington setting of the Surgeon General's Library and the Army Medical Museum, both of which Billings directed, gave additional scope to his broad range of interests. He helped reorganize the marine hospitals, and also reported on army military posts. He called the U.S. Army "the best fed and the worst housed army in the world." He advised the government on matters of vital statistics. In 1880 he suggested that the data compiled from the census "might be recorded on a single card or slip by punching small holes in it, and that these cards might then be sorted and counted by mechanical means according to any selected group of these perforations." His advice was sought on a multitude of matters.

In 1876 the trustees of Johns Hopkins' Fund asked Billings to become their medical adviser. He entered the competition set up for plans for the Johns Hopkins Hospital, and his were accepted. The debt of Johns Hopkins University to Billings is substantial. For many years he lectured there on hygiene, and later on the history of medicine. Professor Tom Cullen took a train car full of students to the Surgeon General's Library annually to see Billings and his monumental collection.

Billings found time to act as Chairman of the Board of trustees of the Carnegie Institution of Washington. The corporation of the projected Peter Bent Brigham Hospital in Boston asked him to draw up suitable plans for their great teaching hospital, which was completed in the year of Billings' death.

In 1895, on retiring from the army,[2] Billings became Professor of Hygiene and Director of the Laboratory of Hygiene at the University of Pennsylvania in Philadelphia. He was induced to leave this post to go to New York to build what is again a monument to his wisdom and ability—the New York Public Library. By welding together the Astor Library—a great reference collection—and the Lenox Library, with the help of the Tilden Trust, Billings created the basis for the modern library services of New York City. The enabling legislation was passed in 1897, the cornerstone laid in 1902 and the great edifice opened in 1911. Billings' imprint is everywhere to be found in the building itself and in the provisions for the use of the books. One important development was the offer to Billings by Andrew Carnegie, of $5,200,000 with which to build 65 libraries in New York.

Many people wondered how Billings found time for all this creative activity. To his friend MacAlister of London he replied: "I will let you into the secret. There is nothing really difficult if you only begin. Some people contemplate a task until it looms so big it seems impossible. But I just begin and it gets done somehow. There would be no coral islands if the first bug sat down and began to wonder how the job was to be done."

No summary of the contribution of John Shaw Billings to medicine has been more strikingly put than that by Dr. William Welch, the doyen of American medicine, quoted by Hume:

> I have been asked on more than one occasion what have been the really great contributions of this country to medical knowledge. I have given the subject some thought and think that four should be named:
>
> 1. The discovery of anaesthesia.
> 2. The discovery of insect transmission of disease.
> 3. The development of the modern public health laboratory, in all that the term implies.
> 4. The Army Medical Library and its *Index Catalogue*, and this library and its catalogue are the most important of the four.

Geoffrey Keynes (1887-1982)

John Farquhar Fulton provides an excellent picture of his friend Geoffrey Keynes, the distinguished surgical brother of Maynard Keynes the economist when he says, "Geoffrey Keynes...is largely responsible for having introduced the personal bibliography, has, since his undergraduate years at Cambridge, maintained a record of almost unparalleled productivity—a productivity characterized by a wide diversity of interests and subjects treated."

During his long life Keynes produced no less than 21 named or personal bibliographies—in 17 individual volumes. These have included Sir Thomas Browne, William Harvey, Jane Austen, John Evelyn, William Blake and John Donne. That on Browne was dedicated to his mentor Sir William Osler.

Fulton explains that Keynes as an undergraduate at Cambridge "developed a great passion for the writings of John Donne" and published the work in 1914. Thanks to Hemingway's story of the Spanish Civil War, Donne has become a household word with his famous phrase "for whom the bell tolls."

When Keynes was pursuing his clinical studies as an undergraduate at St. Bartholomew's Hospital in London he laboured mightily on the bibliography of William Blake. He wrote: "At home in Cowley Street I would close all medical textbooks at ten o'clock and turn to my work on Blake until Big Ben announced that it was midnight. I had been regularly spending Saturday afternoons in the Reading Room of the British Museum and accumulating the material for the massive Bibliography which was to appear in 1921. In 1913 it was being written for the third time, the first and second versions having been condemned by Dr. John Sampson, Librarian to the University of Liverpool." Nevertheless, Sampson, the severe critic, later gave his own copy of Donne's *Poems* (1639) to Keynes, his nearly perpetual pupil.

Keynes' bibliographic thoroughness overflowed into a critical analysis of the portraiture of William Harvey. He obviously relished the opportunity to separate the many forgeries from the few genuine paintings. Sir Geoffrey was overjoyed to attend a small gathering held at the National Portrait Gallery in London to celebrate his ninetieth birthday. Unveiled at this time was the only genuine midlife portrait of Harvey, which had been successfully repatriated from California, where it had been illegally exported a few decades previously. The gallery has, on suitable occasions, loaned this superb painting to one of its rescuers, the Woodward Biomedical Library at the University of British Columbia in Vancouver.

[1] The pioneer educator and physician of the West, Daniel Drake, published his famous geographical study of disease, "Climate and Diseases of Cincinnati," in 1810, five years before he took his M.D. degree at Philadelphia. Though he began his medical apprenticeship at age 15, his formal training at Philadelphia was often interrupted by financial crises. Born in poverty in New Jersey he nevertheless rose to the top of America's medical profession, founded two medical schools, and wrote the finest papers on medical education of the early 19th century.

[2] Billings chose as his successor the brilliant yellow fever researcher Walter Reed, who tragically died of a ruptured appendix one week after taking over the librarianship (1902).

CHAPTER FOUR

Botany

Historically, medicine and botany have been intimately connected, with many of the earliest remedies originating in the world of plants, shrubs and trees. Students of both sciences have made contributions to knowledge—even if botanizing delayed their medical contributions. In this volume there are some undergraduates who contributed in other fields than purely botanical, and their lives are addressed elsewhere.

William Turner (1510?-1568)

While a medical student at Cambridge, Turner published his *Libellus de re herbaria novus*. He is considered by some to be the father of English botany. In the 17 years from 1551 to 1568 he produced, in London, A *New Herball* in three parts. This, his "great Herball," was the only original English herball written in the 16th century, and was produced while Turner was an exile in Germany. He had been imprisoned for preaching without a licence.

He therefore graduated with his M.D. degree in Italy. On his return to Britain, he served both as chaplain and physician, a member of Parliament and Dean of Wells Cathedral. He was next suspended for nonconformity in religion, but remained throughout his life a great botanist.

Valerius Cordus (1515-1544)

Valerius Cordus is often called the father of modern botany. In his all too short life he described more than 500 species in Germany and Italy alone. Like Vesalius he cast doubt on the classical views of his ancient predecessors, and expanded botany to include far more than the plant life around the Mediterranean. He died of malaria contracted in southern Italy while botanizing. His writings were collected and edited by that gifted botanist and student contributor already mentioned, Conrad Gesner.

Otto Brunfels (1464-1534)

Brunfels might be considered a perpetual scholar, for he graduated in medicine at the advanced age of 56 at Basel in the same year that his *Herbarum vivae eicones* was published. His 78-page catalogue, *Illustrious Physicians*, appeared simultaneously, the effort for both which may have hastened his demise four years later.

You will wonder, perhaps to the verge of astonishment, what has driven me, still a beardless youth, and but slightly infected with knowledge of medicine, to publish a book on herbary, when I know there are six hundred of us Englishmen who in this kind of learning would precede me (as the saying goes) on white horses. I confess frankly that I am unworthy to act as bottle–washer to the most learned Doctor Clement. And I readily give place to many other most learned men. But if it had ever been the wish of Doctor Clement or other experts in medicine to bestow such help on their fellow Englishment as Ruellius has done upon the French and Otho [Brunfels] upon the Germans, I should not be going to speak a single word for the present about the names of herbs. But when I saw that those learned men are making no effort of this kind, I thought it best that I should try something difficult of this sort rather than let young students who hardly know the names of three plants correctly go on in their blindness. So my dear reader take this labour of mine with a smile; and if you make any progress in herbarism by me, nothing will give me more pleasure. If I am caught blundering (and this is very easy) I will gladly be corrected by men of learning. For I am not too proud and pleased with myself not to accept gladly the verdicts of the learned. Fare you well.

Dr. C.E. Raven's translation of Turner's preface to his 1538 publication

Carl Linnaeus (1707-1778)

Born the son of a curate, Linnaeus entered the medical school of Lund in Sweden, transferring to Uppsala in 1728. There he encountered the botanic garden that had been developed by Olaf Rudbeck Sr., who will be discussed in the chapter on lymphatics. Linnaeus produced an early manuscript "*praeludia sponsalsovum plantarum*," on the "love life" of the plants. Thanks to Dr. Anders Celsius, the thermometer scale inventor, Linnaeus became a docent, demonstrating the botanical species to medical students, and in 1730 began to develop his treatise, "Fundamental botanica." A grant from the Royal Scientific Society allowed him to visit Lapland in summer and to write, in winter, two papers, "*Systema lapioarum*," and "*Diaeta Naturalis*."

In 1735-38 he pursued his medical studies at the University of Harderwijk, where tuition cost less than at Leyden. He graduated in 1735 with a thesis "*Dissertatio medica inqua exhibitor hypothesis nova de Febrium Causa*." Then he was off to Amsterdam to meet Boerhaave and Gronovius, who offered to publish his undergraduate work, "*Systema Naturae*." Publication of his "*Fundamenta*" and "*Biblioteca Botanica*" preceded his return to Sweden in 1738.

Be not solitary—be not idle.
Caspar Wistar's motto

L'amour—peut-il être guéri par des remèdes tiré des plantes?
Montpellier thesis of F. D. Sauvages (b. 1706)

It is much easier to write upon a disease than upon a remedy. The former is in the hands of nature...the latter will ever be subject to the whims, the inaccuracies and the blunders of mankind.
William Withering

G.C. Reichel (1727-1771)

As a medical undergraduate, Reichel introduced a unique technique into botanical science. He found that by immersing plants in aqueous solutions of Pernambuco wood, he was able to study the distribution of sap within the plants *in vivo*.

William Withering (1741-1799)

Withering was known as "the flower of physicians." As an undergraduate in medicine at Edinburgh, he addressed his fellow students in their Royal Medical Society on hydrocephalus or dropsy of the brain. On returning to Shropshire to practice medicine at the age of 25, he solved the riddle posed by Old Mother Hutton who had a remedy for common dropsy containing 20 components. Withering, with his student interest, pursued the matter and concluded that the powdered leaves of the digitalis plant were the active ingredients. He was proven right when an itinerant tinker selling pots and pans in Shropshire was brought to him vomiting, dizzy and unable to see properly. Withering soon elicited the fact that the traveller's wife had made a herbal tea for him, using many large digitalis or fox-glove leaves picked by the roadside. The patient's pulse rate had been reduced to 40 beats per minute. Withering later wrote: "This good woman knew the medicine of her country, but not the dose of it, for her husband narrowly escaped with his life."

William Woodville (1752-1805)

Woodville was a Quaker who studied medicine and produced his own *Medical Botany* in four volumes—his life's work—in which there appeared 274 finely coloured plates. These were issued over the period 1790-1794. As a student he turned two acres at King's Cross, London, at his own expense, into a botanic garden.

Sir James Smith (1759-1829)

As a medical student, Smith purchased and brought back to England, in 26 packing cases, the valuable collection of natural history objects of Linnaeus. Smith founded the Linnaean Society.

Robert John Thornton (1768?-1837)

This botanically-inclined medical student narrowly escaped from his mother's desire that he study divinity at Cambridge. His father, a well-known doctor, died when Robert John was an infant. While the boy was at school he kept up a small botanic garden and an aviary. He had a menagerie and kept hawks. From Trinity College, Cambridge, he proceeded to Guy's Hospital Medical School in London from which he graduated in 1793. It is said that his graduation thesis was on oxygen; he became a disciple of Professor Thomas Beddoes at the Pneumatic Institution at Bristol, relying on "factitious airs" for the cure of various respiratory diseases.

Thornton inherited a large fortune and set out to produce, in text, engraving and colour, what he called a "national undertaking." He planned this unprecedented venture while a student at Cambridge. He bankrupted himself and squandered his patrimony in producing *The Temple Of Flora, or Garden Of Nature*.

Robert Hooper (1773-1835)

Hooper was born in London and graduated with his Master of Arts and Bachelor of Medicine degrees at Oxford. He was a student of Pembroke College, long associated with Dr. Samuel Johnson of dictionary and conversationalist fame, and more recently with the neurologist Sir Roger Bannister, its Master, who broke the four-minute barrier for humans running the one-mile course. Hooper was a most productive botanist, producing three major publications as an undergraduate. The first was *Observations on the Structure and Economy of Plants* (1797). A year later he published *The Anatomist's Vade Mecum*. He also found time to translate, from the Latin, *Planck's Hygrology, or The Chemico-Physical Doctrine of Fluids of the Human Body*. Later, in 1826, he produced his *Illustration of the Morbid Anatomy of the Human Brain and Its Membranes*, certainly one of the earliest volumes dedicated solely to neuropathology. That must have vied with his masterly description of 4000 autopsies performed at the St. Marylebone Infirmary in London.

William George Maton (1774-1835)

Maton was born in Salisbury and studied medicine at Oxford. He was made a Fellow of the Linnaean Society at age 20. He contributed several scientific papers to the Society and later became its vice-president. A genus of plants has been named for him as were a woodpecker and a shellfish. His clinical work was pursued at the Westminster Hospital and he became physician to the Duchess of Kent and to the infant Princess Victoria.

Edward Frederick Leitner (1812-1838)

Leitner was born in Stuttgart, son of the Royal Court gardener in the Botanical Gardens in that city. His grandfather had been a barber-surgeon in Eckersdorf. Leitner's father died when the boy was four years old. He attended the University of Tübigen and had lectures there in natural science. However, in 1831 Leitner went to a German community

Thornton inherited the family fortune, to which we owe *The Temple of Flora*... He took his heritage and began to think more seriously of an immense work in many volumes which in scope, illustration, paper and typography would surpass anything in any other European country... One hero of his worship was Dr. Thomas Beddoes the strange father of the stranger poet Thomas Lovell Beddoes; another was Dr. Erasmus Darwin, the first of the Darwins. Both were men of distinguished minds, and Thornton quickly followed Beddoes in his curious system of trying to kill one disease and another by making patients inhale different gases. Both were writers and scientific popularizers who used a way of writing which combined a glittering classical pomposity with sentimentality and exoticism... It was from such examples that Dr. Thornton derived his own sugary pomposity of prose and his execrable taste in the species of poem written for *The Temple of Flora*.
Thornton insisted again and again that he was engaged upon "a national undertaking." ... The coloured plates as well were specifically dedicated to Queen Charlotte, consort of King George III—"her Gracious Majesty, the Bright Example of Conjugal Fidelity and Maternal Tenderness, Patroness of Botany and Fine Arts." ... In 1837, Thornton died at his home in London, leaving, apparently, not enough property to dispose of by will, or to make it worthwhile for his heirs to take out letters of administration.
Geoffrey Grigson,
Thornton's *Temple of Flora*
with plates (1972)

near Charleston in South Carolina where he was registered as a student at the Medical College of South Carolina. Within a year he advertised in the Charleston *Courier* that he was willing to give lectures in botany in the Medical College if sufficient interest was shown locally. In this he was backed by six medical doctors. He offered also to give lessons in German, Latin and Greek. A total of 32 signed up for his botanical lectures, but fewer in the language classes. His letters show that he continued to study medicine "regularly."

Leitner had the pleasure and profit of meeting Audubon, the ornithologist. To his auditors in Charleston he explained that he was preparing to take a year off in order to explore Florida, Tennessee and Arkansas. Benjamin Silliman, the editor of the *American Journal of Science and Arts*, published a long letter from Leitner in which he made it clear that he would then finish his medical studies in Charleston.

In 1832, however, Leitner was bitten by a snake. He nevertheless proceeded to cross the Everglades. In this process, as Audubon wrote to his son, Leitner discovered 50 new types of birds. He also collected 700 species of plants. By 1834 he was back in medical school and wrote his doctoral thesis on a botanical subject, "*De Hippomane Mancinella*." He was appointed librarian to the Medical Society of the State of South Carolina. He experimented on buzzards and their reliance on sight or smell in hunting their prey. As a medical man he became the physician to an expedition to Key West on a 1000-mile cruise. By January 15, 1838, he found himself on another expedition of natural history, but was killed by hostile natives near Jupiter Inlet, Florida. His hospital steward was killed at the same time. This came to the notice of the Head of the War Department, Joel R. Poinsett, who had at one time attended the Medical School of the University of Edinburgh. The Mexican flower the poinsettia was named for him.

Some of Leitner's 800 botanical specimens were taken to Berlin where, sadly, they were destroyed by bombs in 1943. He is remembered in Audubon's publications where one species is named for him, *Nymphea Leitneria*. His name also appears on Audubon's beautiful swan plate. The physician-botanist Alva Wentworth Chapman (1809-1899) named a single species for Leitner, the *Leitneria floridana* (cork wood).

CHAPTER FIVE

Cardio–Vascular System

The 13th-century Arab physician, Ibn Nafis has been the subject of at least four medical students' theses concerning his views on the lesser circulation (i.e., from the right side of the heart to the lungs and through the left side's pump, out to the circulation of blood throughout the body). In 1924 a medical student at Freiburg University, M. Tatawi, discovered Ibn Nafis' discussion of this route, while examining several ancient manuscripts in Berlin, and wrote his graduation thesis on it. In 1951, a medical student at the Sorbonne, A. Shehadeh, prepared his graduation dissertation on Ibn Nafis. Thereafter, E. Dante Coppola, at Yale, wrote his thesis on the lesser circulation and credited Realdo Colombo and his student, Valverde, with the discovery of this circuit.

In 1955, E. Edward Bittar, an undergraduate at Yale, working under Professor John Fulton's guidance, wrote a substantial graduation thesis: "A Study of Ibn Nafis." It appended 125 references to the literature, ancient and modern, and was awarded the William Osler Medal for the best student essay of 1955. Bittar's industrious translation of Ibn Nafis' "Epistle" and his "Commentary" was a herculean accomplishment. In the process Bittar found no evidence of a connection between the writings of Ibn Nafis and the anti-Galenic teachings of the Medical School of Padua. Bittar concluded that the "Epistle" was so fragmentary that he could find no suggestion of a pulmonary circuit. As the distinguished Spanish surgeon Josef Trueta writes, the discovery of the lesser circulation belongs to his countryman Michael Servetus (1511-1553), long sought by the Inquisition and burned at the stake, in Geneva, by his one-time classmate John Calvin.

The years from **William Harvey** (1578-1657) to the present are rich in student contributions in the field of the circulation of the blood. In his delightful translation of Harvey's great work *De Motu Cordis*, designed for students, Leake has drawn attention to the fact that William Harvey as a student at Padua assisted his teacher Fabricius of Aquapendente (1537-1619) in experiments. Leake's reference is to observations which Harvey made on chick embryos, about the year 1600, "in the spring season by way of helping out Fabricius" (*De generatione*, exercise 6). Fabricius regarded him as one of his favourite pupils and taught him the virtue of methodical observation. This quality was superimposed upon the background of a basic education at Cambridge at the College of

I profess both to learn and to teach, not from the position of philosophers but from the fabric of nature.
William Harvey

Harvey made their existence a logical necessity; Malpighi made it a histological certainty.
Fraser Harris on the capillaries, 1911

Some of the designs are heraldic, but Harvey's is symbolic, nay, prophetic. A right hand and arm holds up a caduceus, in which, in place of a lifeless staff, the twin serpents are entwined around a lighted candle which throws out beams in all directions. What more fitting emblem could be devised.
Sir Archibald Garrod, on Harvey's stemma, 1924

Johannes Caius, whom Osler called "the first English student of clinical medicine."

From Fabricius, Harvey learned the method of applying ligatures or cords to blood vessels that he later used to ascertain the direction, volume and force of the blood's flow. It was from Fabricius, who in 1600 published his *De formatu foetu*, that Harvey also learned the elements of embryology. Commencing his observations in the chick embryo, as Aristotle had done, with "a drop of blood... which throbs," Harvey came to consider the flowing blood as more important than the heart itself. He refers repeatedly to the blood's primacy, both in time of development in the embryo and in its functions in the body. From this position his generalization logically followed, of "a continual movement of the blood in a circle... caused by the beat of the heart" (1616).

Studious good and honest men do not think it degrading to alter their view if proof and a public demonstration so persuade them, or regard it as dishonest to desert errors.
William Harvey

As I hear in the night the continual rhythm... I am lost in wonder at this perpetual beat of the manifold tides of life. For us... does this shuttle of life throb to and fro. For us in tireless periods this pendulum of man's gravitation tells the seconds which can never return.
Sir Clifford Allbutt, on the pulse

Since, as Michael Foster says, Fabricius "was the first after Aristotle to describe the formation of the chick in the egg," it may be assumed that Harvey's earliest medical thoughts were laden as much with his teacher's experiments on chick embryos as with those on the valves of the veins. The impression which this early association with an embryologist, interested in vascular systems made upon his apprentice may have been crucial in the discovery which Harvey was to make. Evidence in favour of this view is to be seen in the following passage from *De Motu Cordis*:

> I have seen the first rudiments of the chick as a little cloud in the hen's egg about the fourth or fifth day of incubation, with the shell removed and the egg placed in clear warm water. In the centre of the cloud there was a throbbing point of blood, so trifling that it disappeared on contraction and was lost to sight, while on relaxation it appeared again like a red pin-point. Throbbing between existence and non-existence, now visible, now invisible, it was the beginning of life.

Fabricius had a patient helper with his experiments in the year 1600 and the world, 16 years later, was to learn of the helper's new theory of the circulation of the blood.

Jan Swammerdam (1637-1680)

In the year following Harvey's death a pre-medical student in Holland, Jan Swammerdam, discovered the red corpuscles in the blood of a frog. He wrote: "In the blood I perceived the serum in which floated an immense number of rounded particles, possessing the shape of, as it were, a flat oval, but nevertheless wholly regular. These particles, however, seemed to contain within themselves the humor of other particles. When they were looked at sideways, they resembled transparent rods as it were, and many other figures, according, no doubt, to the different ways in which they were rolled about in the serum of the blood. I remarked besides that the colour of the objects was the paler the more highly they were magnified by means of the microscope."

Because of ill-health Swammerdam did not enter the medical course at Leyden until 1663. Within a year he had shown the valves of the lymphatic vessels. In his graduation year he discovered that the lungs of the newborn float if respiration has already taken place. In addition he introduced a method of injecting specimens, using, at first, suet to trace out the blood vessels.

The productivity of this man was unbelievable. He devised microscissors and dissecting devices of great intricacy for his work on insects. He studied the irritability of muscles and their nerves after removal from the body. He vehemently opposed the theory of spontaneous generation.

From his injection syringes he was able to make simple plethysmographs for measuring the volume of the heart in systole and diastole.

After a life of intense activity Swammerdam developed "melancholia," and followed the mystic Antoinette Bourignon to Holstein. He died at the age of 42. *The Bible of Nature* containing his works was lost until Boerhaave published it in 1737, 57 years after the author's death. The *Bible of Nature* set a new standard for biological illustration. There have been few scientists who have accomplished as much as Swammerdam in the 22 years from his discovery of the red cells of the blood to his death.

The outcome of the teaching of today is to hail the student with superior powers of memorizing as a brilliant student, and the one with the great future. The consequence is that his path from the outset is made easy for him. Bursaries and scholarships fall to his share, and before he has acquired any experience, he is appointed to a teaching post. In the absence of any knowledge acquired from the results of his own observations, he is forced to teach that which he himself was taught, and as he cannot discriminate between truth and superstition, he hands both on to his students. As years pass he comes to believe what he has taught is true and may even grow impervious to new ideas which are contrary to the beliefs he has been expounding.
Sir James Mackenzie

Life is a hospital in which every patient is possessed of the desire of changing his bed.
Baudelaire

Adam Christianus Thebesius (1686-1732)

Adam Christianus Thebesius studied medicine at Leyden and there conducted anatomical investigations on the coronary vessels of the heart. By injecting a variety of materials into these vessels he was able to demonstrate their connection with small ostia in the endocardium. His findings were published in his graduation thesis at the age of 22, "*Disputatio Medica inauguralis de Circulo Sanguinis in Corde*" (Leyden, 1708). This "Thebesian System" was confirmed by Abernethy in 1798, using similar injection procedures.

Sir Astley Paston Cooper (1768-1841)

Sir Astley Paston Cooper was the versatile and gifted son of a Norfolk clergyman. He was the wildest of 10 children, and his youthful escapades are said to have interfered with his formal education. Cooper's mother was a descendant of Isaac Newton, and his paternal grandfather was a surgeon. His uncle, William Cooper, was senior surgeon at Guy's Hospital, London, and it was to him that Astley Cooper was apprenticed in 1784, at the age of 16.

In London, Astley Cooper, with his fellow students Holland and Coleman, lived at the home of Mr. Henry Cline, Surgeon to St. Thomas' Hospital. (Coleman later founded the Veterinary College of London.) In company with Coleman, Cooper made many dissections at Mr. Cline's house, and sought to elucidate the problem of collateral circulation. They tied off the femoral and the brachial arteries in dogs, and with the aid of injection techniques followed out the finest collateral branchings of the vascular tree.

Cooper attended and discussed with his student colleagues the lectures of the famous John Hunter, whose spur was constantly driving another contributor, Edward Jenner, with this injunction: "But why think, why not try the experiment?" For a period of seven months Edinburgh was to know the talented Cooper. So highly was he regarded there by his fellow students that, at the time of his return to London, they offered to elect him to their presidency if he ever came again to study.

Back in London, Cooper conducted further animal experiments with Coleman, this time on respiration. As a senior student in 1791, he was asked by Mr. Cline to take over a large share of his lecturing in surgery.

Once launched on his surgical career, Cooper developed, in rapid succession, operations for the ligation of the common carotid artery, the external iliac artery and eventually his heroic ligation of the abdominal aorta (1817). He wrote texts on *Hernia*, *Injuries of the Joints*, *Diseases of the Testis*, and the *Thymus Gland*. Students today still speak of Cooper's fascia.

He had broad social sympathies and was an important figure in the life of London. He was a model of industry, and a great teacher. He gave students an unrivalled chance to learn surgery, and was among the first to lecture from patients rather than didactically. He even took students to help him dissect an elephant that had died in the menagerie at the Tower of London.

Allan Burns (1781-1813)

The meteoric Allan Burns began the study of medicine at age 14 under his brother John who was a lecturer in anatomy and surgery in Glasgow, Scotland. By age 16 Allan was given sole direction of the dissecting rooms of John's establishment. Soon he was studying patients of his brother and friends, and making drawings that later found their way into books he wrote on surgical anatomy, the blood vessels and diseases of the heart.

While he may have lacked a degree in medicine, he was nevertheless invited, at age 23, by the Empress Catherine to take over the direction of a hospital in Russia as well as its surgery. He did not stay long. At the age of 28 he published the work that made him famous: "Observations on Some of the Most Frequent and Important Diseases of the Heart." Burns died at age 31, presumably of a ruptured appendix.

Benjamin G. Hodge and **Thomas Smith**

The thesis requirement for graduation in the medical faculty of the University of Pennsylvania encouraged student research in many fields, as illustrated in the chapter on anaesthesia. In the area of the heart, blood vessels and circulation, there is an interesting candidate known as Benjamin G. Hodge "of the West Indies," who in 1801 submitted his extensive work, "Experiments and Observations on the Absorption of Active Medicines into the Circulation."

He carried out 16 experiments on dogs to assess the amounts of iron, mercury and other substances absorbed by mouth or rectally, as measured in the thoracic (lymph) duct, as well as in the blood and urine.

Hodge waxed eloquent in his consideration of "the rage that has always existed among physicians for finding another and a shorter passage to the bladder than that of the general circulation... but although this new passage has existed so long in the imagination of physicians, yet it has, very unfortunately, never been found to exist in the body."

He was clearly of the cut of other students "of the West Indies" such as Dr. John Coakley Lettsom, founder of the Medical Society of London, and Dr. William Thornton, whose design for the Capitol in Washington, D.C., was selected by George Washington over 14 others.

In 1805, Thomas Smith "of the Island of St. Croix," submitted his graduation thesis at the University of Pennsylvania on "Wounds of the Intestines." His experimental work consisted of the study of 12 types of incision in the small intestine, transverse or longitudinal. He described suturing of the gut, both successful and unsuccessful.

Smith removed two inches of intestine in one case, and three in another, and did an end-to-end anastomosis in both cases, using sutures. Three weeks later the dogs were in good health, and on examining the operative site he reported, "It was with difficulty I could ascertain where the division had been."

Joseph Hodgson (1788-1869)

In 1811 Joseph Hodgson won the Jacksonian Prize offered by the Royal College of Surgeons of London for the best essay on the set subject of "Wounds and Diseases of Arteries and Veins." The quaint preface to his essay, which was later printed (1815) begins: "The diseases of arteries had for some time engaged my attention, when the Royal College of Surgeons in London proposed, as the subject of the Jacksonian Prize for the year 1811 'Wounds and diseases of arteries and veins.' I was happy in the opportunity of submitting the observations which I had collected to the consideration of the committee and had the gratification of receiving a testimony of their favourable judgement in the adjudication of the Prize for my Essay."

Hodgson apologized to the committee that his essay was so long, and noted that the "habits of a draughtsman" enabled him to illustrate many points in this essay. He gave an early, if not the first, description of aneurysm of the aortic arch. As well, he related coronary arteriosclerosis to heart disease.

P.N. Gerdy

In 1823 a remarkable thesis was presented in Paris by a graduating medical student, P.N. Gerdy, on the heart and circulation, with 13 illustrations and extracts from cases of his teachers, Beclard, Ribes and Breshet, all members of the Royal Academy of Medicine. Gerdy's chief interest lay in the early developmental structures of the heart wall. To study the spiral musculature he, like William Harvey, boiled the heart. Later, in 1840, he described with confidence the seat of consciousness in the midbrain.

Richard Bright (1789-1858)

Richard Bright undertook the study of medicine at Edinburgh in 1808 but after two years went off to Iceland with the expedition of Sir George Mackenzie and Sir Henry Holland. He wrote the chronicle of Mackenzie's *Travels in Iceland* insofar as they concerned botanical and zoological elements. On his return he studied for two years at Guy's Hospital in London but in 1812 went back to Edinburgh where he took his Doctor of Medicine degree. He is best-known for his work on the disease of the kidneys bearing his name. He had an incisive mind and an imagination unequalled by his contemporaries.

For his study of kidney disease and its relation to high blood pressure, he was granted, in 1842, by the Governors of Guy's Hospital the use of two wards for a period of six months. The room between the two wards was "fitted up entirely to our purpose" as a laboratory. This constituted the first Clinical Investigation Unit in Britain. For manpower in this research endeavour he pressed into service four "clinicals" whom, he said, he "selected from the more advanced pupils, who had distinguished themselves by their diligence and ability in reporting in the general wards." Tweedie, Barlow and Reese studied the urines of 269 cases of nephritis who passed through the wards in six months, and George Robinson examined microscopically the kidneys of all fatal cases. With this array of talent the nephritic fortress was reduced in a short time. There were no application forms in 18 copies, no security clearances, no public relations departments—just imagination backed by the hard work of dedicated students.

Jean Leonard Marie Poiseuille (1799-1869)

Jean Leonard Marie Poiseuille was born in Paris and there studied medicine. His graduation dissertation of 1828, "*Recherches sur la force du coeur aortique*," describes what he called a "haemodynamometer," which was to replace the Rev. Stephen Hales' arterial cannula for the direct measurement of blood pressure. The introduction of mercury as the registering fluid greatly facilitated clinical and experimental work. This simple instrument was transformed by Karl Ludwig in 1847 into the familiar "kymograph," so omnipresent in the life of medical undergraduates today.

After graduation Poiseuille continued his work in this field, writing in 1830 on "*Recherches sur les causes du mouvement du sang dans les veines*," and in 1839 on "*Mouvement dans les vaisseaux capillaires*." In 1840 he began a series of communications to the Academy of Science in Paris which embraced his other great contributions to the science of haemodynamics. His famous biophysical papers enunciated the direct relationship between the speed of currents in a capillary tube and the fourth power of the tube's radius, the pressure and the viscosity of the fluid—still known as Poiseuille's law.

He was a versatile man, inventing the viscosimeter, and measuring the blood pressure changes occurring with each heartbeat, as well as the degree to which arteries dilate with each systole. He pursued the physics of capillary tubes further. In 1845 he produced a work on the ventilation of ships. He wrote also on respiration, and upon such chemical subjects as the metabolism of glucose and urea. His many contributions to science were recognized by France, and he was fittingly made Officier de la Légion d'Honneur.

So of your questions, don't in mercy try
To pump your patient absolutely dry;
He's not a mollusk squirming in a dish,
You're not Agassiz, and he's not a fish.

If the poor victim needs must be percussed,
Don't make an anvil of his aching bust;
(Doctors exist within a hundred miles
Who thump a thorax as they'd hammer piles;)
If you must listen to his doubtful chest,
Catch the essentials and ignore the rest."
O. W. Holmes
Dean, Harvard Medical School,
1847-1853

Oliver Wendell Holmes (1809-1894)

Oliver Wendell Holmes was born in 1809 into the liberal atmosphere of Rev. Abiel Holmes' and Sarah Wendell's family circle. On both sides of the family tree there were doctors. From his mother he inherited spirit, and from his Yale-taught father an enjoyment of revelry that was to break out repeatedly in The Hasty Pudding Club and in other waggish pursuits at Harvard.

As a boy, O.W. Holmes was in almost daily contact with "The American Jenner"—as their neighbour Dr. Benjamin Waterhouse called himself. Holmes took up dancing and cigars at an early age and, being ready prematurely to enter Harvard, was sent to school for a year at Andover, where he developed a taste for oratory.

At the age of 16, and being all of 157 cm (5'3"), he entered Harvard College, where he became famed for his humorous verse. With his friends he produced an exact copy of the sober Harvard Triennial Catalogue, in which they gave themselves a host of honourary degrees. Rev. Abiel Holmes found it hard to squelch this exuberance since he, in his own time at Yale, had been favoured by parental latitude not often associated with early New England. It is recorded that his mother, Temperance Holmes, sent him off to Yale "with a Dutch liquor case containing six large bottles filled with various kinds of strong waters, probably brandy, rum, gin, whisky, doubtless enough to craze a whole class of young bacchanalians."

O.W. Holmes received his A.B., Harvard, at the age of 20, and his production as class poet stopped the graduation ceremonies for eight minutes, so tumultuous was the applause. He entered upon the study of law but was soon to record that "the temple of the law... seems very cold and cheerless about the threshold." At about this time he read an editorial in a New York paper lamenting the decision of the Secretary of the Navy to dismantle the famous frigate *Constitution*. Holmes blew up. He dashed off three verses entitled "Old Ironsides," sent them to the *Boston Daily Advertiser*, and was famous from one end of the country to the other within a week. He dryly observed that "there is no form of lead-poisoning which more rapidly and thoroughly pervades the blood and bones and marrow than that which reaches the young author through mental contact with type metal."

OLD IRONSIDES

Ay tear her tattered ensign down!
Long has it waved on high,
And many an eye has danced to see
That banner in the sky;
Beneath it rung the battle shout,
And burst the cannon's roar:—
The meteor of the ocean air
Shall sweep the clouds no more.

Her deck once red with heroes' blood,
Where knelt the vanquished foe,
When winds were hurrying o'er the flood
And waves were white below,
No more shall feel the victor's tread,
Or know the conquered knee:—
The harpies of the shore shall pluck
The eagle of the sea!

Oh, better that her shattered hulk
Should sink beneath the wave;
Her thunders shook the mighty deep,
And there should be her grave:
Nail to the mast her holy flag,
Set every threadbare sail,
And give her to the god of storms,
The lightning and the gale!
Oliver Wendell Holmes

Holmes began to attend lectures at the Massachusetts General Hospital, and heard there the famous phrenologist and neuro-anatomist Spurzheim—himself a student investigator of an earlier era. Spurzheim died in the hospital of a "fever" and Holmes was among those who attended the autopsy. He was obviously missing nothing in his new calling. Holmes the versifier kept up his doggerel for some time.

The leaders of the profession in Boston were in the habit of sending their sons abroad for a year's study while undergraduates—a liberal New England tradition that many believe needs reviving on a national scale. John Collins Warren, the surgeon whose name was later to be linked with ether anaesthesia, Nathaniel Bowditch, the navigator and scholar, and James Jackson, the physician-teacher, all sent their sons to Paris. So it was that in March 1833 Holmes sailed to join them, and set himself up in the pension in which Charlotte Corday had murdered the Revolutionary figure Marat in his bath.

But the flamboyant Holmes of the Hasty Pudding Society was beginning to change. He joined the great teacher Pierre Charles Alexandre Louis on the wards of La Pitié every morning from 7:30 to 10:00. He and James Jackson, Jr., were given the rare privilege of free access to Louis' wards and they, along with Henry Bowditch, passed the stiff examinations necessary to enter "La Societé Médicale d'Observation," over which Louis presided. The weekly meetings were compulsory and brought together young men such as Marshall Hall from England, Chomel, and Gabriel Andral, the 33-year-old heir apparent to the chair of medicine. Holmes began to construct in his mind two theories: that most medicines given patients were better given to the fish in the sea; and that puerperal fever could be infectious.

Financially, Holmes put up a running fight with his father and de-

I am too much in earnest for either humility or vanity, but I do entreat those who hold the keys of life and death to listen to me also for this once. I ask no personal favour, but I beg to be heard in behalf of the women whose lives are at stake, until some stronger voice shall plead for them.

I trust that I have made the issue perfectly distinct and intelligible. And let it be remembered that this is no subject to be smoothed over by nicely adjusted phrases of half assent and half censure divided between the parties.... persons are nothing in this matter; better that twenty pamphleteers should be silenced or as many professors unseated, than that one mother's life should be taken. There is no quarrel here between men, but there is deadly incompatibility and exterminating warfare between doctrines.... Indifference will not do here; our journalists and committees have no right to take up their pages with minute anatomy and tediously detailed cases while it is a question whether or not the "black death" of child-bed is to be scattered broadcast by the agency of the mother's friend and advisor. Let the men who mould opinions look to it; if there is any voluntary blindness, any interested oversight, any culpable negligence, even, in such a matter, and the facts shall reach the public ear, the pestilence-carrier of the lying-in chamber must look to God for pardon, for man will never forgive him.

O. W. Holmes

The Contagiousness of Puerperal Fever, 1843

layed his return to Boston until Christmas, 1835. By then he had visited most of Europe's great medical museums, including that of the physician Boerhaave, in Leyden, no doubt to please old Dr. Waterhouse who had graduated there. But it was the spirit of the great Louis which transfixed him. Louis' charm stemmed from his "modesty in the presence of nature." Louis' "Society for Medical Observation" had claimed Holmes' loyalty. The object of the society, as he expressed it, was "to make the problems clear to those who took part in it, to teach them to conquer the difficulties, to make observation really useful by making it exact and precise, and finally to show how one can safely proceed from particular facts to sound generalizations." These were the very methods which Holmes soon applied to the scandal of childbed fever in America. To repeat Pasteur's dictum, "fortune favours the prepared mind"—and the world owes much to the mind prepared so well by Pasteur's compatriot, P.C.A. Louis.

Before leaving Paris Holmes wrote to his family of what may be regarded as some of his discoveries—"I have more fully learned at least three principles since I have been in Paris: not to take authority when I can have facts; not to guess when I can know; not to think a man must take physic because he is sick." "My aim has been to qualify myself... not for a mere scholar, for a follower after other men's opinions, for a dependent on their authority—but for the character of a man who has seen and therefore knows; who has thought and therefore has arrived at his own conclusions."

On returning to Boston Holmes wrote his M.D. thesis on his observations on "Acute Pericarditis" and graduated M.D. Harvard on February 11, 1836. The influence of Louis carried Holmes forward for another two years of writing as he took the Boylston Essay Prizes for 1836 and 1837 on "Malaria in New England," and on "Physical Methods in the Medical Examination."

Soon after graduation Holmes joined the Boston Society for Medical Improvement, doubtless to fill the void in his intellectual life previously filled by the little society in Paris. At one of the Boston meetings he heard of the death of a physician who had assisted at an autopsy a week previously on a woman dead of childbed fever. During the intervening week—the last week of his life—the physician had attended several women in childbirth, and all of these had come down with puerperal sepsis and fever.

This information, coming upon his earlier undergraduate musings in Paris on this subject, produced another outburst of the "Old Ironsides" type. The echo reached to Philadelphia where the pride of the profession retorted with the haughtiness that occasionally characterizes some figures afflicted with "decerebrate rigidity." Thereupon Holmes became the prosecuting attorney in the case, and the sharpening of his wits achieved through his early legal training came to the fore.

Oliver Wendell Holmes the writer had a sharp pen, his real sword. He used it with skill: "Let it be remembered that this is no subject to be smoothed over by nicely adjusted phrases of half-assent and half-censure divided between the parties.... Persons are nothing in this matter, better that twenty pamphleteers should be silenced or as many professors unseated, than that one mother's life be taken."

The forces of opposition that tried to have Holmes sacked from his professorship in anatomy actually propelled him into the Dean's position at Harvard Medical School.

Paul-Louis Duroziez (1826-1897)

Another French physician who contributed to cardio-vascular physiology was Paul-Louis Duroziez. In 1850, while an undergraduate, he was awarded the Corvisart Prize for his essay on "Therapeutic Properties and Physiologic Action of Digitalis." Like Purkinje, Duroziez was interested in the toxic and delirious states encountered in overdosage with digitalis. Graduating in 1851 he chose as his thesis subject an analysis of the cases admitted during the term 1850-1851 to the service of Professor Bouillaud.

Ten years later Duroziez wrote a paper on the subject with which his name is still closely connected: "*Du double souffle intermittent crural, comme signe de l'insuffisance aortique*." In 1877 he published an excellent work on "Pure Mitral Stenosis," its sequelae and sex distribution. His *Clinical Treatise on Diseases of the Heart* was widely acclaimed in 1891, and was awarded prizes both by the Academy of Medicine and the Institute of France.

Duroziez represents the best in general practice in France. He was associated with the clinic at the Charité, but never held a chair nor headed a large hospital service. Nevertheless he is said to have been welcomed universally as a true contributor to medical science. Two years before his death he was made Chevalier de la Légion d'Honneur. His life and works have been chronicled in a student thesis at the University of Paris by Feiga Helfenbein (1922).

Augustus Volney Waller (1816-1870)

The English county of Kent can claim such a student of the heart and blood vessels as William Harvey, just as Shropshire claims clinical observers of the type of Withering. To the name of Harvey should be added that of Augustus Volney Waller, whose early brilliant researches on the smallest blood vessels, the capillaries, led him into that field of degeneration in the nervous system known the world over as "Wallerian degeneration."

Though born in Faversham, Kent, Waller studied his medicine in France, a country with which his life came to be closely linked. His researches, curiously enough, revolved about the tongue of the frog, that indestructible friend of medical research which first showed Malpighi the conversion of venous to arterial blood in the capillaries of its lungs—the missing link in Harvey's great generalization, surmised by him but not demonstrated until microscopes were invented. One thinks of Waller in a long line of investigators dependent for the truth upon the frog: Leeuwenhoek; Swammerdam observing the red blood corpuscles; Pfluger, studying the miracle of oxidation in its tissues; Descartes, the physiologist-philosopher, asking it questions; the brothers Weber, working out the slowing of its heart by stimulating its vagus nerve; Gaskell, finding the nerves that accelerate its heart and human hearts; Johannes Müller and Helmholtz, working out the velocity and direction of nerve impulses in the nervous system; and Joseph Lister, observing inflammation in the web of its foot while he plotted the end of sepsis in surgery.

As a first-year medical student in Paris, Waller watched the coming and going of blood corpuscles through the walls of the microscopic capillary vessels, and he made a beautifully simple drawing of it. This work he published seven years later in *The Philosophical Magazine*. Within three years of this he sent to the Royal Society of London the paper that was to make him famous, on the changes seen in nerves in the frog's tongue when cut off from their mother cells. It was this single fact, more than all others, which eventually caused Ramón y Cajal, Van Gehüchten and Sherrington to grasp the truth now known as "the neurone theory"—that a nerve cell and its fibre processes make up an autonomous unit, which multiplied millions of times gives humankind its nervous system. Waller, by cutting other nerves in the frog, soon discovered the direction of the nerve impulses to the heart, to the blood vessels of the head, and showed that without an intact retina in the eye there could be no fibres transmitting impulses over the optic nerve to the brain. And so a medical student with a frog and a microscope became famous.

Maurice Raynaud (1834-1881)

Few physicians have had such a float through posterity as Maurice Raynaud was to enjoy. The disease described by him in his Doctor of Medicine thesis is still called "Raynaud's disease." Raynaud came from a family of professors and surgeons. In 1860, two years before he was to write his classic graduation dissertation, "*De l'asphyxie locale et de la gangrène symétrique des extrémités*," he saw a 27-year-old female patient in whom all four extremities had spontaneously developed unexplained gangrene. He observed the progress of this patient for a month, and realizing how completely his clinical teachers were at sea as to the origin of this condition, set out to collect similar cases and search for a common denominator. He collected 20 already-recorded cases and five of his own. In view of the modern criticism that many of his cases would not be considered today as Raynaud's disease, it serves well to quote from his thesis:

> I am far from attributing the same importance to all of these cases. Some of them are incomplete, some of them are doubtful.... I would not be truthful if I did not say that I have certain doubts myself, but there is always a certain interest in the collection, into a single bundle, of certain facts scattered throughout science.

The directness of Raynaud's literary style is a pleasant contrast to the sometimes tortured verbiage of modern times. Under the heading, "Local Syncope of the Most Simple Form," he begins:

> Mme. X., at twenty-six years, has never been ill; but she has been the subject since childhood of an infirmity which makes her an object of curiosity to her acquaintances. Under the influence of very moderate cold, and even at the height of summer, she sees her fingers become ex-sanguine, completely insensible, and of a whitish yellow colour. This phenomenon happens often without reason, lasts a variable time, and terminates by a period of very painful reaction, during which the circulation is re-established little by little and recurs to the normal state.... The feet, more impressionable even than the hands, are regularly attacked at meal times and whilst digestion is going on. Menstruation does not appear to

have any influence upon the appearance of the phenomenon, but it is a remarkable fact that the complete disappearance of attacks of local syncope has always been noted by this lady as the first index of a commencing pregnancy.

In 1874 Raynaud published a further extensive paper on this disease and, in fact, maintained his interest in it throughout his all-too-brief life. He died at the age of 47 of a long-evident heart disease.

Raynaud was greatly interested in the history of medicine, and in 1862 wrote a delightful book, *La médecine au temps de* Molière, which is still a great source of information on the rigours of French medical education of that period. He pictures the hapless undergraduate being put through a series of inquisitions every two years, to answer the oddest array of questions imaginable, without having had anything but didactic teaching, and therefore lacking totally in experience.

The defence of theses by graduating students was a great tribulation to many. The student had to swear that he would obey the laws and the customs designed by the faculty, that he would attend the mass said for deceased physicians, and finally that he would wage unremitting war upon irregular practitioners. If the senior student survived the examinations, oaths, and gastronomic exercises, he was registered as a physician.

Willem Einthoven (1860–1927)

Every first-year medical student knows something of the anatomy and possibly the social function of the elbow joint, and of the mechanics of its pronation and supination. Few realize that a first-year student in Utrecht in 1879 made an analysis of this mechanism, under the patronage of Koster, the anatomist, and eventually became—not an anatomist—but the father of electrocardiography.

Willem Einthoven was born in Java, the son of a doctor. When Willem was 10 his father died, and his mother brought her six children to Utrecht for their education. In 1879 Willem entered the University in Utrecht, and as already described, soon became known as a student of great promise. While still an undergraduate, in 1883, he was given an assistantship at the Utrecht Eye Hospital and there worked with Donders and Snellen. Einthoven's graduation thesis was on "Stereoscopic Vision through Colour Differences." While still in his final year he was proposed by Donders for the chair of physiology at Leyden, about to be vacated by Heynsius. The chair was offered to him, but, modest undergraduate that he was, he refused it until his associate Carl Koller, of cocaine fame, finally persuaded him to take it and to give up his plan of returning to Java to practice.

A year later Einthoven published a paper "On the Law of Specific Nerve Energies," which was to bring immediate recognition to his department at Leyden. He spent the next 40 years at Leyden, moving gradually into the physical sciences as applied to clinical problems, and building a great school of able followers.

In order to record the electrical phenomena associated with the heartbeat, Einthoven first employed a galvanometer of the d'Arsonval type. He then moved on to a more sensitive instrument of Ader's design used for recording submarine signals by deflections of a wire suspended between the poles of a magnet. By greatly increasing the strength of the magnet, and by decreasing the weight of the suspended wire he arrived at a much more sensitive instrument. The wire's movement was then magnified by an optical projection system and recorded on a camera. By 1909 Einthoven had a recording system 100,000 times as sensitive as Ader's original model.

In 1903 Einthoven's classic paper appeared on the galvanometric registering of the human electrocardiogram, with the naming of the P, Q, R, S, and T deflections that are still used today. In 1913, with Fahr and de Waart he published the theory of what is still known as "Einthoven's triangle" for deriving the "electrical axis" of the heart.

Einthoven also recorded the electrical impulses passing centrally up the vagus nerve to the brain from the heart. In addition, according to Leonard Hill, he recorded electric variations in the tonus of the sympathetic nervous system. His efforts were all bent to the developing of recording techniques free of inertia and lag. He was able to produce threads of quartz as fine as two millionths of an inch in diameter for use in his electrocardiograph.

As early as 1894, Einthoven and Geluk developed methods for recording heart sounds, and adapted the string galvanometer to register them.

Sir Thomas Lewis has pointed out that the electrical recording of cardiac irregularities brought about an intensive analysis of their mechanism and of the natural history of heart disease. Lewis remarks:

> Einthoven did more than place his wonderful apparatus at the disposal of other workers. He pointed to many of the ways in which it might be employed. Amongst these he called attention particularly to its capacity to portray the electrical events happening in the human heart. Modern electrocardiography, and the analysis of irregular heart action by galvanometric means, may rightly be said to have been inspired by, and in large part founded upon two papers of his published in 1906 and 1908.

Einthoven was a most cultured man, and a great favourite at Leyden—that ancient university that has produced so many brilliant contributors and teachers in medicine. He was awarded the Nobel Prize in 1924 and made a Foreign Member of the Royal Society of London in 1926. His life was one of teaching and fruitful labor, made happy by the universal acclaim and use of his methods.

F. H. H. Akbar Mahomed

A student at Guy's Hospital in London who was to improve the sphygmograph introduced by Professor Marey in Paris, was Frederick Henry Horatio Akbar Mahomed. He was awarded the Pupils' Physical Society Prize in 1870, two years before he graduated. Bright would have been proud of Mahomed, who wrote a classical paper two years after graduation on "The Etiology of Bright's Disease."

Rudolf Magnus (1873-1927)

A method for measuring blood pressure in an exposed artery was reported by Rudolf Magnus, while an undergraduate, to the International

Congress on Physiology at Bern in 1895. He expanded this work for his graduation thesis at Heidelberg in 1898. He later became one of the world's most eminent physiologists, contributing major discoveries in the field of the pituitary gland, peristalsis in the gut, the maintenance of body posture and the effects of stimulation of the semi-circular canals.

Sir Thomas Lewis (1881-1945)

Thomas Lewis, the father of "clinical science" in Britain, was a precocious Welsh medical undergraduate who before the age of 20 began research on the proteins of unstriped muscle, in the laboratory of Professor Swale Vincent at University College, Cardiff. His paper was published in 1901; another on vertebrate muscle chemistry and heat production, in voluntary and involuntary types, followed in 1902.

In the same year his third description, of the haemolymph glands, was later expanded to include the spleen. Not limited to the cardiovascular system, he then wrote a paper on defective development of lateral cerebellar lobes in a dog—all this prior to his graduation at University Hospital Medical School, London, in 1904. A year later his paper on the thymus gland appeared.

Of those years in London he said that to be plunged into clinics, from physiology and anatomy laboratories, was like a student raised in a botany laboratory being confronted with a market garden. His market garden he tamed from his crowded basement laboratory in University College Hospital on Gower Street in London. There he taught British and American pupils in increasing numbers, such as John Parkinson, Jonathan Meakins and Paul Dudley White. The scrapbook of tracings, made on the electrocardiograph (which Lewis personally purchased from Einthoven in Holland), now resides in the Woodward Biomedical Library at the University of British Columbia. In it one can read the tracings made of the above stalwarts in the developing field of cardiology. White's only complaint was that in March 1913 there were only two hours of sunshine in London and he had the misfortune to spend those two hours in Lewis's darkroom in the U.C.H. basement.

Lewis received every medal known to medical science in Britain, and many beyond its borders. He was knighted for his clinical work in World War I. He created and edited the journal *Heart* and its successor, *Clinical Science*, for 35 years.

Frank Donaldson, Jr. (1861-1906)

During the year 1881-82, Frank Donaldson, Jr., a medical student at the University of Maryland worked with the later illustrious William H. Howell (1860-1945) on "the law for the work of the mammalian left ventricle." Donaldson was 20 at the time, having graduated A.B. at Harvard in 1879. Howell was 21.

C. F. W. Ludwig (1816-1895)

Casting back to Richard Bright's era, lived the notable Carl Friedrich Wilhelm Ludwig. John Fulton writes that "one of the greatest physiologists of the nineteenth century, Carl Ludwig was perhaps especially important for his influence on students who included John Burdon-Sanderson (1828-1905) and Henry Pickering Bowditch (1840-1911)...." Throughout his life a vigorous opponent of vitalism, Ludwig became interested in the problem of kidney function while still a student and devoted his M.D. thesis to the elaboration of a purely physical theory of urine formation. This essay, which appeared in 1842, the same year that Bowman published his work, was written in ignorance of the latter's discoveries. In 1844 Ludwig published a new version of his theory, modified to take Bowman's work into account.

Charles Hastings

Roughly contemporaneous with Bright was a meteoric student Charles Hastings. After serving an apprenticeship he went to the University of Edinburgh to take his degree in medicine. He soon joined the Royal Medical Society, possibly the oldest student medical society in the world, and took an active part in its discussions. He assisted a friend in experiments on transfusion, the results of which were published in the inaugural thesis of Dr. Leacock of Barbados. In the spring of 1817 Hastings carried out an experimental inquiry into the action of the blood vessels in health and disease, with a view more especially to demonstrate an independent contractile power in the arterial, capillary and venous systems. It seems that Hastings was the rare student at Edinburgh who routinely used the microscope in physiological and pathological investigations. In the same year he was elected president of the Royal Medical Society. In 1818, when he read an account of his study of the circulation of the frog's foot as seen under the microscope, some speakers in this student society denounced such methods as useless and said that "deductions drawn from experiments on the lower animals were very fallacious and that such investigations were indefensible in themselves" (*Lancet* ii, 182, 1851). When Hastings graduated in medicine in 1818 he wrote his thesis on "*De vi contractili vasorum*."

Though Hastings was offered a teaching post in anatomy, he preferred to take up a vacancy on the medical staff of the Worcester Infirmary. He remained on the staff of the infirmary for 44 years. In one way the major contribution of Charles Hastings, apart from his writing on inflammation of the lungs in 1820, was his establishment of the British Medical Association in 1832 at meetings held in Worcester. The association was an early contributor to funding for medical research in Britain, long before foundations, as they are known today, had been developed.

Karl Landsteiner (1868-1943)

The eminent scientist Karl Landsteiner entered the Vienna Medical School in 1885 and graduated six years later at the age of 23. His first publication was based on his undergraduate work on the influence of diet on the composition of blood ash. He became interested in Paul Ehrlich's 1885 side-chain theory and thereafter spent three years with the distinguished chemist Emil Fischer on the biochemistry of the proteins. By the year 1900 Landsteiner had discovered three blood groups. By 1919 he had published 171 papers on blood agglutination. After World War I Landsteiner, who had left Austria for Holland, came to the United States to the Rockefeller Institute. One of his greatest contributions was made with his colleagues Wiener and Levine in their 1940 description of the Rh factor. Landsteiner was awarded the Nobel Prize for Medicine in 1930 at which time his Nobel lecture was entitled, "On Individual Differences in Human Blood." His title recalls the doctoral thesis of Korver many years earlier on the haemoglobin content of the human placenta as against adult blood.

Peyton Rous (1879-1969)

Peyton Rous, the Nobel Prize winner in Medicine for the year 1966, grew up in Baltimore where, in high school, he entered an essay contest, "On Living Things." A teacher had offered a microscope for the best work by a member of the student Agassiz Society. While Rous wrote a serious piece on "Wild Ferns," he was the lone competitor and the prize was withdrawn with the discouraging news for Rous that there was no contest.

Maintaining his interest in biology he entered, as a college freshman, Johns Hopkins University and gradually gravitated to medicine, which he began to study in 1900. There he worked under the Canadian, John Bruce MacCallum (1876-1906), the fireball who published 27 original papers, mostly on the embryology of the heart, in the 10 years between 1895 and 1906, six of these before graduating in medicine from Hopkins in 1900.

Peyton Rous, the student, was invited by MacCallum to join in his research, but before Rous's graduation in 1904 the tuberculosis which had haunted MacCallum declared itself in earnest, with Rous losing a superb mentor. MacCallum died at age 30. Osler, who taught him as well as Rous, considered MacCallum to be "the most brilliant young man it has ever been my lot to teach.... He caught from Mall... that investigating spirit which has made the anatomical school of the Johns Hopkins University so famous." However, Rous was thrilled to see at first-hand thereafter, Eugene Opie's work on pancreatitis, and Joseph Erlanger's on heart block. Rous's great colleague in the development of the first blood bank, Oswald Robertson, has written about Rous's lonely initial experience at the Rockefeller Institute for Medical Research in New York. Suddenly it was transformed when a New Jersey chicken farmer arrived in the laboratory with a bird which had a large swelling on one leg. Robertson has written that Rous "practically fell on the bird as a heaven-sent answer to his aspirations." The spindle cell sarcoma was removed and its study by Rous opened the gates to what was to become a flood of information on virally caused cancers. When the once-depressed Rous found that the cancer could be transmitted by a cell-free sterile filtrate, he felt that his cup was running over.

Oswald Robertson (1886-1966)

One of the unsung victories of this many-sided researcher was his collaboration with Oswald Robertson and Jay R. Turner of the Rockefeller Institute for Medical Research in developing the banking of blood for emergencies in World War I. When the critically-minded surgeon, Sir Geoffrey Keynes (brother of the economist Maynard Keynes) says of Robertson: "to him a very large number of men indirectly owe their lives" in the first World War, it could well be asked, "Who is this medical hero Robertson?" His close friend, the late J. Garrott Allen, a distinguished professor of surgery at Stanford University, wrote: "The work done by Oswald H. Robertson between 1908 and 1919... particularly that during World War I has long been obscured."

The facts are these: Robertson was born at Woolwich in England.

Eighteen months later his parents moved to California. Oswald graduated from San Francisco's Polytechnic High School and then enrolled in the pre-medical course at the University of California, Berkeley. There, in his first year, as Coggeshall relates, "Robertson did some creditable research on the complement fixation test of rabies." His next research was on a diagnostic test for glanders, for which he was granted the Master of Science degree. He then entered Harvard's Medical School where he won the highly prized Dalton Scholarship Award for his study on pernicious anaemia, at the Massachusetts General Hospital. He interned at the M.G.H. where, a decade later, a treatment for once-forlorn sufferers from pernicious anaemia was pioneered by Minot, Murphy and Whipple.

After his internship Robertson wrote a paper that was published in *California and Western Medicine*, on Ehrlich's test for urobilinogen as an index of liver function. His research fellowship was renewed and this permitted him to do further work on blood dyscrasias.

The year 1915 found Robertson working in Peyton Rous's laboratory in the Rockefeller Institute. His research there on the constituents of blood served him well when Harvey Cushing took the Harvard ambulance overseas in World War I. Robertson jumped at the opportunity to apply the research which he and Rous and J.R. Turner had been prosecuting together on the preservation of blood and of red cell concentrate for transfusions close to the front lines. In some remarkable way, Robertson was able to transfer from the U.S. Medical Corps to the Third Army of the British Expeditionary Force. This took him even closer to the front lines.

George Corner, in his *History of the Rockefeller Institute*, describes Robertson's advanced post. "He built an ice chest out of packing cases and stocked it with flasks of human blood donated by the camp personnel and the walking wounded, and preserved in the Rous-Turner solution. This he used, even after preservation for as long as twenty-six days, in life-saving transfusions of several wounded soldiers fresh from the front lines. His primitive installation was the world's first blood bank."

Robertson was recognized by the U.S. government on leaving the army in 1919 and returned to the Rockefeller Institute to work briefly with Noguchi, and with O.T. Avery who was leading the pneumococcus research—which, years later, yielded the transforming principle—that D.N.A. is the hereditary material. One day Robertson received in the mail a small package from London. In it was the medal and ribbon of Britain's Distinguished Service Order, a highly prized military award for bravery.

Soon Robertson was made professor of medicine at the Rockefeller-inspired Peking Union Medical College. Eight years later he returned to the United States as professor of medicine at the University of Chicago. On retiring to California with a lectureship in biology at Stanford University, Robertson's career had come full circle.

John Bruce MacCallum (1876-1906)

A Canadian who contributed to medical knowledge while still an undergraduate medical student is John Bruce MacCallum. Fortunate in his background, MacCallum fulfilled much of his potential in his 30 short years of life. Considering that he published 27 original scientific papers between 1895 and 1906, five of them before his graduation from Johns

Hopkins Medical School in 1900, it is obvious that he had an unusual personality and intellect. During these same few years, hundreds of letters, many poems and notebooks of memoirs were written which, fortunately, have survived to provide a well-rounded picture of a talented and attractive man and his times.

As a boy, John B. MacCallum was scholastically outstanding and physically healthy. The family did much reading but also enjoyed the pleasures and tasks of the outdoors. In 1892 John followed his brother William to the University of Toronto, enrollling in the class of Arts '96. During his first two years there, he revealed in his letters the gloomy moods which were an integral part of his character, although this was apparent to a lesser extent as he matured. The usual period of self-interrogation in youth was, in his case, rather more prolonged than is common. This probably gave rise to his somewhat melancholy poems, some of which were published in Toronto papers.

It was at Toronto in 1895 that John B. MacCallum published his original scientific work, on "Fresh Water Cladocera," which appeared in the *University of Toronto Quarterly*. In this article he instituted his practice of illustrating all his own work.

It is probable that there is always someone in the life of any research-minded student who inspires the first work and whose encouragement and influence are important to its completion. Such a man, in the case of the younger MacCallum brother, was Professor Ramsay Wright, biologist at the University of Toronto. It would be interesting to know just how the spark is kindled, but records of the events or words between teacher and pupil that lead to the discovery of new things are unfortunately only rarely recorded—the case of Edward Jenner and his mentor, John Hunter, being an exception.

During the term 1895-1896 John MacCallum became better adjusted socially and emotionally to his life at the university. He was fond of dancing and the theatre but took little interest in sports. Each moment of his day was used to advantage, although he never then, nor later, seemed to give the impression of being too busy or pressed in spite of the vast amount of work he accomplished. Sometime in this same term he decided to attend Johns Hopkins Medical School, where his brother had already gone, and he accordingly registered there in the autumn of 1896.

The next four years record phenomenal achievements. He published five important original scientific papers, while creditably passing the required examinations in medicine. He published what is still the classical work on the development and architecture of the muscular wall of the heart. It is said that the work for this paper was completed in three weeks in F.P. Mall's laboratory (the same problem had attracted the interest of another medical undergraduate, Gerdy, in Paris, 75 years earlier). In addition to his own work he proof-read and indexed *The Nervous System and its Constituent Neurones* by Professor Lewellys F. Barker, and maintained a voluminous correspondence with his family and a few friends. Dr. Franklin P. Mall, anatomist and embryologist, and Dr. Simon Flexner who taught pathology, seem to have provided the stimulus for most of his undergraduate research, although undoubtedly the presence of such men as Dr. William Osler, Dr. Welch, and others, was an additional source of inspiration. Four of John MacCallum's five papers were on the anatomy and pathology of the heart; the remaining one concerned the human sartorious muscle. His illustrations for these papers, particularly those of the heart muscle layers, are beautifully drawn and of great value to his readers. All of these publications were of the utmost significance at a time when histology was not commonly used as a basis for the teaching of anatomy. The knowledge of both structure and function was less complete than at present.

John Bruce MacCallum, although aware of his talent, remained modest and unassuming. His research was important to him and, in spite of the apparent ease with which he carried it out, he was under constant strain until each task he set himself was completed. His striving for greater knowledge never ceased and his investigations continued until his death from tuberculosis at the age of 30. Each one he carried out thoroughly and, consequently, his contribution to basic medical knowledge was substantial. As a teacher, both in Denver, Colorado, and at the University of California, he was outstanding and popular, but his scientific research remained always his greatest interest and love.

It is a far cry from Padua to Ontario, and yet the problems faced by Harvey and by MacCallum were similar. Harvey boiled the heart, the better to study its fibrous structure. Gerdy did the same. J.B. MacCallum worked at his problem, with newer methods, but still with the embryologist's approach. What a pity Harvey did not have the distinguished embryologist Franklin Mall at his elbow. Incidentally, they would have had a great deal in common, for Harvey courted unpopularity by thinking about the circulation, and Mall was attacked by some because he used teaching methods designed to make students think.

One cannot leave J.B. MacCallum, the undergraduate investigator, without referring to Osler's great affection for him. In the Osler Library at McGill, there is an unpublished manuscript, "Spirit of Death" by MacCallum, given to Osler by Archibald Malloch, MacCallum's talented biographer. The poem concludes: "Oh come, be swift and take me while I stand,/My work still strong beneath a steady hand."

Malloch, the New York Academy of Medicine's Librarian, summarizes: "When we recall that MacCallum unravelled the heart musculature of the foetal pig in the brief period of a week, conceived his illustrations in a second, and wrote his beautiful paper in a third week, we realize that he was possessed of genius of a high order."

Martin William Flack (1882-1931)

Man's translation into the upper atmosphere in jet-propelled machines during the last half-century has opened a new chapter of human physiology. Today it is assumed that fitness to fly must be proven by any person, in civilian or service pursuits, wishing to pilot or navigate an aircraft through the sky. But the tests of such fitness were not always available—in fact, there were none of a scientific nature before World War I. It was soon after the outbreak of that conflict that Martin Flack of the Medical Research Council of Great Britain was charged with the development of standards of fitness to fly. One such test is still known as the Flack test; in it the candidate blows up a column of mercury 40 millimetres high and holds it with all the expiratory force at his command for as long as he can.

Martin William Flack was born in Kent—that county which has supplied such cardio-vascular student investigators as Harvey and Waller.

Martin's father was butcher and grocer in the village of Borden. Martin made his way in the world through scholarships won at school and at the age of 19 entered Keble College, Oxford, to prepare for a medical career. He was fortunate in the professors under whom he studied—Arthur Thomson and Francis Gotch—and in the friendship of W.H. Jackson, the Radcliffe Librarian, himself a Fellow of Keble.

In the summer of 1903, the village of Borden witnessed the arrival of the great anatomist and teacher, Arthur Keith, at Mann's Place, which delightful spot was to prove a weekend refuge from the unceasing round of London. The butcher's delivery man announced proudly that his master's son, Martin Flack had recently come down from Oxford and was to commence the clinical part of his training in London. For Arthur Keith this was stimulus enough, and in a twinkling he had Martin Flack enrolled at the London Hospital, and, of course, headed for undergraduate research with Keith.

This partnership was to lead to the discovery of the important pacemaker or sino-auricular node of the heart. The work was conducted during the summer of 1906 at Keith's cottage in Kent, where he had assembled 130 hearts, a microscope, and a microtome for cutting thin sections through small blocks of tissue. One evening on returning from a bicycle ride Arthur Keith found that Flack had come upon a new structure in the right auricle of a mole's heart. It had the microscopic composition of an electrical conducting system but was located far from the then-known auriculo-ventricular conducting fibres. A review of the already prepared slides of other hearts showed this newly found structure to be present consistently. This was indeed a new discovery in the terra incognita of the heart. By Christmas 1906 the student and his professor had their report ready for publication. It appeared in the *Journal of Anatomy* early in 1907 entitled, "The Form and Nature of the Muscular Connections between the Primary Divisions of the Vertebrate Heart."

This productive student research bears out the value of close personal collaboration between pupil and professor in an unhurried setting. What was the setting? Sir Arthur Keith's wonderful autobiography recounts the story of their consultations over games of golf:

> Going to a neighbouring chalk ridge on which sheep were grazed [we] laid out a course of nine holes without asking the leave of anyone. With the help of James Braid's manual and our mother wit we set out to learn the great game. We both became infatuated; we would drop our work on the heart to fight out many and many a game. The ridge on which we played was fringed by a belt of wood. That wood swallowed up our supply of balls at an amazing rate.

Flack's reputation as an investigator naturally spread along the corridors of the London Hospital and before long Sir Leonard Hill snared him for physiological pursuits. Together they investigated many problems in respiration and circulation, in athletes especially, until 1908 when Flack graduated. The following year a Radcliffe Travelling Fellowship enabled him to study with Kronecker and Asher in Switzerland. He returned to work with Hill in London and moved to the Applied Physiology Laboratory of the Medical Research Council with Hill when it was established in 1913.

The First World War saw Flack seconded to the embryo Air Service. From then until his death in 1931 his life was full to overflowing with contributions to aviation medicine. His Milroy Lectures of 1921, delivered before the Royal College of Physicians of London, have preserved, for all to read, the great volume of observations made by trained observers in the First World War. Present-day problems of anoxia and hyperventilation and motion sickness were recognized as cardinal problems then. Flack's energy as an investigator and teacher became a legend in the Royal Air Force. Great was the grief of his colleagues in medicine and in aviation when he died of septicemia in 1931 at the age of 50.

Martin Flack's career illustrates the value of close informal relations between students with fertile minds and teachers filled with the spirit of scientific adventure. His basic researches and his planning of research establishments in aviation medicine left mankind in his debt a short nine years after his death. The pilots who served in the Battle of Britain, the "few" to whom the world owed so much, in turn owed much to Martin Flack.

Carl John Wiggers (1883-1963)

After attaining a degree in pharmacy Carl John Wiggers entered the University of Michigan and graduated with the M.D. degree in 1906. In 1905 he described the action of adrenalin on cerebral blood vessels. He demonstrated and communicated his work to an Ann Arbor meeting of the American Physiological Society in 1905. He conversed there with Joseph Erlanger and Yandell Henderson. As a medical student he enjoyed a paid assistantship in the physiology department.

From 1905 to 1911 he published 13 papers on cerebral, coronary and pulmonary blood vessels and their responses to electrical or chemical stimuli. He developed new apparatus to measure blood flow and reported on the effects of haemorrhage. During the next 40 years he continued his studies in depth, in the field of cardiology. Western Reserve Medical School now has a Wiggers Prize in Physiology. In the year 1910 the new professor of medicine at the University of Michigan, who had just come from Stanford University, A.W. Hewlett, advised Wiggers to demonstrate to first-year students how physiological information could be applied to clinical problems and to the interpretation of signs and symptoms of disease. Hewlett, one of William Osler's favourite pupils at Johns Hopkins University, had told him of his recent visit to Munich where he had discovered the new methods devised by Professor Otto Frank. Wiggers was so impressed with Hewlett's description that he went to see these new methods in 1912 because he found that the pressure recorders available in the United States were not as reliable as he wished. Later Wiggers succeeded J.J.R. Macleod at Western Reserve University when Macleod went to Toronto where he encountered Banting and Best as they set out on their discovery of insulin.

BLOOD TRANSFUSIONS

The use of transfusions of blood has been bedevilled for centuries by the problem of coagulation. Several scholars, including Christopher Wren at Oxford, are said to have initiated blood transfusions in whatever type of recipient.

The story of human blood transfusion begins with a needy student, Arthur Coga, who, on November 23, 1667, was given by Dr. Lower and Dr. King, at Oxford, a transfusion of 14 ounces of sheep's blood. This event took place before a group of bishops and parliamentarians, and for his part, the student was paid one guinea. He made no complaint of any kind, and it is recorded that "his pulse and appetite [were] better than before." The same performance was repeated before the Royal Society of London on December 12, 1667, also in a painless fashion. It is difficult to say precisely when the idea of blood transfusion was first published, but one reads in Aubrey's *Lives* in 1649 that Francis Potter, "a man of startling skill in mechanics," originated the "notion of transfusion of blood." Aubrey says:

> He told me his notion of curing diseases by transfusion of blood out of one man into another, and that the hint came into his head reflecting on Ovid's story of Medea and Jason, and that this was a matter of ten years ago [thus in 1639]. About a year after, he and I went to try the experiment but 'twas on a hen and the creature too little and our tools not good.

By June 1666, as the Royal Society records show, Lower in Oxford was successfully transfusing blood from the jugular artery of a mastiff to the jugular vein of an exsanguinated greyhound. In the same year sheep's blood was being transfused into a mastiff. Before long lamb's blood was being transfused into a youth and an adult, in Paris, before the Académie des Sciences.

Although the student Arthur Coga survived in England, there was one fatal outcome in Paris, which led to a decree, in 1668, virtually putting an end to transfusion for several hundred years.

The decree in France came partly as a result of a letter written by a medical student, Guillaume Lamy, on June 8, 1667. The letter protested vigorously against the transfusion done one month previously by Professor J.B. Denys of sheep's blood into a youth in Paris. Lamy's letter was written to Moreau, the King's physician, and he castigates "the pretended usefulness" of transfusion in curing diseases of any kind. Prophetically, Lamy cautioned against diseases produced by impurities in the blood. He knew of the importance of the correct temperature of the blood, and he warned of the danger of coagulation. At his age, not unnaturally, he believed that transfusions were better for old people than for young. The Royal decree against transfusion, which stemmed from Lamy's extensive letter, permitted blood transfusion only when approved by a member of the Faculty of Medicine of Paris.

The apparatus required for transfusion was not lacking, for Boyle gives an excellent description of Christopher Wren's ingenious brass device for lining up a vein under the tip of a syringe so that substances could be injected into the blood stream of a dog, in the year 1656. Boyle speaks of Wren as "our dexterous experimenter" and adds that one of Wren's dogs was given a warm solution of opium in sack, "whereupon the dog began to nod with his head, and falter and reel in his pace.... After some time he began to come to himself again." It remains only to say that the dog grew fat and was stolen. Nearer to the present, Norman Dott, known to all as the distinguished Scottish neurosurgeon, actually designed some of the early equipment for transfusion in human beings from artery to vein while he was still a young medical student. Another Scottish student who assisted his teacher, Dr. James Graham, of Edinburgh, with the first organized group of blood donors was none other than Sir James Learmonth, well-known both in America and in the United Kingdom for his work on the surgery of the sympathetic nervous system and its effect upon peripheral blood vessels.

The cardiovascular field has been the happy hunting ground for many undergraduate investigators. At age 19, Eduard Friedrich Wilhelm Weber, the younger of the two famous brothers, measured the pulse velocity for the first time and was able to show that Bichat's theory that the pulse wave was felt simultaneously in all arteries was fallacious. Four years later, in 1829, the younger Weber took his degree in medicine at Halle.

Jay McLean (1890-1957)

Almost a century later, in 1916, a second-year medical student at Johns Hopkins University, Jay McLean, discovered the anticoagulant, heparin. McLean's story symbolizes the grit and determination of some medical students in this field. McLean wrote, "The discovery of heparin came as a result of my determination to accomplish something by my own ability." His story begins with the San Francisco earthquake, in which his family lost everything. This catastrophe did not rob McLean of his ambition to study medicine at Johns Hopkins University, however, and one finds him, even as a high-school student in California, reading Simon Flexner's great study, *Medical Education in the United States*. As a premedical student he worked in a gold mine in the Mojave Desert at 25 cents an hour. He learned to do blood counts and urinalyses at an infirmary to pay his way as an undergraduate science student at the University of California, and at one time even scrubbed the decks of the San Francisco Bay ferries to support himself. After completing one year of the medical course at the University of California he sought to transfer to Johns Hopkins University, but the dean at San Francisco miserably wrote ahead to Hopkins to say that McLean was "not the kind of man Hopkins sought."

McLean, however, was not to be downed, and spent the next 15 months as an oil driller to accumulate enough money to attend Johns Hopkins Medical School despite the fact that he had already been refused there once. He arrived in Baltimore just as classes were beginning and was lucky enough to find a vacancy in the second year. He made straight for the laboratory of Professor Howell, whose textbook in physiology he had read while a student in California. Howell shuddered in his shoes as he faced this one-man tornado from the west and thought that he was sending him on a suitably long goose chase when he put him to work on a search for clotting substances in the blood. Although the result was not premeditated, it is typical of the contrary nature of Mclean in so many ways that he ended up not with a clotting substance, but with the important anti-clotting substance, heparin. His ability to recover it from the dog's liver was a most important factor in making it available for use in transfusions. His predecessor Lamy, in Paris, had clearly seen, 250 years earlier, how important anticoagulants would be.

Wilder Penfield (1891-1976)

Long before Wilder Penfield became one of the world's leading neurosurgeons and brain researchers, he plunged into the sea of war-emergency blood substitutes. As a Rhodes Scholar at Oxford during the First World War studying physiology in Sherrington's laboratory, he spent the generous Oxford vacations working at a hospital in Paris for wounded French soldiers. The difficulties encountered under fire near the front lines in blood transfusions increased the need for readily available infusions of blood substitutes. Solutions of sodium chloride, gum arabic with glucose, gelatin, and sodium bicarbonate were all under study.

When his Rhodes scholarship came to an end, Penfield joined Professor W.H. Howell at Johns Hopkins Hospital in Baltimore to carry out research under the committee on surgical shock of the National Research Council. He submitted his findings to the *American Journal of Physiology* in 1918: "The blood pressure of experimental animals was kept at a shock level for various lengths of time by progressive bleeding so that their condition resembled that which must frequently exist in wounded men at the front who have sustained severe and continued loss of blood.... I have not been able to show that gum-sodium bicarbonate solution or gum-glucose solution is more efficacious in saving life than is an isotonic solution of sodium chloride." He added: "All dogs in which the venous pressure rose while the arterial pressure was falling, for a period of twenty minutes or more, died regardless of treatment." This was a far cry from the problem which Sherrington had set Penfield at Oxford—the nerve pathways mediating the severe pain of kidney stones passing down the ureter. The little man with the pince-nez had admonished him, smiling, "You would be wise to limit your research to one ureter."

Penfield's subsequent conquests in studying the human cerebral cortex at operation contain a faint echo of his vascular work at Hopkins when he came to the study of vasoconstriction on its cortical vessels. He was, par excellence, a great believer in research opportunities for medical students, which made the Montreal Neurological Institute a mecca for young researchers—most of whom became university professors who, in turn, encouraged another generation of student investigators.

In fifteenth-century Leipzig the master set the following penalties: (1) fine of ten new groschen for lifting a stone or other missile with a view to throwing it at a master but not actually throwing; (2) for the throwing and missing, eight florins; (3) for wounding without mutilating, eighteen florins and compensation to the master; (4) for actual mutilation, expulsion.

Wilder Penfield,
The Second Career

Cecil K. Drinker

Drinker has been described as one of the most brilliant students ever to attend the University of Pennsylvania Medical School. He spent the summer of 1913 as a student assistant to Professor A.N. Richards as did many other medical students who found Richards to be an excellent mentor in research as well as in his own subject, pharmacology. Drinker had great skills in metal work and he built for Richards an improved mechanical perfusion pump. Together they were able to keep a mammalian brain functioning by perfusion for an unprecedented time. Thereafter Richards used it very successfully to perfuse the mammalian kidney. Richards also spent a year in Henry Dale's laboratory at the National Institute for Medical Research in the United Kingdom and on his return established the first course in clinical pharmacology in the United States. His powerhouse was joined by H. Cuthbert Bazett in 1921, coming from Sherrington's laboratory at Oxford following wartime research on head injuries. Richards became an expert in the microscopic study of the flat kidney of the frog. His laboratory attracted over the years Howard Florey of penicillin fame, Comroe, Dripps and Eugene Landis.

Dickinson Richards Jr. (1895-1973)

Another Richards took his Bachelor of Arts degree at Yale in 1917, saw war service and in 1919 entered the College of Physicians and Surgeons at Columbia University in New York. He did a research degree, Master of Science, in physiology in 1922 and graduated M.D. in 1923. He was a pupil of Lawrence Henderson at Harvard and of Henry Dale in London. He was awarded the Nobel Prize in 1956 for his work on heart catheterization.

HAEMOPHILIA

As far as I was concerned the story started when I was a medical student, and one of the patients assigned to me was a case of haemophilia. He was a young man, with a small cut on his chin, which bled persistently. We tried dressings and bandages and strapping, the blood just went on oozing through everything. The cut was sewn up, with the result that he got an enormous haematoma and the stitches burst. Then it was cauterized, but after a day or two a large slough separated and he was bleeding from a wound much larger than the original cut. We tried adrenaline, ice packs, hot packs, pressure dressings and things got steadily worse. Meanwhile he had lost so much blood that he had to be transfused, quite a major proceeding in those days. The bleeding stopped, but it went on intermittently for weeks between transfusions. He survived, but only just, and the whole case made a deep impression on me. I read up as much as I could about haemophilia, and it seemed a bizarre and fascinating condition. It had an aura of mystery connected with Rasputin, the Tzars of Russia and the royal families of Spain and Britain. Its inheritance seemed extraordinary at a time when genetics was a closed book to most medical students, and the transmission of so devastating a disease by apparently normal women to their sons seemed particularly strange. The

Arnold Rice Rich (1893-1968)

Arnold Rice Rich was another young man in a hurry and after only two years at the University of Virginia he took his bachelor's degree. A year later he achieved his master's degree in zoology, publishing his thesis on flatworms while he was a medical student. Entering Johns Hopkins Hospital Medical School in 1915, he published two undergraduate papers in his own name in 1917 on the nature and properties of metathrombin and on "The Changes in Clotting Power of an Oxalated Plasma on Standing." It is said that "he did not allow the school curriculum to interfere with his research to any great degree." Following military service as an army sergeant, Rich decided to specialize in experimental surgery. However, the professor of surgery, Halsted, told Rich that he must first do a year in pathology. Rich never left pathology and fell under the influence of the Canadian professor, W.G. MacCallum.

Apart from one year of postgraduate work in Vienna, Rich spent the rest of his life at Johns Hopkins. He was made professor of pathology in 1944 when he succeeded MacCallum. He was a great teacher and researcher and enlivened clinico-pathological conferences by taking on William Thayer and McGhee Harvey to the delight of large audiences. This violinist and chamber music aficionado was awarded the Kober Medal of the Association of American Physicians.

Some of these young researchers had unusual qualities. For instance, when **James Learmonth**, already mentioned, returned from the World War I to the University of Glasgow Medical School, he exhibited such visual memory that his examiners in anatomy thought his reproduction of the brachial plexus on his examination was so close to Gray's *Anatomy* as to suggest that he had "cribbed" the entire examination from some source. He answered the charge by offering to reproduce any plate that the examiners wished to select from Gray's great textbook. That settled the matter. While he was an undergraduate he called on his wartime experience as he measured the relationship of wind velocities to the spread of gases in warfare. He also wrote on the inheritance of blood groups before he graduated. On that occasion he was awarded the Lauder Brunton Prize. Eventually he was named Regius Professor of Surgery at Edinburgh. One of his interests, the surgery of the autonomic nervous system, he pursued while on a Rockefeller Fellowship. He was for some years on the staff of the Mayo Clinic in Minnesota. His contemporary, **Norman Dott**, on returning from war service became so active in skiing that he broke his femur. As a result he lost two inches from the fractured leg. He immediately had his colleagues resect two inches from the opposite femur so that he could walk on a level keel.

Kenneth James Franklin (1897-1966)

Franklin went up to Oxford as a student of the classics before World War I. After serving in the Royal Field Artillery in France and Belgium, he returned to Oxford to study medicine. As an undergraduate he assisted Professor J.A. Gunn in a research on the pharmacology of the sympathetic nervous system that was published in 1922.

After graduating in medicine in 1924 and serving as one of Sherrington's demonstrators in physiology, he put his classical education to good use in translating the cardiovascular works of Fabricius of Aquapendente and his Paduan pupil William Harvey. As a college tutor at Oriel College, dean of Oxford's medical school and vice-chairman of the Nuffield Institute for Medical Research, Franklin led, by Oxford standards, an unusually busy life. He avoided the rarefied atmosphere, so frequently described by aspiring writers as "port and prejudice" as the mainspring of the dons' activities. The work which he and Peter Daniel, Josep Trueta, Marjorie Pritchard and others carried on in illuminating renal circulation was performed in the observatory built by Dr. John Radcliffe about the year 1785, next door to the Radcliffe Infirmary.

Franklin, together with the Regius Professor of Medicine, Sir Farquhar Buzzard, and with the neurosurgeon Hugh Cairns and his Australian fellow Rhodes Scholar Howard Florey, supported clinical teaching "for credit" at Oxford, resulting, after W.W.II in a full school.

Eugene M. Landis (b. 1901)

Landis was born in Pennsylvania in 1901 and took his bachelor's and master's degrees there prior to his M.D. degree in 1926. His magnificent contribution to cardio-vascular science, made while an undergraduate in 1925, was the direct measurement of the blood pressure within the capillary circulation. Several papers in the *American Journal of Physiology* were required in 1926 to report this important development. Landis carried his researches further and in 1927 was awarded his Doctor of Philosophy degree.

Werner Forssmann (1904-1979)

Forssmann graduated in medicine in 1929 from Friedrich Wilhelm University, Berlin. His doctoral thesis was based on the studies that he and a small group of his classmates made in the previous year on the effects of feeding liver upon the circulating blood. That critical year, in his preparation for great events to follow, included assistance that he rendered Rudolf Fick (son of Adolf, of the Fick principle) in measuring blood flow. This was, likewise, a preparation, unrecognized no doubt, for cardio-vascular research which brought Forssmann the Nobel Prize for Medicine or Physiology in 1956. The story of Forssmann's later daring research on his own cardio-vascular system can be condensed by simply stating that without the approval of his superior in surgery at the Red Cross Auguste Victoria Hospital in Eberswalde near Berlin, he anaesthetized his left elbow, opened the vein and through it ran a narrow, flexible catheter until he felt it was sufficiently stable to allow him to walk down-

symptons were all referable to the failure to stop bleeding after even slight injuries. This bleeding might be from cuts or injuries to the skin or mucous membranes, as in my case, or into the tissues. Patients might get enormous haematomas almost anywhere. The worst feature was haemorrhage into the joints which caused great pain, and, since this often recurred, led to final destruction and crippling. Why these patients bled in this way and what could be done about it were the subjects of considerable and fruitless argument.

At that time ideas on haemostasis were, in general if not in detail, much the same as they are today. People stopped bleeding because the blood clotted, or the platelets agglutinated, or the vessels contracted. The only laboratory test of haemostatic function which was abnormal in haemophilia was the clotting time of the blood. If you took blood from the vein of a normal person and put it in a glass tube it clotted in 5 or 6 minutes, if you did the same thing with blood from a severe haemophiliac, it would not clot for half an hour or more, and it was a pretty poor clot which formed even then. Since nothing much wrong could be demonstrated with the platelets or vessels in haemophilic patients it was assumed that bleeding was due to a failure of blood coagulation. But the nature of this failure was mysterious.

R. Gwynn Macfarlane (1967)

stairs to the x-ray department. There, his astounded colleagues urged him to give up the idea of catheterizing his own heart. However, once the fluoroscope showed that the catheter had entered the right ventricle the attitude of his colleagues changed considerably. On November 5, 1929, the *Klinische Wochenscrift* carried the first news of this incredible and courageous advance under the arresting title "Probing the Right Ventricle of the Heart." The rest of his history, unfortunately, shows a pathetic local medical ostracism. The Nobel trustees, however, recognized the fortitude of the man and awarded him, and his American colleagues in this field, the Prize for Medicine or Physiology in 1956.

Robert Gwyn Macfarlane (1907-1987)

Macfarlane entered St. Bartolomew's Hospital Medical School in London in 1926. His student researches on haemophilia were published in December 1931 in the hospital's *Journal*. His interest began earlier, however, when he was assigned to study a young boy who had entered hospital with non-stop bleeding. The unravelling of the haemophilia conundrum was Macfarlane's life work. Even his onerous duties in World War II could not deflect his interest. As clinical pathologist to the Radcliffe Infirmary at Oxford he covered many fields—some of them of extreme urgency, as in the case of gas gangrene which he studied as a Major in the Royal Army Medical Corps. He was made a Fellow of the Royal Society of London and a Fellow of All Souls College, Oxford. He wrote definitive biographies of both Florey and Fleming.

Sisvan William Gunn

Gunn was born in Cyprus and educated at the University of Marseille's medical faculty and at the University of Geneva. He has become one of the world's experts on "disaster medicine" and has written books and dictionaries on that growing specialty. After years of editorial service at the World Health Organization and at the International Red Cross in Geneva, he has travelled to crisis areas in most of the world to study them in detail. As an undergraduate in the renowned medical school in Geneva he prepared, in 1952, his M.D. thesis on the prophetic topic of "*Expériences sur l'hémostase biologique en neurochirurgie et investigations du problème d'antigénicité de la thrombine*." His experimental results showed that there were no untoward effects from the use of thrombin preparations on the brain or other tissues—a great boon to haemostasis where clips or sutures cannot be applied.

Graham Travis Schuler, while a medical student at Queen's University in Kingston, Ontario, in 1958 conceived the idea of an electronic recorder which would register visually the electric manifestations of a heart attack just as it was beginning or after it was well established. With 70 electrodes recording the activity over the heart from all dimensions of the organ he was able to identify minor attacks, leading hopefully to earlier treatment. Schuler then developed a foetal electrocardiograph capable of recording a heartbeat at the twelfth week of pregnancy.

Thomas J. Fogarty, born in 1934, began a lively career in heart surgery by developing, while a medical undergraduate at the University of Cincinnati, instruments and procedures for the extraction of emboli and thrombi. In the 30 years following his graduation in 1960 he produced 106 publications stemming from improvements in the understanding of embolic crises and in their rapid resolution. There is no limit to his ingenuity in this field which began in his undergraduate years.

L.H. Peterson, when a medical student at the University of Pennsylvania, devised a method, along with colleagues, for recording directly the arterial pressure pulse and blood pressure in man. He found that the earlier use of lead tubing limited greatly the flexibility needed in this operation. He therefore used synthetic polyvinyl and resin tubing, which he said was "intended for such application as electrical insulation." He heated this for 72 hours in an oven at 110° centigrade and then was able to draw it out to any desired length and diameter. This was introduced into the artery through a removable needle and plunger. This unusual tubing was made by a varnish and insulator manufacturer. Peterson graciously acknowledged the help which he had from Professor H. Cuthbert Bazett, previously described as one of Sherrington's pupils.

A pre-medical student at the University of British Columbia, Patrick Bosley, presented his work on the capillary arterio-venous anastomoses in the human finger nailbed to the joint meeting of the British and Canadian Medical Associations in Toronto in 1955. He completed his medical education in England.

CHAPTER SIX

Chemistry

Joseph Black (1728-1799)

Joseph Black was the son of an Irish wine merchant who lived in Bordeaux—the home of the physiologist, François Magendie. At the age of 12 Black was sent to grammar school in Belfast, and at the age of 18 he entered the University of Glasgow. Upon the completion of his pre-medical studies he enrolled in the medical faculty of the University of Edinburgh in 1751.

The rival views of two of his professors, Alston and Whytt, on the treatment of kidney stones, intrigued Black, and in the second year of his course he approached his teacher William Cullen with a plan of investigation. In simplest terms, Black sought a treatment for kidney stones that would be superior to the then-used lime water. Cullen welcomed him. As Professor Robinson has stated it: "No professor took a more lively interest in the progress of an emulous student than Doctor Cullen. It was his delight to encourage and assist their efforts, and therefore he was not long in attaching Mr. Black to himself, in his most intimate co-operation."

There is perhaps no other instance of a graduation thesis so weighted with significant novelty as Black's.
Osler

Black commenced work on magnesia alba and it was in heating this substance that he discovered that it lost "a remarkable proportion of its weight in the fire." This fact was more important to him than any cure for kidney stones and thereafter his "attempts were directed to the investigation of this volatile part."

At this distance in time it is hard to appreciate the significance of Black's work on carbon dioxide. The gas had been named "gas sylvestre" by van Helmont a century earlier, because it could be produced by burning wood. But now Black appeared with something more than a name for the substance—he called it "fixed air"—he derived it in such a manner that he sounded the death knell of the traditional phlogiston theory. That theory held that when a substance was heated something was added to it. Black, by using a fine balance—and thus starting quantitative chemical analysis—proved that some substances when heated lost weight. Taking lime as an example, he heated it, driving off carbon dioxide or "fixed air."

Black showed this gas to be incapable of supporting life. He knew also that the expired air from animals contained his "fixed air." He wrote:

> Quicklime therefore does not attract air when in its most ordinary form, but is capable of being joined to one particular species only which is dispersed through the atmosphere either in the shape of an exceedingly subtle powder, or more probably in that of an elastic fluid. To this I have given the name of "fixed air."

Black's undergraduate work dating from 1752 was embodied in his graduation thesis, "*De humore acido a cibis orto, et magnesia alba*," which was presented to the medical faculty in Edinburgh on June 11, 1754. It was read in amplified form before the Medical Society of Edinburgh on June 5, 1755, and published in 1756 under the title "Experiments upon Magnesia Alba, Quicklime, and Some Other Alkaline Substances." It was twice reprinted, in 1777 and 1782.

Black's later description of these years full of discoveries is informative. He wrote:

> Here a new and boundless field seemed to open before one. We know not how many different airs may be thus contained in our atmosphere, nor what may be their separate properties. This particular one has evidently very curious and important ones... I fully intended to make this air and some other elastic fluid the subject of serious study. A load of new official duties was laid upon me [i.e. he was elected Professor of Medicine and Chemistry of the University of Glasgow in 1756]. In the same year, however, in which my first account of these experiments was published... I had discovered that this particular kind of air, attracted by alkaline substances, is deadly to all animals... And I convinced myself that the change produced on wholesome air by breathing it consisted chiefly, if not solely, in the conversion of part of it into fixed air. For I found, that by blowing through a pipe into lime water, or a solution of caustic alkali, the lime was precipitated and the alkali was rendered mild... In the same year I found that fixed air is the chief part of the elastic matter which is formed in liquids in vinous fermentation. Van Helmont has indeed said this, and it was to this that he first gave the name "gas sylvestre."

Black's essay on fixed air has been classed by some as approaching Newton's *Optics* as a model for investigators. He is still a model for investigators. He is also known for his discovery of "latent heat" and his theory of "specific heat," which together provided the basis for the later discoveries and generalizations of Mayer, Joule and Helmholtz in thermodynamics.

Black was widely known as a great and sympathetic teacher. Among his pupils he numbered James Watt of the steam engine, who never failed to acknowledge the training he had received from Black. The medical student-poet, Oliver Goldsmith, also studied with Black. Daniel Rutherford, another pupil, was to discover nitrogen while still an undergraduate.

In 1766 Black succeeded to the chair of chemistry at Edinburgh, and retired in 1797, a beloved and revered teacher. He died in 1799, as Stirling relates, while eating his frugal meal. He was found by his servant "with his cup—which contained milk diluted with water—on his knees which were joined together, and kept it steady with his hand in the manner of a person perfectly at ease."

Daniel Rutherford (1749-1819)

Daniel Rutherford was born in Edinburgh, November 3, 1749, the son of Dr. John Rutherford, one of the founders of the Edinburgh Medical School. Daniel graduated in arts at Edinburgh and then embarked on a medical course there, graduating in 1772. After extensive study and travel in Europe he took up practice in Edinburgh, where he became president of the Royal College of Physicians. In 1786 he succeeded Dr. John Hope in the chair of botany. He died at the age of 70, having long suffered from gout.

As a medical undergraduate Rutherford was attracted to Joseph Black's laboratory where he was given the problem of finding what remained of the atmosphere after combustion, followed by absorption of the "fixed air" thus produced. Seventeen years after Black had presented his graduation thesis on "fixed air," Rutherford published his graduation essay, "*Dissertatio Inauguralis de aëre fixo dicto, aut mephitico*," thus anticipating Priestley's work.

Rutherford's method, basically, was to remove the oxygen from a sample of air by the burning of charcoal, phosphorus or a candle. He then removed the carbon dioxide with lime or alkali, leaving a residue of what is today known as "nitrogen." The name "nitrogen" was used by the French chemist Chaptal to signify the capacity of this gas to produce nitric acid when electric sparks were passed through it.

Rutherford also established the fact that nitrogen would not support life. He established its exact proportion in air. Lavoisier called this gas "azotic gas" because it would not sustain life.

Johann Jacob Berzelius (1779-1848)

The future distinguished chemist Berzelius studied medicine at Uppsala in Sweden, graduating in 1802. Two years before graduation, however, he published his first paper on an analysis of mineral waters. His graduation thesis in 1802 was "On the Action of Galvanism on Organic Bodies." He went on to appointments as assistant professor of botany and of pharmacy at the University of Stockholm. By 1815 he had been made professor of chemistry at the Caroline Medico-Chirurgical Institute. There he added to his discoveries such elements as cerium, selenium, silicon, zirconium, titanium and thorium.

Jarvis Roebuck "of the Island of St. Croix," for his Doctor of Medicine thesis at the University of Pennsylvania presented on June 8, 1801, chose the title "Experiments and Observations on the Bile." This showed remarkable tenacity by a student trying to find out if there are differences in the bile of different animal species. He studied, with the pioneer chemical processes then available, the bile of oxen, dogs, humans, and the sturgeon. He sought to prove that bile can exist in the blood vessels with impunity. He completed 10 detailed experiments and followed patients on the wards. In one of his experiments he injected dog bile into the external jugular of a dog which animal "a few hours after appeared very dull, would not quit the place where he lay... gradually recovered his appetite and is now perfectly well." He concluded his thesis with the words: "In embracing an antiquated doctrine, I am sanctioned by experiment. This surely ought not to be deserted for the deceptive flushings of a diseased imagination."

In 1803 a botanical and pharmacological thesis was presented at the University of Pennsylvania by John M. Walker of Virginia. The title was "An Experimental Inquiry into the Similarity in Virtue between Cornus Florida and Sericea, and the Cinchona Officinalis of Linnaeus." He made the point that the War of Independence of 1778 had cut off the supplies of cinchona bark from the United States and that the only available material was very expensive. He became interested in therapeutic tests, comparing cinchona with native dogwood. He reviewed 37 cases as to the effects on the pulse and noted that the French Army surgeons in America used Cornus Florida as a substitute for Peruvian bark.

John Davy (1790-1868)

While still a medical student in the year 1811, Davy, brother of Sir Humphry, published his first paper upholding his brother's views on hydrochloric acid and its structure. John Davy's graduation thesis was concerned with the blood, and his "Physiological Researches" was published in London in 1863. He is best-known for his two-volume work, *Memoirs of the Life of Sir Humphry Davy*, published in London in 1836, seven years after the subjects' death.

James Blake (1815-1893)

The discovery of gold in California brought together restless and vibrant figures from all parts of the world, none more so than Dr. James Blake. Born in Gosport, England, on July 14, 1815, his education in the medical field was pursued at University College, London, and probably in France also, for his early publications mention the use of instruments obtained in Paris. Throughout his life he was an admirer of Claude Bernard.

At University College he studied under Thomas Graham and the physiologist William Sharpey who was to inspire other undergraduate contributors such as Joseph Lister. In 1838, at the age of 23, Blake, the medical student, read a paper before the British Association on the effects of certain salts on the body's metabolism. It was published a year later in the *Edinburgh Medical and Surgical Journal*. This student paper is a milestone. In it Blake recounts what must have been the first determinations on the circulation time of the blood. The burden of his communication was the physiological effect of intra-arterial and intravenous injection into animals, of various chemicals, including strychnine and the recently isolated alkaloids, morphine and nicotine. He published this work in French after communicating it to the Academy of Sciences in Paris. His theory was that the effect produced by drugs was determined by their chemical structure.

He saw his experiments as shedding light in two directions by showing first, what physiological reactions followed certain chemical injections, and second, what physico-chemical properties of the reacting tissues might be deduced from the results.

While a senior medical student in 1839 Blake also experimented with the obliteration of veins in animals, and communicated his results to the editor of the *Lancet* in a discussion of the treatment of varicose veins. He wrote:

> By arresting the circulation in the vessel for a few hours (twelve to sixteen); by passing a couple of needles under it and using the twisted suture; and by the application of gentle external pressure, the slight degree of irritation thus produced will be sufficient to cause such an effusion of lymph and serum in the sheath of the vessel as to lead to its permanent obliteration.

While Blake practised medicine in Conduit Street and Pall Mall in London and qualified as a Fellow of the Royal College of Surgeons, his interests were largely along the line of thought of his undergraduate researches. By 1846 he had come to three important conclusions, that: the electro-positive element of an injected salt was the determining factor in the resultant physiological reactions; an increase in toxicity paralleled an increase in the atomic weight of the electro-positive element in inorganic compounds; and the effects attributable to the electro-positive elements reappear as one ascends the scale of atomic weights. He thought, too, that crystal structure was concerned in these physiological effects. Valence was thought to determine the direction and range of action, with monovalent elements acting specifically on the pulmonary circulation, divalent on the heart, and the higher valences on the central nervous system.

Blake showed that the electro-negative elements, also, could be arranged in order of their physiological reactions. His grouping of all the elements tested is remarkably similar to that developed 20 years later by Mendeljeff in his "Periodic Table."

The restless and sceptical mind of Blake drove him to seek the western plains of the United States. In 1847 he became professor of anatomy and surgery at the St. Louis University Medical College. He wrote on abnormal distribution of the thyroid arteries and on filaria in dogs' hearts. By 1850 he had reached Sacramento, California, where he set up in practice near the busy wharves and undoubtedly treated the miners as they passed into the gold country. By 1856 he was contributing articles on diphtheria and on gun-shot wounds to one of California's first medical journals. In 1860 he wrote on the ineffectual drug therapy of pulmonary tuberculosis, and quoted his own cases who had gained more from his prescription of rest, sunshine and fresh air. This was 20 years before recognized authorities in the field proposed just such a method.

In 1861 Blake moved to San Francisco, becoming editor of the *Pacific Medical and Surgical Journal* and professor of midwifery and diseases of women and children in the Toland Medical College, later the Medical School of the University of California. He served as president of the California Academy of Science for four years and delved into all manner of analyses on drinking waters, ores, fish and grapes. He believed that grapes which had the highest organic acid and aldehyde content would make the best wine. He also interested himself in the geology of California and Nevada, in local anthropology and in earthquakes. He set up a meteorological station in the Sierra Mountains and one in Southern

California and put forward some original hypotheses based on his recordings. He eventually returned to his researches on chemical composition as related to physiological effects, but in 1876 put it aside to open a tuberculosis sanatorium in the Mount Saint Helena area of California, not far from the Toll House in which Robert Louis Stevenson and his bride lived after their marriage in San Francisco.

Four years later he gave up his hospital and moved to Middletown, California, where he began spectroscopic studies to further extend his chemico-physiological thesis. He travelled to Europe to present his work in England, France and Germany. One of his communications concerned the toxicity of thallium compounds.

The versatility of this physician may have proved his undoing, but he has most surely been overlooked by medical historians when they have been apportioning credit for the discovery of systems like the "Periodic Table," and for the supposedly modern rest-and-fresh- air treatment of tuberculosis. His medical student interest in "biochemorphology," to use Leake's term, remained with him until the time of his death in 1893.

Friedrich Wöhler (1803-1882)

Wöhler is remembered as the man who synthesized an organic compound from inorganic materials. He lived into his eightieth year and died five months after Charles Darwin. He had seen Napoleon enter his native city near Frankfort-am-Main. In his youth he had been interested in minerals and in drawing and sketching from nature, especially bird life. His father had been a student at Marburg University so Wöhler started his medical training there. His research as a student was on the passage of waste materials into the urine—his and his dog's. He won a prize for this report. He synthesized cyanogen iodide. Some of his professors were more critical than supportive.

Wohler transferred to Heidelberg where he could work with Leopold Gmelin, who was pleased with Wöhler's discovery of cyanic acid. He completed his Doctor of Medicine degree at Heidelberg. Thereupon he wrote to the great chemist Berzelius in Stockholm who told him that he would welcome him in his laboratory. There he prepared silver cyanate. Liebig, another youth headed for fame in chemistry, prepared the "isomer" of it, a term later coined by Berzelius.

Wöhler not only astounded the chemists but also the philosophers by producing an organic substance from an inorganic beginning. He had an excellent education and was keen on music and the arts. One of his students at Göttingen was the American Frank Jewett of Oberlin College. He brought home with him news of Wöhler's isolation of aluminum. A student at Oberlin, Charles Martin Hall, learned of this and on February 23, 1886, handed Jewett a pellet of aluminum. Hall patented the process the same year and a huge aluminum industry was born. The odyssey of Wöhler's professional life was remarkable and began when he conceived of the idea that the food's benzoic acid could be the source of hippuric acid in the urine. This research began the era of synthesizing important organic chemicals.

Alfred Smee (1818-1877)

Plaster of Paris bandages for splinting injured limbs have been known to medical students for over a century. The forerunners of these surgical aids were splints composed of chalk and gum devised by a London medical student Alfred Smee. He was a gifted undergraduate and in 1840, the year in which he qualified to practice medicine, he also published a fundamental book, *The Elements of Electro-Metallurgy*. For his work in this field he was made a fellow of the Royal Society in the following year, at the age of 23.

One wonders how this medical student found the time, and especially the space, in which to carry on such large-scale experiments as he did. The fact is, that he accomplished this work not in any university setting, but within the walls of the Bank of England. How "The Old Lady of Threadneedle Street" came to house such bizarre affairs has been told by J.A. Giuseppi, the archivist of the Bank of England, in his account of "Families of Long Service at the Bank of England."[1]

Alfred Smee was the son of the distinguished Chief Accountant, William Smee, who resided in the vast premises of the bank. On the recommendation of the surgeon, Sir Astley Cooper, the recently graduated Alfred Smee was made the first surgeon to the bank, and spent some of his time in attending staff porters and clerks. In 1842 he developed the famous ink known as "Bank Black," which is still used for the writing of the Court Minute Books in England. Twelve years later he joined with others of the bank staff in introducing a new system of printing bank notes and cheques. He was an innovator all his life and even in his retirement in Surrey carried on an experimental garden.

Albrecht von Graefe (1828-1870)

This future leader in the field of ophthalmology studied at the University of Berlin where he had the benefit of some of the greatest teachers in medical history: Müller, Virchow, von Brücke, Du Bois Reymond, Remak, Traube, Dieffenbach, Romberg and Schönlein. Von Graefe graduated in 1847 with a thesis based on original experiments—"*De Bromo ejus que praecipuis preae paratis*." He died at age 42 of overwork, which it is thought brought on tuberculosis. His contributions to ophthalmology have probably never been exceeded, as he dealt with new descriptions and new work on iridectomy, glaucoma, lid lag, cataract and retinal artery embolism.

Johann Luwig Wilhelm Thudichum (1829-1901)

This "chemist of the brain," so styled by his biographer Drabkin, began the study of medicine at the University of Giessen in 1847. He was already writing about the town of Budingen and its festival. He was offered the editorship of the local paper but pressed on with his medical studies. He took his last year of medicine at the University of Heidelberg and then returned to Giessen for his medical degree. At Heidelberg he had such famous teachers as Henle, Gmelin, Bunsen (who originated chemical spectroscopy and spectrophotometry), Kekule and Kussmaul.

At Heidelberg the medal-winning essay Thudichum wrote was entitled "Urea in Amniotic Fluid." This was based on his own undergraduate researches in which he disagreed with Wöhler. He made careful observations on urine volume after beer-drinking, a field in which he would have had broad scope at Heidelberg.

During the political uprisings in Germany in 1848 Thudichum was very active, so that by 1853 he had to take refuge in London. He became a British citizen in 1859. By then his first book in English had appeared, *A Treastise on the Pathology of the Urine, Including a Complete Guide to its Analysis*. This was published by Churchill in London in 1858 and ran to 429 pages. Thudichum was a pioneer in the chemistry of the brain. He was an excellent pianist and singer. Among other things he invented was a nasal speculum. The chemical substances that he characterized in the brain were in the dozens. He was a chemist who dealt in analytical methods for gall stones, liver pigments and carotenoid pigments. These were a long way from the subject of his medical thesis of 1851 at Giessen—"Fractures of the Upper End of the Humerus."

Thomas Lauder Brunton (1844-1916)

This alert student graduated in medicine at the University of Edinburgh in 1868 at the age of 24. His graduation dissertation was on digitalis and its uses. A year earlier the *Lancet* in London published his work entitled, "On the Use of Nitrite of Amyl in Angina Pectoris." This arose from his witnessing some experiments by Dr. Arthur Gamgee on the use of this chemical in animal experiments. Brunton wrote that "it occurred to me that a substance which possesses the power of lessening [the arterial tension] in such an eminent degree as nitrite of amyl would probably produce the same effect [as bleeding the patient]." Brunton was not only an observant student, but also senior president of the Royal Medical Society of Edinburgh.

He was a pioneer in another field, that of surgery of the heart, and in the *Lancet* of 1902 he published a "Preliminary Note on the Possibility of Treating Mitral Stenosis by Surgical Methods." He wrote in part, "One is impressed by the hopelessness of ever finding a remedy which will enable the auricle to drive the blood in a sufficient stream through the small mitral orifice, and the wish unconsciously arises that one could divide the constriction as easily during life as one can after death." He then made various experiments on the possibility of reaching the mitral valve surgically, first on cadavers and later on animals. He added, "The good results that have been obtained by surgical treatment of wounds in the heart emboldens one to hope that before very long similar good results may be obtained in cases of mitral stenosis."

In reply, the editor of the *Lancet* spoke out against Brunton's "heroic therapeutic suggestion" and accused him of an attempt "to incite others to pursue a path into the unknown which must be beset with very grave difficulty and responsibility." Brunton replied that his work in his laboratory on animals, in which he had punctured or wounded the heart, had gone on for the past 35 years.

So great was the effect of Brunton's innovative work on the medical world that he was one of those considered as a possible head of the department of medicine at Johns Hopkins Hospital. For many years he had known William Osler, who was eventually given the position. In fact J.S. Billings, who made the eventual selection, had a high regard for Brunton. Some of the finest books in the Surgeon General's Library were gifts from Brunton in his earlier days. Brunton had carried on most of his early pharmacological experiments in a laboratory 12 feet by six feet in extent.

Paul Ehrlich (1854-1915)

Paul Ehrlich's name is known alike to chemists, bacteriologists and clinicians as a great contributor in these fields of science. Rarely is it appreciated, however, that his prophetic discoveries in the chemistry of tissues and their staining reaction and the associated fields of blood diseases, immunity and bacteriology, actually began during his undergraduate period in medicine.

Ehrlich was born on March 14, 1854 in Upper Silesia, into a prosperous Jewish family. His father was an innkeeper who loved cigars. His mother was a woman with great organizing ability. Any scientific interest in his family setting might be said to stem from his grandfather, who, in the fashion of those times, cultivated an interest in popular science.

One can say that the two major contributions of Ehrlich to contemporary science were the observant eye and the indomitable spirit. The unique characteristics of Ehrlich [were] vision and determination born of a sense of social responsibility.... These characteristics were able to achieve revolutionary medical advance because of a public conviction that advance was possible; because of facilities which permitted single-minded concentration upon that advance; because of an industry which could and did assist liberally; and because of a medical organization steeped in the tradition of investigative medicine."
Cornelius P. Rhoads

In one field at least, Paul Ehrlich appeared precocious. At the age of eight he set the town chemist to compound cough drops to his own boyish prescription. Paul was sent to school in Breslau, where his interest in chemistry was so stimulated that he brought home many ideas and problems to be worked out in the vacations, in the laundry of his home. He had also in school a very good record in Latin. One of the early scientific influences was undoubtedly that of his cousin, Karl Weigert, who was nine years his senior.

After one term at the University of Breslau, Ehrlich moved to the University of Strasbourg, where Professor Waldeyer was just beginning to introduce chemistry into medical studies as a special discipline. With the early development of the German aniline dye industry, Ehrlich had a ready supply of staining agents to apply to tissues. Waldeyer encouraged this early interest of Ehrlich and permitted him to work in his laboratory after the classes were over for the day. It was here that Ehrlich discovered the new type of cell which he called a "mast cell." Having completed his basic sciences, Ehrlich returned to Breslau on Karl Weigert's advice and was there given space to work in the laboratories of the famous Cohnheim and Heidenhain. One of the visitors to the laboratory was Robert Koch, in Breslau to lecture on the anthrax bacillus.

At the age of 23 and while still an undergraduate, Ehrlich published in the *Archives of Microscopic Anatomy*, an outline of his theory of histological staining. He was preoccupied throughout with the "idea of a chemical binding of heterogeneous substances to the protoplasm." This concept he developed into his famous side-chain theory, which he was to exploit during the rest of his life. The facility with which Ehrlich was able to conjure up a three-dimensional picture of the arrangement of the atoms in a particular molecule was one of his greatest assets. As he said, "I can picture the chemical formulae in my mental vision and I believe that this fact has been of the greatest value to me in my studies." Of his earliest childhood, this vivid visual imagery had been a noticeable characteristic.

When Ehrlich graduated at Leipzig with his M.D. degree in 1878 at the age of 24, his thesis was an amplification of his undergraduate work. It was entitled: "Contributions to the Theory and Practice of Histological Staining. Part l, the Chemical Conception of Staining. Part 2, the Aniline Dyes from Chemical, Technological and Histological Aspects."

Having passed his state examination as a physician soon afterwards, Ehrlich began as an assistant and later as a senior house physician at the Charité Hospital, Berlin, in the service of Professor von Frerichs.

This most sympathetic Chief encouraged Ehrlich in his staining of blood films and his daily use of the diazo-reaction on the urines to be examined in the clinic. The crudeness of the surroundings that von Frerichs was able to offer for this clinical laboratory work in no way discouraged Ehrlich.

In 1882 Ehrlich heard the distinguished country doctor, Robert Koch, lecture before the Berlin Physiological Society on tuberculosis. After the lecture Ehrlich rushed to his laboratory and set up slides covered with tuberculous sputum. These he stained and left overnight on the laboratory stove, long-since cold. In the morning the charwoman in the laboratory started the fire, which so promoted the staining that, when Ehrlich arrived, the tubercle bacilli were everywhere to be seen. On communicating this information and on showing the slides to Robert Koch, the latter became so impressed that he turned his investigations towards the causes underlying the disease rather than to mere descriptions of the effects of tuberculosis.

With von Frerichs' death in 1887, years of hardship and disillusionment began for Ehrlich. The new chief of the service, Professor Gerhardt, sought to force Ehrlich into the rigid routine of clinical medicine devoid of any laboratory interest. Ehrlich became depressed, ill and developed tuberculosis. He wisely left Berlin and went to Egypt, where he stayed for two years. There he wrote: "When I felt so miserable during the time with Gerhardt, I often stood before the cupboard in which my collection of dyes was stored and said to myself, 'These are my friends which will not desert me.'" On returning to Berlin in 1889, Ehrlich was invited by Robert Koch to join him in the new Robert Koch Institute for Infectious Diseases. Here again, Ehrlich's great ability to analyze tissue constituents or foreign substances in tissues, through the use of dyes, brought great reward. He sought to develop chemicals that would attach themselves to bacteria in such a way that the bacteria would be immobilized or killed, and thus laid the groundwork for chemotherapy. He developed the standards still used today for measuring diphtheria antitoxin in units.

His later discoveries in the field of chemotherapy against syphilis are well-known. Consistently, the threads of Ehrlich's undergraduate studies on blood, lead poisoning and histological staining with aniline dyes run through all his life's work. The therapeutic vistas opened by this kindly, unworldly and absent-minded professor know no parallel in recent times.

On his death, *The Times* of London carried the following obituary notice: "The vast number of problems he set himself bears witness to the strength of his imagination. He opened 'new doors to the unknown' and the whole world at this hour is his debtor." Ehrlich shared the Nobel Prize in Physiology or Medicine in 1908 with Metchnikoff. Among his students was a later Nobel Prize winner, Sir Henry Dale.

Sir Frederick Gowland Hopkins (1861-1947)

Frederick Gowland Hopkins was born at Eastbourne, June 20, 1861. His father died when Frederick was a child. He was privately educated up to the age of 17, when he took his first paid job as a clerk in an insurance office. He did not particularly like the work and only stayed for six months. He then served as an assistant in a commercial analytical laboratory. He wrote of this time: "These years taught me something perhaps which might not have been learned elsewhere, for instance, how to obtain results in the shortest possible time; intellectually, they were nearly sterile years."

Hopkins became restless in this atmosphere and as a result undertook to attend a course of lectures at the Royal School of Mines. He was fortunate enough to hear two or three lectures on chemistry from the elder Frankland, which, as Hopkins says, were "the only lectures on chemistry to which I have ever listened." After completing this course, Hopkins joined Dr. P.F. Frankland in a new private laboratory, remaining there only six months, again because of the routine nature of things. Through attendance at University College, London, he prepared himself to pass the examinations required for candidates for the Institute of Chemistry. Having come to the notice of Sir Thomas Stevenson, who was a medical expert to the Home Office, Hopkins was invited to become his assistant in a laboratory devoted to medical jurisprudence at Guy's Hospital. In this laboratory, Hopkins was able to earn his living while at the same time studying for the medical qualification of the University of London. Once started in medicine he never turned back and his intellectual curiosity was greatly stimulated by each successive phase of the medical course. Though his undergraduate studies kept him hard-pressed for time, he nevertheless did his best to "keep some sort of research going."

I have memory of an address given by him [Sir Frederick Gowland Hopkins] at a British Association meeting. In an uninviting, gaunt lecture-room he decanted for nearly an hour on the cell as the theatre of chemical processes. Without any deliberate attempt at eloquence ... he conjured up for his audience ... a picture of the cell as a tiny sponge containing perhaps a thousand foci of different actions cooperatively confined within a unitary whole. An organized factory manifoldly hydrolysing, pulling to pieces, and contemporaneously constructing and reconstructing. And this unity bounded outwardly by a mosaic of countless chemical pores and leaking like a sieve. As I listened I felt I was being privileged for the time to see something of the microcosmic world in which my friend's scientific thoughts took shape and did his bidding. One mental factor which, it seemed to me, such thinking must demand, was a peculiar intensity of visual 'imagination, continuously checked in factual knowledge.'

Sir Charles Sherrington in an obituary note on F.G. Hopkins

Hopkins had already become a contributor to scientific journals and at the age of 17 published an article in *The Entomologist* dealing with the bombardier beetle. In 1889, while working in the analyst's laboratory, he published a report on the chemistry of the pigments in the English brimstone butterfly. This communication was later amplified and the pigments discussed in detail in the *Philosophical Transactions* of the Royal Society. In a way, this work was the starting point for much of Hopkins' future research on nitrogenous compounds. He showed that the pigment isolated from the butterfly's wing was a uric acid derivative. Typically, Hopkins came up with an improved method for estimating uric acid, which was later to be the key with which he opened several doors in medical research.

In 1894 he qualified under the Conjoint Board and received his London M.B. degree. In 1898 he was invited to join Sir Michael Foster at Cambridge in the teaching of "chemical physiology," and to assist in research being undertaken in Foster's laboratory. Though he went in fear and trepidation, he remained and spent his very productive life there.

To revert to his work on uric acid estimation, Hopkins became interested in studies of dietary protein and its supposed influence on the amount of uric acid excreted by the body. This led him to experiments on purified proteins to be included in artificial diets. By 1901 he had isolated and identified, with the help of S.W. Cole, the key substance tryptophane. Progressing in the same logical sequence, he, along with Edith G. Willcock, started to work out the nutritionally essential amino acids, showing among other things that zein could be improved upon by the addition of tryptophane. In turn this led to his theory of "unidentified accessory food factors," which were highly essential in any diet, no matter how rich it might be in proteins, carbohydrates, fats and minerals. His interest in pathological physiology then led him to a survey of deficiency diseases arising from a protracted lack of his accessory food factors, now called vitamins.

In 1929 Hopkins shared the Nobel Prize with Eijkman, well-known for his work on the deficiency disease, beri-beri.

It would be wrong to imply that Hopkins' entire life centred about the discovery of accessory food factors for, in fact, he did pioneer work in many unrelated fields. For instance, he, along with Walter Fletcher, was the first to accurately determine the lactic acid production arising from muscular work. Hopkins was greatly interested in the cell catalyst glutathione, which he believed to be a dipeptide. When Blythe Eagles and Hunter, much younger Canadian workers in the field, showed that glutathione was actually a tripeptide, Hopkins set out to improve his method of isolation of the compound and hastened to confirm their results.

Hopkins' work came at an opportune time in the history of cell chemistry, especially in tissue oxidations and in reductive processes. He produced 132 papers in his lifetime, many of them landmarks in biochemistry. He was made a fellow of the Royal Society in 1905 and became its President in 1931.

This much-beloved teacher became professor of biochemistry at Cambridge and Head of the Sir William Dunn Institute of Biochemistry. He was knighted in 1925 and the Order of Merit was conferred upon him in 1935.

With his distinguished white head and flowing mustache, this slight figure was the most magnetic of men. He did not live isolated from the world, but like Rudolf Virchow, was part of the world and knowledgeable about it. As early as 1896 he helped to establish in London the Clinical Research Association which offered a pathological service to practitioners and involved a great deal of night work for Hopkins. In his later years and despite his blindness, which was gradually handicapping him, he remained the patron saint of modern biochemistry, ever-kind, ever-tolerant of youth, and ever-humble. His North American students included J.H. Quastel, F.R.S., a brilliant researcher at McGill and at the University of British Columbia.

No account of Sir Frederick Gowland Hopkins would be complete without a reference to the spirit of the laboratory around him at Cambridge. From 1923 to 1931 a group of brilliant editors, associated with Hopkins in his biochemical work, produced an amazing annual called *Brighter Biochemistry*. For the year 1924-25, J.B.S. Haldane contributed to this annual a "report," which commenced:

Sir, on the upper floor the classes
Included genii and asses,
the former got out tryptophane,
The latter poured it down the drain etc.

Hopkins always gave a hand with the comic annual and produced the following masterpiece on "Biochemical Equipment—A Glance into the Future," in which he contrasts the rude equipment of 1898 with that of the present and of the supposed A.D. 2000 version. The 1898 portion of the dialogue between himself, as "Aminophilus," and Sir W.B. Hardy, the colloid expert as "Collophilus," is reproduced overleaf:

Acids and alkalis are terms originated and employed by chemists, consequently absurd and improper enough, for certainly among the hordes of men they are the most stupid, ignorant and foolishly biased of all mankind. They are the pest of Germany and the vermin of all Europe.
Dr. Gideon Harvey (1640-1700)

It is to be observed where men are most in the dark their impudence reigns most. They are not content fairly to dissent, but to insult everybody else.
Dr. Martin Lister

There is only one proven method of assisting the advancement of pure science—that of picking people of genius, backing them heavily, and leaving them to direct themselves.
Dr. James Conant, President, Harvard University

BIOCHEMICAL EQUIPMENT—A GLANCE INTO THE FUTURE

A.D. 1898.

(A small room in the building which still adorns Corn Exchange Street)

Collophilus: Pray lend me your test tube, Aminophilus; my own is under repair.

Aminophilus: Most certainly, Collophilus; I know that it will receive your customary care in the handling of apparatus. You find me, as it happens, in a philanthropic mood; Charles has just captured a mouse in the cellar.

C. Felicitations. You will at last be able to proceed with your Nutritional Investigations. Let me confess that I, too, am in expansive mood. Before leaving my house this morning, I was able to purloin an egg (I think a fresh one) from the domestic store. I may say that the yolk, and part of the white, are very heartily at your service.

A. Too generous. I am, it is true, in need of a source of amino acids; but nothing must interfere with your important Colloidal Studies.

C. Believe me, it is impossible for me to employ, at the moment, all the material represented by a whole egg. The Laboratory, I find, lacks any source of polyvalent ions. I possess sodium chloride, which, like the egg, is of domestic extraction; but can you, I wonder, provide me with a minimal quantity of, say, ammonium sulphate?

A. Fortunately, owing to the generosity of the Professor of Agriculture, I possess a specimen of that useful salt. A portion is at your command.

C. Encouraging in the very highest degree. You embolden me to mention, though with much hesitation, my need for metallic ions of high valency. I possess a solution of pen-nibs in hydrochloric acid, but—

A. If, my dear Collophilus, you are venturing to think of salts, of, let us say, Cerium or Thallium (I mention them with awe), then indeed you are, as you claim, in expansive mood. We must, you know, be reasonable. May I suggest a possibility? I am thinking of the domestic store. Could you not try alum?

C. An inspiration. Tomorrow the coagulation potency of a trivalent ion shall be explored.

(On the morrow Collophilus opens a new Chapter of Science.)

Wilhelm His, Jr. (1863-1934)

Wilhelm His, Jr. (the son of the Leipzig anatomist Wilhelm His [1831-1904]), is best- known for his recognition in the embryonic heart of the auriculo-ventricular bundle. His student work first came to notice in 1893, when he studied medicine at the University of Strasbourg. His graduation dissertation in 1889 was on the metabolism of pyridine. Soon after his discovery of the A-V bundle His showed that cutting this bundle caused dissociation of the auricular and ventricular beats of the heart, which Fulton has called "undoubtedly one of the outstanding disclosures in the history of cardiology."

A future professor of pharmacology, **Alfred Joseph Clark** (1885-1941) prepared himself thoroughly at Cambridge and at Barts Hospital,

London. His undergraduate research was on small haemorrhages in gastric ulcer and in bowel carcinoma. He tried many tests, such as the benzedine, guiacum, and spectroscopic examinations in patients who for three days had been kept off meat, green vegetables and iodides of any kind. He gave thanks in his paper to Archibald Garrod for chemical advice, and to such other outstanding clinicians as Osler, Thomas McCrae, and C.F. Martin of McGill University.

Clark became, as a pharmacologist, a brilliant advocate of universal and equalitarian medical service in Britain.

Otto Loewi (1873-1961)

This Nobel laureate had one ambition at university, the study of the history of art, but his parents persuaded him to take up medicine. He began this study at Strasbourg. The anatomy lectures he could tolerate, but the rest of his course drove him to audit lectures in the history of architecture and in general philosophy. In fact, he transferred to the University of Munich Medical Faculty for one year in order to enjoy the art galleries, the opera and the theatre in that great city. However, in 1894 he returned to Strasbourg for his fourth year and there enjoyed the teaching of Naunyn, who was interested in diabetes and liver disease particularly. Schmiedeberg was the distinguished pharmacologist with whom Loewi began research on his thesis topic. He was also developing an interest in biochemistry, thanks to his professor, Hoffmeister.

The thesis topic assigned to Loewi was the study of hydrocyanic acid, arsenic and phosphorus on the isolated frog heart. In the laboratory were Oscar Minkowski, of fame for his work on diabetes following pancreatic pathology, and Arthur Cushny, who was working on the pharmacology of heart action.

Loewi's thesis in 1896 was a great preparation for his later work on the isolated heart of the frog, where he proved that vagal nerve stimuli affected the heart by discharge of chemicals at the nerve endings involved. Sir Henry Dale, who shared the Nobel Prize with Loewi in 1936, gave an amazing account of Loewi's productive dreams. On the first night of dreaming Loewi plotted out in his mind the precise experiment which would prove the chemical transmission of nerve impulses. He scratched a few notes on a pad of paper, but in the morning could not interpret them. Luckily, he had the same dream on the second night, by which time he was prepared and wrote down the procedures exactly as he was to perform them with such success.

Charles Arthur Lovatt Evans (1884-1968)

Lovatt Evans took his medical qualification in 1916. By then he had published singly or with some of Britain's leading physiologists 20 papers.

Born in Birmingham, he attended a school in which the only chemistry taught was by an itinerant master once per week. However, he called the experiments "wizardry." At age 14 he left school to become a technical assistant to this master for one year.

Evans had an insatiable appetite for education and took correspondence courses at the Birmingham Municipal Technical School until age 16. He then joined Professor Wace Carlier at the department of physiology in what was then called Mason Science College. He developed a small home laboratory and his time spent there was characterized by several explosions. However, at the age of 17, in 1901, he left school with many prizes and certificates and for the next nine years supported himself by giving tuition and lecturing to prepare University of London matriculation students. He demonstrated in physiology at the Birmingham Midland Institute and gave interim lectures in physiology at the University of Birmingham. By 1907 he was able to matriculate as an external candidate for a degree at the University of London. All the while he assisted the professor of physiology at Birmingham. At that time physiology in England included histology, or the microscopic study of tissues. Such was their excellence, that the microscopic slides which he prepared then were in use 20 years later.

His ink-pot career began in 1903 when he published his first paper along with Professor Carlier, "A Chemical Study of the Hibernating Gland of the Hedgehog." His professor referred to him in those years as "an experienced analytical chemist." That paper was followed by four on the action of enzymes. At the age of 26 he sat the University of London bachelor of science examination and was told to remain after the completion of the test, when he was introduced to Professor Starling and his brother-in-law, Professor Bayliss. Five days later these world-class scientists offered Lovatt Evans the prestigious Sharpey Scholarship worth £150 per year. For added income he was encouraged to do coaching in the evening. In 1912 Starling sent him to Freiburg University for several months of laboratory study.

With the First World War on, he qualified in medicine and joined the Royal Army Medical College staff to work with Professor Starling on anti-gas projects, and accompanied him to Italy to prepare the troops for possible gas attacks. For his manifold researches he was made a Fellow of the Royal Society of London in 1925 and became a pillar of the British physiological establishment.

Rudolph Albert Peters (1889-1982)

Peters entered Gonville and Caius College, Cambridge, in the year 1908, when its great figures in physiology and biochemistry were at the top of the tree worldwide. His teachers included Barcroft, Langley, A.V. Hill, Anderson, W.B. Hardy and the great Gowland Hopkins. With Barcroft's help Peters embarked on the study of "The Chemical Nature of Specific Oxygen Capacity in Haemoglobin," which appeared in the *Journal of Physiology* in 1912. He also wrote upon "The Effect of Exercise on the Dissociation Curve of Blood." Then he joined the distinguished A.V. Hill in studying the heat and the lactic acid produced in frog muscle after stimulating the appropriate nerve. Commenting on the heated discussion which followed his paper, Peters said, "I have found more lactic acid than Meyerhof's people liked and consequently, of course, they all said it was wrong. Actually, my results were right."

Peters qualified as a medical practitioner in 1915 and went directly to the World War in Europe. He was soon in the thick of the struggle at Vimy Ridge, where the losses were horrendous. For his bravery he was awarded the Military Cross and Bar. Post-war, when he was trying to establish biochemistry as a separate subject, he fortunately had the support of Sir Charles Sherrington. They both felt that biochemistry was crucial in the future of medical research and treatment.

At Oxford, Peters was keen on clinical biochemistry and worked closely with the nearby Radcliffe Infirmary. He was also keen on the future of microbiology. His work on the deprivation of vitamin B-1 in pigeons was a classic. However, less was reported about one of the B-deficient animals, in this case a goat, who, fed up with his diet, jumped through the glass roof of biochemistry. His B-deficient diet consisted, among other things, of newspapers, but it was made clear to us that the paper being eaten was not the *Times* of London.

Peters was elected a Fellow of the Royal Society of London in 1935. During the Second World War he was as active as he had been in the First, and lived a very productive life up to the time of his death in 1982.

Hans Adolf Krebs (1900-1981)

Krebs was born in Hanover, Germany, and at age 15 decided to follow his father into medicine. He completed his army service in 1918 and was discharged within two months of the Armistice, entering the University of Göttingen in 1918 for his preclinical studies and then to Freiburg to complete them. There he had lectures at first-hand from research-minded professors who related their discoveries. In 1920 he spent the summer semester working as an anatomist under Professor William von Möllendorff. His project was the staining of striated muscle with a wide selection of dyes. He thought he could identify the constituents of tissues by studying the physical chemical properties of the stains used to produce good microscopic images. His first publication was on the staining of skeletal muscle with such dyes.

After completing the summer semester of 1920 he moved to Munich, where he studied with clinicians who were heavily involved in medical research. Even after receiving his Doctor of Medicine degree in 1925 Krebs, in his hospital internship in Berlin, kept up his research by injecting various dyes into the bloodstream and picking them up in the cerebrospinal fluid. He produced several papers at that time and attended many courses in medicinal chemistry. Krebs' subsequent course can be summarized briefly. In 1926 he was an assistant in Otto Warburg's laboratory at the Kaiser Wilhelm Institute for Biology in Berlin. In 1930 he went to Hamburg and then returned to Freiburg, where he worked on the synthesis of urea. By 1931 he was publishing, with Kurt Henseleit, papers on their joint discovery of the amino acid ornithine. A year later they formulated a cyclic process for the synthesis of urea. In April 1933 the Nazis simply abolished Krebs' post and within two months he joined the laboratory in Cambridge of Sir Frederick Gowland Hopkins, thanks to a Rockefeller Foundation grant.

Krebs received the Nobel Prize in Medicine in 1953. When he retired from the chair of biochemistry at Oxford he was invited by Dr. Paul Beeson, Nuffield Professor of Clinical Medicine to organize a new laboratory at the Radcliffe Infirmary. In the subsequent 14 years Krebs published 100 papers, making him a good subject for a volume on *Old Endeavour*. His colleagues in the same Metabolic Research Laboratory published even more than 100 papers during those years.

Carl Ferdinand Cori (1896-1994) and **Gerty Radnitz Cori** (1896-1957)

Cori and Radnitz both were born in Prague in 1896. On returning from World War I, Carl Cori resumed his clinical studies at Prague and worked in the Pharmacological Institute on the physiology and pharmacology of the heart during excitation from the sinus node. He shared a laboratory with another future Nobel laureate, Albert Szent György. Radnitz, on the other hand, worked on the influence of the thyroid on body temperature regulation, especially in congenital myxedema. She continued work on her animal studies after the removal of both the thyroid and spleen.

Bernardo Alberto Houssay (1887-1971)

Houssay was born in Buenos Aires of French parents. At the age of 13 he entered the school of pharmacy of the University of Buenos Aires and completed his degree with honours. He then enrolled in the medical faculty of the university and in 1910 graduated with the M.D. degree with honours. His research as an undergraduate had concerned the physiology of pituitary extracts, and foreshadowed a career in endocrinology. Also as an undergraduate, he was appointed as an assistant in physiology at the university and became a full professor in the School of Veterinary Sciences on graduation. Gradually he built up a great volume of research on such things as coagulation and hemolysis of the blood. His appointment as full professor in the University of Buenos Aires Medical School came in 1919 and thereafter he developed an Institute of Physiology, which became his base for future studies in fat metabolism, the pituitary hormones and their relation to diabetes. Then he went on to thyroid and adrenal hormones which brought him both local and international fame. He had come a long way from his graduation thesis of 1910, which he did entirely on his own, since at that time in Argentina one had clearly to be self-educating. The thesis was published in 1911, as "*Estudios sobre la accion de los extractos hipofisarios*."

In 1943 Houssay and his university colleagues attempted to bring to an end the military regime of General Juan Perón, but for his trouble on behalf of a democratic country he was dismissed from all his university posts. However, he kept up his opposition to the military junta as did his other colleagues, and eventually they won. He was invited to join the National Institutes of Health in Bethesda, Maryland, but returned to his country in 1955 after the Perón years were brought to an end. He was fond of saying that science had no country but scientists did. One might say that starting with his thesis publication he became both an Argentinean and an international scientist of the first rank, and was awarded the Nobel Prize in Medicine in 1947. He contributed to 2000 scientific papers in his lifetime.

Yngve Zotterman

Zotterman was a Swedish student at Cambridge University, where he graduated with his bachelor's degree in 1922. However, he had been already publishing in the *Journal of Physiology* as early as 1920. Returning to Sweden he studied medicine and graduated in the year 1925. By then he had half a dozen student papers published, some in the *Acta Obstetrica* and in the *Acta Pediatrica*. His student work was related to calcium and the pH of milk. Thanks to his preparation at Cambridge, he pursued very fundamental work in sensory receptors as in single taste receptors in the tongue. He extended this with his colleagues Liljestrand and von Euler, both of whom became Nobel Prize winners in Medicine.

Together, the three Swedish physiologists clarified the activities of chemoreceptors in the carotid body. Zotterman is best-known for his research with Adrian at Cambridge in 1926 on adaptation of receptors to various stimuli in the nervous system.

Axel Hugo Theodor Theorell (1903-1982)

Theorell was born in Sweden the son of a practising physician. His mother was descended from a Peruvian Indian. At the age of three, Theorell was stricken with poliomyelitis and was given a muscle transplant that enabled him to walk extremely well. Raised in the state schools he began the study of medicine in 1921 at the famous Karolinska in Stockholm, graduating in 1924. He published several papers on research done as a medical undergraduate. He has been credited by Irving Page with discovering the lipoproteins, but he always said he found that hard to believe. His very early interest was in the possible influence on the sedimentation of red blood cells brought about by the lipoproteins. Never afraid to combat error in medicine, Theorell's work made it clear that enzymes were made up of proteins, thus dismissing the famous German chemist Willstatter's views which had reigned supreme for too long. The man whose muscles had been crippled by a virus went on to isolate crystalline myoglobin. He won the Nobel Prize in 1955.

Theorell, right into his eightieth year, was a great organizer in medical research and in state policy. He was one who spearheaded the development of the Axel Wenner Gren Foundation's building in Stockholm, wherein most of Sweden's health-related charities and associations could be brought together in offices and at mealtimes. On another issue, he was closely associated with Professor Zotterman, who happened to head the driving safety groups in Sweden and was aided by an enormous black dog who sat in the seat beside him. Any scientific visitor was relegated to the rear seat of his car, and the hair-raising driving exploits of this alleged safe-driving crusader were legendary.

Alfred Vogl

This third-year medical student in Vienna was assigned to a case of post-war malnutrition and syphilis. For this highly infectious disease Novasurol was prescribed and as a result there was a great outpouring of urine on each day that the substance was injected intravenously. From an early collection of 500 ccs daily, the post-injection amount rose quickly to 1200 ccs. The presiding nurse was given to the construction of beautiful charts that showed that the next daily injection produced 2000 ccs of urine.

Vogl's next case was also a syphilitic, a very large man with heart disease in advanced congestive failure. Vogl injected two ccs of Novasurol with the result that 10 litres of urine were passed. Vogl wrote later, "We were convinced that we had witnessed the greatest man-made diuresis in history."

Thereafter, a boy with a greatly enlarged rheumatic heart, in failure, was admitted to the wards with no urine being passed. In desperation Vogl injected intramuscularly the standard amount of Novasurol whereupon the boy passed three litres of urine. His death the next day from the enlarged rheumatic heart did not, however, signal the end of the Vogl chapter in diuretics. Thus did a third-year medical student bring about a new chapter in renal disease treatment.

Earl Wilbur Sutherland, Jr. (1915-1974)

Earl Sutherland, Jr., was the fifth of six children born in Kansas. At the age of 18 he entered Washburn College in Topeka, Kansas, where, after four years, he was awarded the Bachelor of Science degree. He then entered the distinguished Washington University School of Medicine, at St. Louis and, as he wrote later, he "was intrigued and puzzled by the actions of hormones." He already knew a considerable amount of medicine from his apprenticeship as a hospital orderly in Kansas. On entering the medical school he was hired by Carl Cori as a student assistant in the department of pharmacology. Sutherland's first two papers, with S.P. Colowick, involved the use of purified enzymes in polysaccharide synthesis from glucose. Fifteen years later this interest in the synthetic process stimulated and guided Sutherland to the discovery of cyclic AMP when he was professor at Western Reserve University at Cleveland, Ohio. By then, he was the head of the department of pharmacology at that superior institution.

Following his graduation as a Doctor of Medicine at St. Louis, Sutherland became an intern at the celebrated Barnes Hospital where he undertook, despite protests from his clinical heads, additional research. Thereafter he served his two years' military service as a battalion surgeon in Patton's Army in Europe. For eight years after the end of the Second World War he served as associate professor in biochemistry in St. Louis, publishing on glycogen synthesis with Cori and with C. DeDuve on glucagon. Returning to Western Reserve University in Cleveland, Sutherland held the chair of pharmacology for 10 years. He was awarded the Nobel Prize in Medicine in 1971. His biographer Lawrence Sherman wrote, "Earl Sutherland has spent his entire investigative life following up his youthful work." Ira Pastan added, "One of the most impressive aspects of Sutherland's contribution is that it is truly unique. Today important discoveries are often made simultaneously in different laboratories. In the case of Earl Sutherland, the rest of us were years behind."

Arthur Kornberg (b.1918)

Arthur Kornberg was born in Brooklyn, New York, and attended the Abraham Lincoln High School in that city. His father was a sewing machine operator in the sweatshops of the Lower East Side of New York, so Arthur earned his way through the College of the City of New York, graduating with honours in the Bachelor of Science group in 1937. A scholarship took him to the Rochester School of Medicine in New York State where he qualified with the M.D. degree in 1941.

As early as his college days in New York he had been interested in regulators of life processes, and his first scientific paper at the University of Rochester, while a medical student, concerned these processes. He studied with a distinguished Spanish enzymologist Severo Ochoa in New York and later with the Coris in St. Louis. His early work led him logically to a study of DNA polymerase and this in turn to the elucidation of the enzymic mechanism involved in DNA replication and eventually to the biological synthesis of DNA. At the age of 41 he shared with Ochoa the Nobel Prize for the year 1959. He never forgot his roots, as is demonstrated by his important publication, "Latent Liver Disease in Persons Recovering from Catarrhal Jaundice and in Otherwise Normal Medical Students, as Revealed by the Bilirubin Excretion Test."

Daniel Carleton Gajdusek (b. 1923)

Born in Yonkers, New York, Gajdusek as a teenager worked at the Boyce Thompson Institute for Plant Research in that city. His interest was in the synthesis of potential pesticides. None was ever put to use for that purpose, but one became a commercially important weed killer.

Gajdusek's father had been a butcher in Slovakia and his mother was a first-generation American of Hungarian origin. He took his undergraduate degree at the University of Rochester and then proceeded to take his Doctor of Medicine degree at Harvard. With a fellowship from the National Foundation for Infantile Paralysis he entered the laboratory of John F. Enders at Harvard, where he spent three years. He did his draft service with the army at Walter Reed Institute for Research in virology, which prepared him for a new life in the study of epidemic disease in the Middle East. After two years in Iran, he worked with the well-known Australian scientist and future Nobelist Sir Macfarlane Burnet at the Walter and Eliza Hall Institute of Medical Research in Melbourne. Off he went to the highlands of New Guinea where, among the Fore people in an isolated setting, he first came in contact with kuru, a neurological disease of doubtful origin. This was but the first of many visits that Gajdusek made from his National Institutes of Health Laboratory in the USA. The story of the development of his research, with skilled colleagues, is unique in the history of medicine. The perpetuation of the disease kuru in the Fore people seemed clearly to depend on the eating of the brains of those dying of the disease. From this point on, undergraduate interest in methods of killing pests was transferred to a far more complicated search for the basis of kuru and similar neurological diseases.

For his manifold and basic discoveries in this field Gajdusek was awarded the Nobel Prize in Medicine in 1976.

Bengt Ingemar Samuelsson (b.1934)

Samuelsson was born on the shores of the Kattegat at Halmstad, Sweden. He began his medical training at the University of Lund, with his mentor there, Sune Karl Bergström. However, Bergström was given a senior appointment at the Karolinska in Stockholm, so Samuelsson went with him to study the newly discovered prostaglandins. He achieved his doctorate in medical science in the field of biochemistry in 1960 and graduated in medicine at the Karolinska in 1961.

Samuelsson's early work was done in this field well before he graduated in medicine. Much of the development that Bergström and Samuelsson did was based on the pioneer work of Ulf Svante von Euler. Samuelsson was following in the footsteps of one of the world's best trained and most productive medical scientists, whose path was strewn with Nobel Prize winners. Ulf's father shared the Nobel Prize for Chemistry in 1930 and his godfather Svante Arrhenius won a similar Nobel Prize in 1903. For years von Euler was the secretary to the Nobel Foundation.

After holding a research fellowship in chemistry at Harvard University, Samuelsson returned to Sweden, where he became assistant professor of chemistry at the Karolinska. In 1972 he became chairman of that department. By 1978 he was dean of the faculty of medicine and five years later was made Rector of the Royal Caroline Institute. He shared the Nobel Prize in Medicine with John Vane in Britain and with his old mentor, Bergström.

Aaron Bunsen Lerner

In October 1947, Aaron Lerner reported on an "Unusual Purpura Associated with the Presence of a High Concentration of Cryoglobulin" in the *American Journal of Medical Sciences*. While a student in the Ph.D.-M.D. combined program at the University of Minnesota, Lerner encountered a patient in the university hospital in Minneapolis, in whom there was a severe sensitivity to cold. The patient had already been studied at the Mayo Clinic in 1942 where a diagnosis of cold allergy had been made.

In the words of Professor Cecil Watson, Lerner "observed a white precipitate in serum ... after it had stood overnight at room temperature. This [led] to an extensive study of protein, which was eventually named for the first time a cryoglobulin." Watson described Lerner's Ph.D. thesis, written on the way to his M.D. degree as "a little classic. I remember when Aaron showed me the tube with the white precipitate. He had not yet found that this would go back into solution very readily on warming, but he was to find that out later in the day. The patient had a remarkable acropurpura, and the thought naturally occurred to us that he might be precipitating this protein out in the periphery where the temperature went down to some extent, as in fingers, toes, and ears. This was borne out by the fact that the protein precipitated quite rapidly as the temperature was lowered from 37° down to 32°... . Aaron's finding made it quite clear that this was a physical phenomenon unrelated to any ordinary allergy."

After qualifying for his Ph.D. degree, Lerner went on to take his M.D. degree and thereafter to join the biochemistry section of the Army Chemical Centre in Maryland.

A.C.A. Smith

Between May and November of 1966 Smith as an undergraduate at the poison treatment center of Edinburgh's Royal Infirmary studied 127 patients in whom it was essential to estimate the concentration of barbiturates in the blood. Smith devised a simple method that could be used in the side room of a ward. His method did not give false positive results for the common non-barbiturate hypnotics, tranquillisers, and anti-depressant drugs. It was ideally suited to performance by clinicians. This very neat undergraduate contribution was made during Smith's elective term which he took in the toxicology laboratory.

Patrick Anthony Merton

Merton was completing his medical training at Cambridge and at St. Thomas's Hospital in London when, in 1945, he completed a study on the source of urinary ammonium. He had been a pupil at Cambridge of W.A.H. Rushton at Trinity College. During the year of his qualification to practice medicine he began research at the National Hospital, Queen

Square on myasthenia gravis and familial periodic paralysis. From lecturer in physiology at Cambridge in 1957 he became reader and then professor in the year 1984, keeping up research at Queen Square as well as being a Fellow of Trinity College, Cambridge. With H.B. Morton he pioneered the stimulation of the motor cortex in intact human subjects. This has produced a great deal of research activity in clinical and physiological work around the world.

[1] *Genealogists' Magazine*, 10:12, 1949.

CHAPTER SEVEN

Digestion

Gentlemen,
Instead of promising that I shall satisfy your curiosity in what relates to the Anatomy of the Brain, I begin by publickly and frankly owning that I know nothing of the matter. I wish I were the only Person under the necessity of talking in this manner, because I might in time become acquainted with what others know; and it would be a great blessing to Mankind if this most delicate Part, and which is liable to so many dangerous Diseases, were as well understood as the generality of Anatomists and Philosophers imagine it to be. It is very certain that it is the principal Organ of the Soul and the Instrument by which it works very wonderful Effects. The Soul...is nevertheless utterly at a loss to describe its own Habitation, and is nowhere more to seek than at home. We need only view a Dissection of that large Mass, the Brain, to have ground to bewail our Ignorance. On the very Surface you see varieties which deserve your admiration; but when you would look into its inner Substance you are utterly in the dark, being about to say nothing more than that there are two Substances one greyish the other white, which last is continuous with the

The study of man's digestive processes is replete with names of student contributors. Among them are: Stensen, de Graaf, J.R. Young, Claude Bernard, Pavlov, W.B. Cannon and others.

Niels Stensen (Steno) (1638-1686)

Niels Stensen was the son of the court jeweller in Copenhagen, who unfortunately died when his son was six years old. Raised by his grandparents, Stensen had a private tutor who taught him Latin, German, Dutch, French, Italian, English, Hebrew and Greek. At grammar school he came under the benevolent influence of Ole Borch whose interests ranged from medicine and natural science to chemistry and philology, and whose proficiency was to lead him to a chair in the University of Copenhagen.

At the age of 18 Stensen entered the university after a boisterous initiation ceremony. He chose as his preceptor Thomas Bartholin, the famed anatomist. Stensen had been at university two years when the armies of Sweden overran Denmark and laid siege to Copenhagen. The student regiment, 266 strong, took its place on the barricades, with Stensen as a corporal in charge of 86 of them. Twice in the 18th and twice in the 19th century students were called to defend their beautiful and cultured city. In Stensen's day it was the Dutch fleet that broke the siege and ended the famine.

Bartholin sent his pupil to Amsterdam to continue his undergraduate medical studies under his friend Blasius. It was in his laboratory on April 7, 1661, that Stensen made his first great discovery. He had purchased a sheep's head for dissection and was working on the veins of the face when, to his surprise, his scalpel slipped through a cavity and struck the teeth with a metallic sound. Stensen had really been working inside the duct which leads the saliva of the parotid gland into the mouth. This is still called Stensen's duct.

Blasius dismissed this as a freak of nature, and patiently explained to Stensen that the true function of the parotid gland was to warm the ear. Then he pretended to have known about the parotid duct for years, so that Stensen, having confirmed the existence of the duct in the dog also, wisely moved on to Leyden, to work with Sylvius and van Horne. There in July 1661 he gave his famous "Disputation" on his discovery. Within a short time Stensen discovered the duct of the lachrymal gland, the ducts of the sublingual gland and the buccal glands, thus adding to his student reputation.

In 1662 he published his findings in *Observationes Anatomicae*. Two years later, in Copenhagen, he published his "*De musculis et glandulis observationum specimen*," dedicated to King Friedrich III. He propounded the theory that the glandular secretion was manufactured in the glands themselves and was secreted through the ducts. He discovered the follicles in the ovaries, and Peyer's patches of the intestine.

Concerning the muscles Stensen's views created a sensation second only to that which followed Harvey's publication of 1628. He wrote: "The heart has been considered the seat of natural warmth, as the throne of the soul and even as the soul itself. Some have greeted the heart as the sun, others as the King; but if you examine it more closely, one finds it to be nothing more than muscle."

Stensen travelled to Paris where he addressed Thevenot's circle of savants (including Swammerdam) in a philosophical discourse on the brain. This was published in the work of his grand-nephew Winslow, "*Exposition anatomique de la structure du corps humain*." Recently the Danish neurosurgeon Edward Busch has translated this discourse into English. Doubtless under the patronage of Thevenot, Stensen visited Italy, and in Florence, with the backing of Viviani, Galileo's biographer, was appointed physician to Ferdinand II, Grand Duke of Tuscany, a patron of the sciences. Stensen was given a pension, a residence and a connection with the ancient Hospital of Santa Maria Nuova, founded in 1288. At least in Florence Stensen had more opportunities for work than Vesalius had enjoyed in Madrid.

In Florence Stensen was converted to Catholicism. Five years later, King Christian V of Denmark asked him to return as professor of geology, a subject in which he had developed a great interest in Italy. In fact he is regarded as the father of scientific geology. Once home in Denmark, however, he became embroiled in religious differences and after two years left to become a bishop in Germany. He died in the service of the church in 1686.

An echo of Stensen's student work comes to us in Albrecht von Haller's graduation thesis in 1728 at Leyden wherein the erroneous view of Coschwitz, the surgeon and professor of anatomy at Halle, that the lingual vein was the true duct of the submaxillary gland, was disproved by this brilliant student.

Nerves distributed all over the body; that the greyish Substance serves in some places for a Cortex to the White, and that in other places it separates the white Filaments from each other. For, to say that the white Substance is only an uniform Body like Wax without any Art concealed in it, would be to think too meanly of this great Masterpiece of Nature. If this Substance is everywhere Fibrous, as it appears in many places to be, you must own that these Fibres are disposed in the most artful manner; since all the diversity of our Sensations and Motions depends upon them. We admire the contrivance of the Fibres of every Muscle, and ought still more to admire their disposition in the Brain, where an infinite number of them contained in a very small Space, do each execute their particular Offices without confusion or disorder.

From Niels Stensen, *Dissertation on the Anatomy of the Brain*, read in M. Thevenot's house in the year 1665 in Paris. Translation by Professor E. Busch, Copenhagen.

Regnier de Graaf (1641-1673)

Another contributor in the study of digestion was Regnier de Graaf. He was born in the town of Schoonhaven, which lies between Rotterdam and Arnheim. His father was a man of keen intellect and was interested in architecture and in the development of hydraulic machines. De Graaf embarked upon the study of medicine at Utrecht under van Diemerbroeck whom he called, "An excellent professor to whom I owe the progress I have made in the study of the human body." During the year 1663, de Graaf transferred to the University of Leyden where he studied under such stimulating teachers as John van Horne and François de la Böe (Sylvius). He was a contemporary of the students Stensen, Frederick Ruysch and Jan Swammerdam.

In 1664, at the age of 23, de Graaf published his first scientific work, the preparation of which had occupied a considerable amount of his time as a medical student. It was entitled "*Disputatio medica de natura et usu succi pancreatici*." It was 90 pages long and contained three excellent plates, describing his method of collecting pancreatic juice by a temporary fistula.

The book began with a dedication to his father, to relatives and to the senators and councillors of Schoonhaven. Looking back on his early trials as a student researcher, he later said, "After racking the brain and putting the spirit to all sorts of torture to find a proof that would completely satisfy us, we found a method by the grace of God." The method, which worked so successfully, employed the quill of a wild duck, which he states to have been longer and thinner than that of any other bird. He fashioned a small retractable wooden plug on a thread to be passed through the hollow of the quill until it stopped up the narrow distal orifice. Taking a fasting animal, he performed a tracheotomy and opened the abdomen. He tied off the duodenum at the pyloric junction and washed out its contents. He placed the quill in the pancreatic duct and passed the attached thread through a telescoping paper tube that was to conduct the juice to a flask. The flask had an air escape hole in it through which the thread finally passed. When all was in order he pulled the thread and started to collect the precious pancreatic juice. He managed to collect as much as an ounce of the juice in a seven-hour period.

De Graaf canalized the pancreatic duct and the parotid duct simultaneously in one animal in order to show that the two juices were different. He tested the juice by tasting it and noticed periodic variations in its apparent acidity and salinity. Sometimes he classed it as "insipid." At Angers he had an opportunity to dissect out the pancreas of a sailor who had just been killed by a falling mast. He also tasted and made other observations on the juice encountered in this case.

In the fashion of the times, physiological theory far outdistanced observable facts. De Graaf's views on the pancreatic juice largely reflected the teaching of Sylvius who believed that "effervescence" was a main feature of digestion and was parallel in some manner to physiological fermentation.

De Graaf listed the uses of the pancreatic juice as the promotion of effervescence with the assistance of the bile, in order to dispose of the mucus inside the intestine. This in turn was to allow the lacteals to absorb the chyle of the digested food; the pancreatic juice had also the important function of separating the usable part of the food from the useless.

A French edition, considerably enlarged, appeared in Paris in 1666, in which de Graaf referred to the works of Stensen, Wirsung, Rudbeck, Bartholin, Wharton, Harvey and others. Bartholin had imagined that the pancreas was the excretory organ of the spleen just as the bile duct was considered the excretory organ of the liver. However, de Graaf disproved this quickly when he splenectomized a dog and later collected pancreatic juice through his temporary fistula.

On July 23, 1665, de Graaf received his Doctor of Medicine degree from the University of Angers. He then travelled in France for a considerable time, never neglecting his anatomical studies. As he says, "In my journeys in France, I put all my energies to the dissection of bodies which I found there in sufficiently great quantities; I preferred most to dissect the pancreas and the genital parts since I found there consistently new things, unremarked by anatomists before me."

For a time in 1666, de Graaf returned to practise in Delft. However, the year 1667 finds him back in Paris as the centre of interest in a coterie collected by Dr. Bourdelot, to whose home, de Graaf records, "the most curious wits of the University do frequently resort." On one occasion de Graaf depancreatized a dog before Dr. Bourdelot's gathering. Though the doctor told his servants to watch the dog carefully, it later succumbed. Two and one half centuries later another young student, Charles Best, working with Frederick Banting in Toronto, was to learn the reason why.

De Graaf returned to Delft where, in 1668, he published his three remarkable treatises in one volume: "*De virorum organis generationi inservientibus*"; "*De clysteribus*"; and "*De usu siphonis in anatomia*." His hydraulically-minded father had nothing on Regnier de Graaf who used a length of bird's intestine with a quill at either end to permit blood transfusions between animals. The design of a syringe developed for anatomical injections, using a silver or copper barrel and a leather plunger, resembles modern instruments.

In 1672 de Graaf's greatest work was issued. It is that for which he is chiefly famous today. Its title was "*De mulierum organis generationi inservientibus*." A translation of its subtitle would read, "A new treatise wherein it is demonstrated that man and all those animals that are called vivipara, these no less than the ovipara, derived their origin from the egg."

A year later de Graaf was dead, a victim of the plague, at the age of 32.

His work, "*De virorum*," established the tubular nature of the testicular tissue. He was at great pains to put down fantastic theories about certain vital elements in the blood being miraculously transferred to these tubules. With his newly invented syringe, he injected the spermatic blood vessels with mercury and showed them to be quite distinct from the semen-bearing tubules. He never discoursed on his anatomical findings without stating the generalization deriving from them. Hence he said, "Man, then, cannot be immortal on this earth, but he has the consolation in dying, of living again in his children, and God has given him the means of generation, not only for a thousand years but even for a species of Eternity—and for this purpose there are certain organs of the human frame fashioned with a structure so delicate that the hand of Providence may therein be witnessed."

The basic and well planned research that preceded his publication of "De Mulierum organis generationi" demands admiration even today. De Graaf left excellent drawings of the rapidly developing embryo examined at predetermined times in the best experimental tradition. His supply of experimental animals encompassed 100 rabbits, 40 goats and many other assorted species. In addition to the stages of embryonic development he offered the first description of the corpus luteum.

De Graaf was ever-thorough and called on his former colleagues at Leyden for supplementary proof of his own theories. He wrote: "One can assert that the females of all sorts of animals have eggs, since they are found not only in birds and in oviparus and viviparus fish, but also in quadripeds and in women. We have found eggs in rabbits, hares, pigs, sheep and cows... . I begged Stensen to apprise me of his observations in species that I lacked. He did not neglect to reply frankly, saying that he found eggs of different sizes in deer, guinea pigs, badgers, roe deer, wolves and asses; in mules even and in other animals."

In the nine-year period between the publication of his student research on the pancreatic juice and his death in 1673, historians found a rare record of resourceful industry. The combination of manual dexterity and ability to plan an experiment, evidenced in his student work, is even better exemplified by his later and greater works on the organs of reproduction and their function.

From this brief consideration of the works of Regnier de Graaf, two important themes emerge. First, it was a time for discovery—with his contemporaries Stensen, Swammerdam and Ruysch all making great names for themselves. Second, there was a common denominator running through the careers of these men—and that is the sagacity and the helpfulness of the great teacher Sylvius. He believed in his students and this belief, as history shows, was justified.

Johann Nathanael Lieberkuhn (1711-1756)

Under family pressure Lieberkuhn began his studies at the University of Halle and Jena in the field of theology. However, three years later he decided upon medicine and the natural sciences and continued his studies at Jena and thereafter at Leyden. At Leyden he was taught by the unrivalled Boerhaave as well as Siegfried Albinus. Lieberkuhn's Doctor of Medicine thesis at Leyden in 1739 was entitled, "*De valvula coli et usu processus vermicularis*." After a visit to London he was made a Fellow of the Royal Society for his work. He is perhaps better-known for his dissertation in 1745, "*De fabrica et actione villorum intestinorum tenuium hominis*." Even before his 1739 dissertation for his M.D. degree, he had designed (1738) the so-called solar microscope.

An immediate contemporary, **John Fothergill** (1712-1780), wrote his inaugural dissertation on "Emetics" at the age of 24. His many contributions were brought together in three volumes by his fellow Quaker, John Coakley Lettsom (1744-1815), born on Little Jost van Dyke Island in the British Virgin Islands group. Together these forceful men founded the Medical Society of London in 1773. Each has been memorialized with an annual oration at that ancient society, which still inhabits its classical and beautiful building at 11 Chandos Street in Cavendish Square in London. Sir William Osler gave the Fothergillian Oration there in 1917.

Edward Stevens

In 1777 Edward Stevens presented a dissertation at Edinburgh for his M.D. degree, "*De alimentorum concoctione*." Stevens is said to have first isolated the gastric juice and performed digestive experiments outside of the body. Michael Foster in his admirable *History of Physiology* notes that Stevens took advantage "of a man of weak understanding who gained a miserable livelihood by swallowing stones for the amusement of the common people." Stevens was quick to see the investigative possibilities of this man's stomach and had him swallow small perforated spheres made of silver, within which he had inserted foods both raw and cooked, and even specimens of bone. Forty-eight hours later the spheres were examined after they had been voided, whereupon it was found that whole grains of legumes and wheat were hardly digested at all. Experiments were done on dogs and sheep as well as on oxen, and in the case of the latter animals the vegetable foods were readily digested. Meat was not so well digested. From a dog's stomach, however, a fluid was withdrawn which readily digested cooked meat outside of the body without any suggestion of putrefaction. In this, Stevens was answering the long-held theory that digestion was a form of putrefaction. The early American physiologist Young came to the same conclusions. In fact, the views of Stevens and Young were very close to those of the Italian experimenter and philosopher Spallanzani.

Benjamin Rush (1745-1813), while a student at Edinburgh, also wrote his thesis on the digestion of food, and carried out a number of unusual experiments on his own stomach in the process. His degree was granted in June 1768.

John Richardson Young (1782-1804)

The next student pioneer is John Richardson Young from western Maryland, who in 1803 wrote his graduation thesis at the University of Pennsylvania School of Medicine on "An Experimental Inquiry into the Principles of Nutrition and the Digestive Process."

Young opens his essay by rejecting the teachings of William Cullen of Edinburgh—that vegetables possessed food value because of their acid content, along with their contained sugar and oil. Young also held that water went into the formation of the body solids. He discussed the association between salivary secretion and gastric juice secretion with great insight.

Young experimented chiefly on animals that swallowed their food without breaking it up by physical means. The large American bullfrog (rana ocellata) was therefore used, and the rates of dissolution of field mice, spring frogs, ground beef and veal, in the frog's capacious and easily-entered stomach, were recorded. Snakes were also used, and into their stomachs a great variety of things were forced, such as lizards and small frogs. Fleshy parts were dissolved and bones and teeth were softened, but only at one half the speed of the process already observed in the bullfrog. All food retracted from their stomachs, by threads previously tied to it, showed a red or acidic reaction on litmus paper.

To compare human digestion with that already studied, he swallowed the condyles of the thigh bone of a chicken, and observed their greatly softened state and their weight loss four days later. He also placed in frogs' stomachs little linen bags containing bread, peas, beans and wheat. After 30 hours only the bread was gone. The intact peas, beans and wheat had resisted "the gastric menstruum." However, when these were broken up, as they would be by the jaws of animals, Young found them dissolved, after a suitable time in the stomach of the frog. For good measure Young's thesis even quotes Morgagni's story of a young lady, living on vegetables in Lent, who vomited a fully developed plant "with perfect leaves and roots!"

As further proof that the gastric juice acted with impartiality on animal and vegetable foods, Young cited the relevant literature, mentioning two polar bears who grew fat on a vegetable diet only, and a pigeon that was trained to eat meat, even to the exclusion of grain from its diet.

With ingenious experiments upon himself and upon his bullfrogs he concluded that digestion was not analogous to the fermentation of wine nor the putrefaction of food. His friend Mitchell "avoided his usual breakfast, in the place of which he took, between the hours of eight and ten, twelve ounces of sugar. Nothing more was taken until one o'clock. Having the power to ruminate, it was at this hour thrown up; the mass was sweet ... no disengagement of air was to be perceived ... there was not the least eructation of air during the whole period the experiment was going on. If ever a vinous fermentation took place in the stomach, we expected to have found it in this experiment as this viscus was plentifully supplied with saccharine matter, which passes so readily to this state; but as nothing of the kind occurred, we conclude the vinous fermentation had nothing to do with the digestive process."

Against the theory of digestion as putrefaction he wrote: "On an empty stomach I made a light dinner, on chicken pye, and drank simple water; in half an hour, by irritating my fauces, it was thrown up; at this time it was plentifully supplied with gastric fluid, as well as saliva, as the quantity of food was but small. It was then exposed in a tumbler to a heat equal to the human temperature. For the space of nine hours there was not ... any disengagement of air. As digestion is performed sooner than this period, it was not attended to any longer."

Young was able to place litmus paper in the stomach of a bullfrog which had no food for two days. On retraction it was coloured red, as by an acid. Young made experiments upon himself, taking meat on an empty stomach. After regurgitating it, he established the fresh and non-putrefied nature of the meat and the acid nature of the juice enveloping it. He concluded: "We have little hesitation, therefore, in saying that the acid so constantly found in the stomach of man, and almost, probably all animals, is to be referred to their gastric fluid."

The rudimentary chemical methods at hand led Young, incorrectly, to suppose that the acid was phosphoric acid. But the main content of his thesis was first-class in every respect. He speculated on the possibility of using gastric juice to dissolve large kidney stones, and even experimented with human kidney stones placed in the stomach of a bullfrog, pulled out and weighed every two days.

Young's attempt to synthesize a theory of digestion to replace that which he had demolished was very thorough. He wrote, in part: "Aliment is dissolved by the gastric menstruum; it then passes into the duodenum and meets with bile and pancreatic liquor; after being united with these, a heterogeneous mass is formed called chyme, and from this the lacteals secrete chyle." He was a good clinical observer too, and mentioned the fact that "nutrition goes on when the biliary ducts are obstructed, and also when the pancreas is scirrhous."

Young was the son of Dr. Samuel Young and Ann Richardson Young of Hagerstown, Maryland. The father, a graduate of Trinity College, Dublin, and an M.D. from Edinburgh, was to live to the age of 108. His wife died, probably of tuberculosis, at 31. Their son died in 1804, one year after graduating in medicine at the University of Pennsylvania. He was not only a good investigator, but a literary man. He had been active in the Cliosophic Literary Society at Princeton University where he graduated in 1799.

Howard Kelly was interested in Young and wrote of his life in the

Johns Hopkins *Hospital Bulletin*: "Young's name will shine with an even brighter luster, as the one who first effectively introduced and patiently followed out in this country the modern laboratory methods. Young was our first real scientist in the field of medicine."

Claude Bernard (1813-1878)

While a few of the researches by students already described in this work would seem to concern relatively trivial subjects, such could not be said of the two undergraduate works of Claude Bernard, the father of experimental medicine.

Claude Bernard was born at Saint-Julien (Rhone) near Villefranche, on July 12, 1813, the son of a small estate proprietor and wine grower. The parental home was so situated that on a clear day one could see the Alps in the distance. Claude Bernard was to use it later as a summer cottage.

The village curé taught the boy music and Latin, until it was time to attend the Jesuit college at Villefranche. After leaving the college Claude Bernard went to Lyon, where he worked for approximately two years as a pharmacist. The quackery and subterfuge that he found in the business there thoroughly sickened him and he gave it up. However, he found time to write a vaudeville comedy, *La Rose du Rhone*, which was performed. In addition, he composed a prose drama, *Arthur de Bretagne*. This was published posthumously in 1886 in Paris.

Armed with these literary works, he set off with two companions for Paris at the age of 21 and sought there the advice of the dramatic critic at the Sorbonne, Saint-Marc Girardin, who advised him to study medicine, despite his talent in the theatre.

The decision made, Claude Bernard threw himself into his studies in anatomy and physiology especially. In order to support himself he opened a course of lectures in a little experimental laboratory, which he set up opposite the Collège de France. Unfortunately, it soon closed for lack of students. Bernard was not a distinguished student; in fact he was rather inattentive. This may be accounted for by the numerous serious flaws which he detected in his professors' lectures. Fortunately, however, in his fifth year he became preparateur to the famous Magendie, professor of medicine in the Collège de France, actually occupying Laennec's old chair.

Despite the fact that Bernard had to continue to give private tutoring and lectures in order to cover his student expenses, he pioneered with his undergraduate researches. By May 1843 he was ready to publish his first paper describing work that he had done on the distribution of the chorda tympani, his interest having been stimulated by a case of facial hemiplegia which he had seen as a student on the wards. In his later years he showed an oft-recurring interest in this subject.

In the same year Bernard published his doctoral thesis on his undergraduate researches on gastric juice. His excellent basis in anatomy and great manual dexterity were evident from the thesis. He described his work on the intravenous injection into an animal of cane sugar and of his finding it unchanged in the urine. When, however, it was injected after the contents of a fresh stomach had acted upon it, the sugar recovered in the urine was no longer cane sugar. This was the germ of his later enquiry into the glycogenic function of the liver. The changing of cane sugar into blood sugar by the gastric juice was one of the things which stimulated his life interest in nutrition.

Also in 1843 he became interested in the role of the pancreas in digestion, and again his ability as a dissector led him to see that the pancreatic duct entered the gut in almost the same area in which he had noticed the filling of the lacteals in the dog after a meal. To further his studies, he improved upon the pancreatic fistula devised by Regnier de Graaf (1662). He hypothesized a three-fold action of pancreatic juice. This was revolutionary teaching in a world that regarded all digestion as being accomplished by the stomach alone. Bernard set out originally to study carbohydrate metabolism and that of fat and protein as well. His interest in diabetes caused him to begin with the carbohydrates and he never progressed beyond that stage of his plan.

Still turning over in his mind the problem of diabetes, Claude Bernard decided to find out where the dextrose in the blood was destroyed. His friend, Barreswil the chemist, had just devised the copper sulphate test for dextrose. And with this key Claude Bernard set out on his hunt. He found instead where glucose is produced. He discovered that the hepatic vein carrying blood away from the liver was loaded with glucose, even in a dog fed on meat only and with no sugar in the diet. He then thought of the liver as an organ or gland which "secreted" sugar.

Bernard was faced with the additional theory that the liver existed only to put out bile, an idea reminiscent of the functions assigned to the parotid gland, that of warming the ear, before Stensen's work. Bernard found that when the liver was washed out with water and was entirely free of sugar it would, if kept warm, produce sugar from some "glycogenic substance." Boiling the liver stopped this. But a combination of boiled liver and a little raw liver would once again produce sugar. So it was that Claude Bernard came to elaborate his theory of "internal secretions."

Again, from wrong premises, Claude Bernard came up undismayed with the discovery of the vasomotor nerves. He was soon back into the chorda tympani problem and discovered the difference between vasoconstrictor and vaso-dilator nerves.

In 1846 Claude Bernard quite independently found that when stimulated, the vagus nerve slowed the heart—something that the brothers Weber had first communicated orally at Naples in 1845. Starting in 1844, Bernard set out to analyze the physiological action of the drug curare, first brought back from the New World by Sir Walter Raleigh in 1595. It was shown that the drug was harmless when swallowed because it does not diffuse into the body but that it is fatal when even the smallest amount is introduced into a surface wound of the body.

During Bernard's undergraduate days, he had already observed in 1842 the peculiar colour of the blood in cases of carbon monoxide poisoning which he had seen. By 1855 he had time to proceed with fundamental work on the problem and published on it in 1857. In the course of his work he had to develop a method for measuring the available oxygen in blood samples and was not long in reaching the conclusion that oxygen and the iron of the red corpuscles are intimately related in respiratory functions.

In 1868 Claude Bernard relinquished his chair at the Sorbonne to his pupil, Paul Bert, and moved to fine laboratories built for him at the

Museum of Natural History by Napoleon III. He was made a senator in 1869. He was admitted to the Académie Française and took Flourens' seat there. Such great figures as Renan, Pasteur and Gambetta numbered among his friends. In 1877, in the last year of his life, he returned to his two earlier themes, the gastric juice and the glycogenic function of the liver.

Claude Bernard's wife and two daughters turned against him and left him, becoming anti-vivisectionists. Bernard was given a state funeral at the urging of Gambetta. His successor in the Académie Française was none other than his friend Renan. The Collège erected a bronze statue to him in 1886, as did the faculty of medicine and science in Lyon in 1894.

Ivan Pavlov (1849-1936)

"This is in truth an amazing fact—that a recently graduated science student, who had not yet finished his medical course, became the director of scientific investigations in the most famous clinic of internal diseases in Russia," wrote Pavlov's biographer, Boris Babkin, in his introduction to one of the most influential student investigators of all time.

Ivan Pavlov was born in 1849, as was William Osler. At the age of 12 the "liberation of the serfs" made a great impression on him. He was educated in a church school at Ryasa and its library became one of his chief haunts. As a boy Pavlov had read a translation of G.H. Lewes' *Practical Physiology*, which was followed by I.M. Sechenov's *Reflexes of the Brain*. These two volumes he kept beside him in his library for the rest of his life. Sechenov had been greatly influenced by Darwin's *Origin of Species*, which appeared just as he was graduating in medicine in Vienna.

Pavlov was attracted to medicine because of the exact methods which were just beginning to be applied in research. Sechenov's work on the organs of sense undoubtedly influenced his decision. It was the professor of physiology in the general course, Ilya Cyon, who first suggested a problem to Pavlov, and as a pre-medical student he carried on a time-consuming research on the nerves of the pancreas. For this he received a gold medal at the time of completing his pre-medical studies.

On commencing his medical student life Pavlov became an assistant in the physiological laboratory of the Veterinary Institute of the Medico-Chirurgical Academy. It was there that he did his first work on the role of nervous influences in the circulation of the blood and on the physiology of digestion.

During the summer vacation in 1877 he had the good fortune to work in the laboratory of Professor Heidenhain in Breslau, and as a result published in 1878 a paper on the effect of tying off the ducts of the pancreas in rabbits. Before he graduated, in December 1879, he published a remarkable paper on his own method of making a permanent pancreatic fistula. This method allowed him to collect the digestive juices in an active, healthy animal. This was but one of the results of the animal clinic that the young Pavlov set up, where the operating theatre and after-care were organized as if for human surgery. Impressed by this, the distinguished clinician Botkin asked the undergraduate Pavlov to direct his research laboratory for him.

After graduation Pavlov was able to travel for two years, thanks to a fellowship. He worked in Carl Ludwig's laboratory and, for a time, in

Heidenhain's laboratory again. He returned to Russia to find a new Institute of Experimental Medicine ready, and plunged into further researches on digestion. He was given a chair at the Military Medical Academy that he continued to hold for 34 years. With Bowditch in Harvard and Pavlov in St. Petersburg the influence of Carl Ludwig's pupils was to be dominant for several generations of medical students. Almost contemporaneously with Cannon, Pavlov began to report on psychical factors influencing digestion in animals. In the old log buildings in the village of Koltusky Pavlov laboured, despite war and revolution, and was eventually installed in beautiful quarters in the neighbouring settlement of Pavlovo. There physiologists from all over the world, including Banting came to see him and to admire his unrivalled facilities for the care of experimental animals.

Pavlov is best-known for his work on conditioned reflexes, first in association with the gastro-intestinal tract and later in the sphere of psychiatric problems. He had great faith in the explicable nature of human behaviour as the following quotation suggests: "The time will come, even if it be remote, when mathematical analysis, based on natural scientific analysis, will embrace in its magnificent formulae all these equilibria, including finally life itself."

The later declamatory state of Russian physiology, of an official caste, did violence to Pavlov's life-long scientific activity and should not be allowed to obscure the virile life of a great discoverer. His pupils inside and outside Russia carried on his tradition of hard work. Pavlov's "will" had this to say to students:

> From the very beginning of your work train yourself to strict consistency in the acquirement of knowledge... .
> Learn the ABC of science before you attempt to scale its peaks...
> Learn to do the heavy work that science involves. Study, compare, accumulate facts... Without facts, your theories are labour in vain.
> Do not turn yourself into a museum custodian of facts. Try to penetrate into the secret of their origin.
> Never think that you already know everything.
> Do not allow pride to take possession of you.
> Remember that science demands a man's whole life.

Pavlov died in his eighty-fifth year, still at work in his laboratory. He was probably the best-known figure in science in post-revolutionary Russia. Pavlov's great teacher Cyon, famous for his work on the depressor nerves to the heart, suggested Pavlov's first research wherein Pavlov studied the secretory innervation of the pancreas. Unfortunately, this was never published. Sadly reminiscent of the anti-Semitism of the Nazi era, Cyon was removed in the Czar's time from his professorial chair and left Russia. Pavlov reacted violently to this and refused to continue as an assistant to the "pompous ass" who was installed in Cyon's place. Pavlov's successor, the Cambridge-trained Orbeli, was to meet a similar fate, with Moscow pseudo-scientists.

Charles Robert Richet (1850-1935)

Richet was born in Paris where his father, Alfred Richet, was professor of surgery. His father insisted that he should study medicine, though he wanted, in his heart, to pursue a career in literature. However, after entering medical school he published his first paper on somnambulism in 1875. He managed to pursue his medical studies as well as those in physiology conjointly, taking his M.D. in 1877 and his Doctor of Science degree a year later. For these two degrees he presented his theses, "*Recherches Expérimentales et Cliniques sur la Sensibilité*" and "*Du suc gastrique chez l'homme et animaux, ses propriétés chimiques et physiologiques*." As Stewart Wolf relates in his superb biographical note on Richet in *Nobel Laureates in Medicine or Physiology*, both theses were based on "a rare opportunity to study stomach function in a young man who had acquired a gastric fistula, a surgical opening into his stomach through the skin of his abdomen. The fistula was required because his oesophagus, or gullet, had been seared shut when he accidentally swallowed lye." Richet fell on his work in physiology as a tornado. He began in 1879 by publishing the first French translation of William Harvey's *De Motu Cordis*. Richet proceeded to work on respiration and body temperature regulation in dogs, the involvement of a small centre in the brain sensitive to bacterial toxins and foreign proteins initiating fever. There was no stopping him.

In 1888 Richet joined an engineer in an attempt to build and fly a primitive aircraft. Two teen-aged boys, Jacques and Louis Breguet, produced such a plane but the Wright brothers in the United States had beaten them by a few weeks. However, Richet's name remained on the aircraft manufacturing group for some time before he dove into the world of physiology again.

Richet's work on metallic poisons was soon replaced by huge bibliographic undertakings, and his *Dictionnaire de physiologie* remained the standard work between 1895 and 1913. He produced a play that was performed at Monte Carlo in which Sarah Bernhardt played the lead role. Soon thereafter he began the work that was to win him the Moscow Prize and, in 1913, the Nobel Prize. His next prize was for a poem about Louis Pasteur in 1922. From the end of the first World War in which he was a well-known pacifist Richet began his work on blood plasma and blood transfusion. He was honoured with the Grand Cross of the Legion of Honour.

At the age of 75 Richet decided to retire as a professor but kept up his physiological interests.

This many-sided man died in 1935. Thirteen years before that event, Sir Charles Sherrington, O.M., wrote of Richet: "To honour him is to honour the spirit of physiology in its most graceful, most eloquent and most inspiring presentment—physiology poetized so to say. May we not say that there is not one whose physiological writings and speaking display such imaginative power without allowing imagination to add to or subtract from scientific truth by one iota."

Christian Bohr (1855-1911)

The distinguished physiologist Christian Bohr was the father of the world-famous physicist Niels Bohr. Fritz Buchtal of Copenhagen says that even as a medical student Christian Bohr was interested in physiology. He published his first paper on the effect of salicylic acid on digestion at the age of 22. He received his doctor's degree in medicine after submitting his thesis on fat in milk. At age 26 Bohr had the opportunity to work in the laboratory of Professor Carl Ludwig in Leipzig, and while there branched out into the physiology of blood and respiration. His first paper, published by the Danish Royal Academy of Science when he was 22, was entitled "*Sur la respiration pulmonaire.*"

Walter Bradford Cannon (1871-1945)

Human beings, in a rather automatic way, swallow a great deal of food in the course of their lives—taking the process wholly for granted. In 1896 a medical student at Harvard University was puzzling over the mechanism of swallowing when he overheard a conversation in a tram, to the effect that a machine had been invented in Germany for looking right through a person.

The student, Walter Cannon, lost no time in getting to the door of his professor of physiology in the medical school, Henry Bowditch, with a request that he be allowed to try out these new x-rays in a study of swallowing.[1] He had come to the right man—for Bowditch had studied in Germany under Carl Ludwig who had encouraged generations of undergraduates in research projects.

With a primitive x-ray machine Cannon began his studies, knowing nothing of the dangerous radiation burns he was likely to develop in the process. He was so fearful of the sparks shot off by the machine that he shielded his body with a large sheet of lead, thus minimizing the frightful effects that many of the early workers elsewhere suffered.

He began on December 6, 1896, by watching pearl buttons pass down the oesophagus of a dog. Twenty days afterward he was asked to demonstrate the process in a goose, before the annual meeting of the American Physiological Society. The demonstration of the orderly and rhythmic contractions of the muscular walls of the oesophagus was of great interest, since the prevailing theory was that air taken into the mouth was in some way compressed, thereby driving the food down into the stomach.

Cannon as a premedical student was influenced by C.B. Davenport in Harvard College, and had begun investigative work there in a small way on determining the influence of light on the direction and rate of movement of organisms. On entering medical school he depended for his financial support on assisting with a class in comparative anatomy at nearby Radcliffe College, and in his final year of medicine conducted this course single-handed.

Walter Cannon came of French Canadian stock on his mother's side. His great-grandfather, Jacques de Noyon, escaped the Indian massacres at Deerfield, Massachusetts, in 1704 and with his bride, Abigail Stebbins, settled on the south bank of the St. Lawrence River near Montreal, the shore which furnished medicine with another man of gastro-intestinal fame—Alexis St. Martin, the subject of William Beaumont's classical investigations on the stomach.

One of de Noyon's granddaughters, Sarah Wilma Denis (as the name became contracted) migrated to Wisconsin, settling as a teacher at Prairie du Chien. Here she married Colbert Cannon, a descendant of Samuel Carnahan (later Cannon) of Boston. Laura Cochran Cannon had walked beside her husband Samuel's covered wagon from Massachusetts to Ohio, as her great-grandson loved to tell his medical class. To Colbert and Sarah Cannon was born Walter Bradford, in October 1871, in Prairie du Chien, which was the site of William Beaumont's second series of observations on the ever-absconding Alexis St. Martin.

Raised in St. Paul, Walter Cannon was encouraged in the use of tools by his father. One is reminded of Harvey Cushing's boyhood and of the high opinion he held of learning to use tools early in life. He said it forced one to learn to make decisions and to get on with the job.

Cannon's biological interests became apparent in high school and he was greatly influenced, as was his entire generation, by the writings of Thomas Huxley. Cannon collided with a narrow-minded family parson over such matters and withdrew from the church.

He won a freshman scholarship to Harvard, and with $180 from his family set out upon his career, being fully self-supporting from that day on. At Harvard College, as he has related in his interesting autobiography, *The Way of an Investigator*, Cannon was, at first, at a loss to know what notes he should take at lectures. A classmate with more beef than brains advised him to take down nothing until the professor began to shout—and then to write that down verbatim.

Graduating with his B.A. degree summa cum laude in 1896 Cannon completed his M.A. degree and his first year of medicine together in 1897. The philosopher William James dissuaded Cannon from his one-time desire to read philosophy saying, "Don't do it, you will be filling your belly with east wind."

Cannon's work as a medical student found him perfecting a gruel of bismuth sub-nitrate that could be easily swallowed by animals in association with their normal food. His advances were communicated to the American Physiological Society, and by the time of his graduation in 1900 he was an authority on the motion of the food through the gut. (Rieder's oft-quoted paper in the German literature on the "bismuth meal" was published five years later.) Four papers were published by Cannon as an undergraduate, two of them with the assistance of another medical student, Albert Moser. There is one significant exchange recorded between Cannon, as an undergraduate, and one of the laboratory dieners or preparators. Cannon once entered the laboratory at an hour when there was no prescribed class exercise and was rudely told that no student was allowed therein. Six years later Cannon, as Bowditch's successor in the chair of physiology, had a chance to change this—and change it he did. There is nothing so discordant in an institution dedicated to the pursuit of knowledge as the display of usurped authority by non-teaching staff. The educational process, as the term implies, is "to lead out." Unfortunately, students—the *raison d'être* of medical schools—are still occasionally considered as recurrent nuisances by department officials.

Cannon was a student's professor and his election in 1906 to Bowditch's chair an occasion for mutual satisfaction. Bowditch had held it for 35 years; Cannon was to hold it for 36, so that for a total of 71 years the benign spirit of Carl Ludwig, and his interest in student investigators, was to preside over the physiological laboratory at Harvard. Dr. Joseph Aub has recounted the fact that in his class alone, six men in their first year were so inspired by Cannon's instruction that they completed investigations worthy of publication while still undergraduates. At about the same time Cannon's friend Sir Arthur Hurst was being assisted by four London medical students in an x-ray survey of the intestinal tract in normal humans. They joined him in authorship of a resulting paper, which was published in Guy's *Hospital Reports*. All four students later distinguished themselves in separate medical specialties.

In order to help his students find their feet, Cannon wrote an exemplary laboratory manual for them. His lectures always contained stimulating questions or suggestions for future investigation, and many fell on receptive ears. Since the year of Cannon's birth—1871—when the first physiological laboratory in the country was organized by Bowditch, as George Higginson Professor at Harvard, fresh ideas have been welcomed and new minds stimulated in this famous school, to the great benefit of the American people.

By the year 1912 Cannon had completed his key work on the production of adrenalin in the bloodstream by such stresses as pain, low blood sugar and cold, on the rhythmic movements of the walls of the digestive tract, and on the muscle in the gut and its intrinsic and extrinsic nerve supply. He had probed the origin of "hunger pains" and surmised the psychic forces that played upon the motions and secretions of the stomach. In this connection Walter Meek has drawn attention to Michael Foster's words concerning the great physiological investigator, Claude Bernard: "The chiefest sign of genius in inquiry [was] to leave the road at the right turning and to follow a bye-path which brought him to a great result."

Cannon's career turning point came when one of his experimental cats became angered with him—as some cats do with experimenters occasionally—and all gastro-intestinal movements stopped, as demonstrated by x-rays. Cannon set out to find the reason, and spent his next 20 years on this phenomenon. As a result the world now knows a great deal more than it did about the emotional origin of some of its digestive upsets. Medical literature was greatly enriched by the appearance in 1915 of Cannon's book, *Bodily Changes in Pain, Hunger, Fear and Rage*, and in 1932 of *The Wisdom of the Body*. He came to regard the medulla of the adrenal gland as part of the nervous system, as first suggested by a graduate student at Cambridge University, T.R. Elliott. In these golden years Cannon displayed the spirit of Carl Ludwig and of Purkinje, in having many of his own discoveries published by the students assisting him.

As an internationalist in science Cannon was saddened by the First World War. He was not long in joining the British workers under William Bayliss, however, at the laboratory for surgical research set up at Dijon.[2] They looked for possible "toxic factors" in traumatic shock, and eventually Cannon described the condition as "toxic exemia," a view not far removed from that widely held today. For his services he was made a Commander of the Bath by King George V, and was awarded the Distinguished Service Medal by the American government. Cannon and Bayliss also suggested the use of a gum acacia solution intravenously to combat shock, much as plasma is used today.

In 1940 the National Research Council in Washington called Cannon to be chairman of its committee on shock and transfusion, to see if preserved blood could be made available for front line use.

Between the wars Cannon served as exchange professor in Paris, in 1929, and in Peiping in 1935. He visited Russia at the time of the International Physiological Congress in 1936 and formed a great affection for the Russian people.

No man of science in modern times has received so many honorary degrees, medals, and been called to so many lectureships, and yet remained so unaffected, so painstaking in his work. Cannon was partial to the needs of the dispossessed in Spain and China. He travelled widely abroad, but also knew his homeland intimately. With his inspiring wife and five children and an indestructible Ford car he went annually to the mountains of the west for years. One of these in Glacier Park was called Mt. Cannon in his honour.

Professor Cannon died in 1945 of a white blood cell disease that first became evident in 1929. He typifies the best in American education and medicine. He was the 20th century's Claude Bernard. His influence has been unique for no one has so fired the imagination of medical students with a belief in their worth as investigators. His pupils from almost every country in the world have taken back with them something of this spirit. As Robert Morison said in a memorial tribute: "More enduring is the feeling he left in all of us that it is possible for men throughout the world to live and work together for the common good." Generations which could not have known him will long enjoy his candid and intriguing autobiography.

Virgil P. Sydenstricker (1889-1964) and **George Lindor Brown** (1901-1971)

Virgil P. Sydenstricker was born in Hamilton, Montana. He qualified for his bachelor of arts and master of arts degrees from Washington and Lee University and then proceeded to Johns Hopkins in Baltimore, qualifying there for his M.D. degree in 1915. When he was a medical student he wrote and published his first paper with the famous George Hoyt Whipple, who was already a well-known researcher in the field of intestinal studies bearing on nutrition. In 1919 Sydenstricker became resident physician to the university hospital in Augusta, and in 1922 was appointed professor of medicine in Georgia's Medical College. One of his good works was the effort he put into the elimination of pellagra from the southern United States. Sydenstricker also gave a classic description of sickle-cell anaemia.

George Lindor Brown entered the University of Manchester at the age of 18 on a scholarship and was taught by such outstanding physiologists as A.V. Hill, H.S. Raper and B.A. McSwiney. After taking his bachelor of science degree with honours, he worked from 1924 to 1925 in McSwiney's laboratory on the effect of drugs on the mobility of isolated strips of the stomach. For this work he received his master of science degree. He did further research on the gastric muscle of cats, dogs and rabbits and then studied the reversal of the action of adrenalin in this situation. In all, Lindor Brown had published five papers before he graduated in medicine at the University of Manchester in 1928. He moved to the University of Leeds and eventually to Oxford, where he worked with J.C. Eccles and Hebbel Hoff. He then proceeded to the Medical Research Council Laboratories where his work on the chemical transmission of the nerve impulse made him an outstanding scientist. He was awarded the fellowship of the Royal Society of London in 1946. Thereafter he became professor of physiology at University College, London, and eventually Waynflete Professor of Physiology at Oxford.

[1] Visualization of the outlines of the human stomach by x-rays was pioneered in America by J.C. Hemmeter (1864-1931) in the spring of 1896 in the physics laboratory of the State Normal School, Baltimore, Maryland.

[2] Cannon was a member of the 'Harvard Unit,' which went to France long before the United States entered the war. He worked with Cuthbert Wallace at a Casualty Clearing Station and later joined the research group in London which included Bayliss, A.N. Richards and H.H. Dale.

CHAPTER EIGHT

Endocrines

Jean Conrad Brunner (1653-1727) has been already mentioned in connection with his view that the duodenal glands he had discovered in 1672 were, in his words, "a secondary pancreas." His later removal of the pancreas in a dog, producing diabetic symptoms, was an early indication of the role of that organ in diabetes.

Théophile de Bordeu (1722-1776)

In 1742 at the age of 20, this medical student at the University of Montpellier in southwest France published his thesis entitled "*Dissertatio phisiologica de sensu generice considerato*." He had no use for Galenic theories of "vital spirits." The hypothesis he formulated was that every gland and probably every tissue and cell discharges products into the bloodstream, which in turn influence other glands and tissues. He was eventually made professor of anatomy at Pau in the Basse Pyrennes. He was highly critical of the distinguished professor of medicine Joseph Lieutaud at Aix en Provence, though Lieutaud described quite clearly the pituitary-portal system of veins passing between the hypothalamus and the hypophysis. Lord Zuckerman, the distinguished Oxford anatomist has drawn attention to Lieutaud's possible prevision of secretion of hormones by the brain.

Anders Adolf Retzius (1796-1860)

Retzius was a student of medicine at the University of Lund, though he spent one year at the University of Copenhagen. On graduating at Lund in medicine in 1819, he wrote his doctoral thesis on the anatomy of the chondro-pterygious fishes, but more importantly he described his discovery of the adrenal glands in elasmobranchs. While still a medical student he also instructed at the Royal Military Academy of Veterinary Science. He went on to be the distinguished professor of anatomy at the Karolinska, Stockholm's great medical school.

Paul Langerhans (1847-1888)

Paul Langerhans excelled, as a medical student in 1867, when he began an investigation into the microscopic structure of the pancreas. Virchow had been quick to recognize unusual qualities in this student, who came from a long line of doctors, and had enabled him to work in his Institute in Berlin.

Two preliminary papers came from Langerhans' pen, on the nerves of the human skin as shown by Cohnheim's gold staining method, and on the changes seen in the tactile corpuscles in the skin during central nervous system disease. Physicians still speak of "Langerhans' granular layer" in the skin; and of "Langerhans' stellate corpuscles" or nerve terminals in the epidermis.

In the summer vacation of 1867 Langerhans began a thorough study of the cell types encountered in the pancreas. This organ was long regarded as an abdominal salivary gland of some kind. After detailing eight already known types of cells, Langerhans, in his graduation thesis (1869) embodying his student work, described a new cell that did not conform to the assumed salivary gland picture. He saw "a small irregularly polygonal structure. Its cytoplasm is brilliant and free of any granules, its nucleus distinct, round and of moderate size.... These cells lie together, generally in considerable numbers, diffusely scattered in the substance of the gland."

His 31-one page dissertation began: "There is indeed hardly another organ in which there is such glaring contrast between the brilliant results of physiological research and the complete darkness in the realm of anatomic knowledge."

Langerhans developed a Berlin blue and glycerine mixture for the retrograde injection of the pancreatic duct, and this showed up the widely ramifying collecting system. However, his newly discovered cells bore no apparent relation to the duct system. He could see the "islets" even in a fresh rabbit pancreas, so thin were the layers in it.

This inquisitive medical student concluded his thesis with the humility that comes of hard work in the laboratory, often with meagre results: "I cannot in any way put forth the conclusive results of a completed investigation. I can describe at most a few isolated observations which suggest a much more complicated structure of the pancreas than hitherto accepted. The purpose of these lines can therefore at best be to help draw greater attention to the pancreas than has hitherto been given by anatomists."

Langerhans has been sympathetically memorialized by Dr. H. Morrison of Tufts Medical School, Boston, who has translated his thesis into English. Langerhans began his career amid the medical and political lore of a family long immersed in the life of Berlin. After a year at Jena he began the study of medicine in Berlin in 1866. After graduation he continued on in Virchow's laboratory in order to work on what is now called the reticulo-endothelial system. Within a year he wrote to Virchow about the things he was encountering on a trip to North Africa and Asia Minor—all anthropological, for that was one of Virchow's great interests.

Medical research is the most truly international commodity we possess. It knows no protective tarrif, no embargo, no boundary line to prevent its free dissemination for the good of all. At present it is the common language and common spirit among the nations.
Sir Frederick Banting, F.R.S.,
Victoria, B.C., 1926

While Langerhans was made a professor of pathology in Freiburg he was forced, by a bout of tuberculosis, to give it up and to retire to Madeira. Though he continued to contribute researches on the spread of the tubercle bacillus in the body, and on leprosy, he died of his disease at the age of 41.

Five years later the generous Laguesse attached Langerhans' name to "the magic islands" discovered in the pancreas, which islands soon were credited with having an internal secretory activity, in close association with capillaries. In fact Laguesse started off the series of events that led Von Mehring and Minkowski, Opie and Ssobolew, W.G. MacCallum, and finally Banting and Best into the study of the islet cells, which in 1921 resulted in the harvesting from them of life-giving "insulin."

Langerhan's short dissertation started off a chain-reaction of inestimable value.

Ivar Sandstrom (1852-1889)

When Santiago Ramón y Cajal visited Stockholm to receive the Nobel Prize in medicine he remarked that gray matter flourished under gray skies. This was certainly true in the case of Ivar Sandstrom, who, as a student in the pre-clinical course at Uppsala in 1877, discovered the parathyroid glands.

Today it is known how important these minute structures are for the regulation of calcium metabolism in the body. Fatal muscle spasms or tetany may follow their accidental removal during thyroid operations. In 1877, however, no one knew of this connection. It took a dogged medical student three years to round out even the anatomical picture, so hard-pressed was he with his prescribed studies. It was to be an erstwhile student discoverer—William G. MacCallum, of avian malaria fame—who worked out the calcium regulating role of the parathyroids in 1905 at the age of 31.

The thoroughness of Sandstrom's gross and microscopic observations was such that his descriptions have hardly been bettered over the intervening years. Dr. Carl M. Seipel has translated Sandstrom's account into English. With engaging simplicity this student began:

> About three years ago (1877) I found on the thyroid gland of a dog a small organ, hardly as big as a hemp seed, which was enclosed in the same connective tissue capsule as the thyroid, but could be distinguished therefrom by a lighter color. A superficial examination revealed an organ of a totally different structure from that of the thyroid, and with a very rich vascularity.... The existence of a hitherto unknown gland in animals that have so often been a subject of anatomical examination called for a thorough approach to the region around the thyroid gland, even in man.... It was exclusively with the purpose of completing the investigation, rather than with the hope of finding something new that I began a careful examination of this region. So much the greater was my astonishment therefore when in the first individual examined I found on both sides at the inferior border of the thyroid gland an organ of the size of a small pea, which, judging from its exterior, did not appear to be a lymph gland, not an accessory thyroid gland, and upon histological examination showed a rather peculiar structure....

The great vascularity of this possibly endocrine or hormone-secreting tissue had greatly impressed Sandstrom. As he prepared to show some microscopic slides of his early work to his sympathetic teacher, Professor Edward Clason, Sandstrom looked into Clason's microscope, which was at that moment focussed on a section of the pituitary gland. Struck by the similarity of the glandular tissue shot through with myriad blood vessels, Sandstrom cried out in amazement: "Have you already seen the gland I was going to show you?"

Sandstrom's description was thorough and painstaking. In fact it was too thorough for the editors of a German scientific periodical to whom it was submitted, unsuccessfully, for publication. For this reason the world knew little of the work except for Retzius' review in a German yearbook. In 1892 Gley rediscovered the glands, and brought Sandstrom's work before the world. Actually, Richard Owen in 1850 read a paper to the Zoological Society of London on the parathyroid glands of the great Indian rhinoceros that died in 1849, having been bought for 1,000 guineas in 1834. Of course, Sandstrom's microscopic work on the gland was his real contribution, which is not to diminish his own independent finding of the glands in the much-dissected dog.

Sandstrom knew what he was about, and he knew his limitations. He concluded: "While working on the above description of these hitherto unrecognized organs, I have tried to go through the older as well as the newer literature in order to find out whether these glands have been previously known and then forgotten again—but unfortunately, the literature which I have had at my disposal has been too scanty and too hard of access for these studies to pretend to be complete." He then quoted Remak and Virchow, who had given rudimentary descriptions of the gland but nothing as detailed as Sandstrom's material.

Sandstrom's student paper shows a good grasp of general anatomy. He mentions, for instance, the signs and symptoms that one might expect from a tumour or swelling of the parathyroids, as judged from their proximity to the oesophagus and to the recurrent laryngeal nerve supplying the vocal cords. Again, Sandstrom looked for, but did not find, some close relation between the gland and the lymphatic vessels. He was obviously testing out its possible role as a lymph gland. The volume of work undertaken and completed by this medical student was exhaustive. He dissected out the glands of a large variety of mammals and examined their position and minute structure in 50 humans.

The thoroughness demonstrated in this work also is to be found in Sandstrom's method of teaching histology or microscopic anatomy. His later students at Uppsala studied histology at the microscope, while he lectured to the class. They became literate in the subject by actually making the slide their textbook, there being no intermediary.

Sandstrom came of a family of public servants and scholars. In his short life of 37 years he accomplished much, despite recurrent mental illness. His contribution provided not only the framework for the future physiology of calcium regulation in the body, but also for an understanding of some of the hazards of thyroid surgery. His work, too long unrecognized, is a tribute to all medical students who have pioneered and to the sympathetic teachers who have encouraged them.

Pierre Marie (1853-1940)

Neurologists the world over claim Pierre Marie as one of the most brilliant founders of their specialty. Why then is he included in a chapter on endocrinology?

As a medical student Marie became interested in the tremor, especially visible in the extended arms and fingers, in cases of thyroid disease in which an excess of this hormone is released into the bloodstream. His graduation thesis in 1883 first graphically presented this sign, which every medical student today searches for in doing a physical examination. Under the tutelage of the great clinician Charcot he grew up in the wards of the Salpêtrière in Paris, observing clinical abnormalities and then pursuing them to the pathological laboratory for an explanation.

It was in this manner that Marie, with Charcot, described the disease known as peroneal muscular atrophy in 1886, just three years after Marie had qualified in medicine. This work took him on an excursion into pathology, the laws of heredity, muscle diseases and electrophysiology. In the same year, Tooth, in his Cambridge M.D. thesis, described the same features of the disease, and his name is today coupled with those of Marie and Charcot in its definition.

Marie's fame as an endocrinologist rests upon his thorough description of acromegaly, the disease that Marie may have seen as he walked through the streets of Paris—the large head and the enormous extremities. As he studied these people in hospital he learned that they also had large tongues, headache and increasing visual difficulty, an intense thirst with a great outpouring of sugary urine, and with either amenorrhoea or impotence. In reviewing an autopsy performed when he was a student in 1882, Marie found that the acromegalic patient, Henri Honrot, had hidden within the pituitary fossa in the base of his skull a tumour resembling a hen's egg in size. The enlarged pituitary fossa of another case of Marie's was later described by the ever-enquiring Broca and gradually the pituitary origin of acromegaly came to be established. Finally in 1921 the patient and pioneering work of Herbert Evans and Long showed that the growth hormone found in the anterior part of the pituitary gland was definitely responsible for the production of gigantism.[1]

As Sir Henry Cohen has shown in his paper read to the Royal Society of Medicine in 1953, Pierre Marie's life is one of extraordinary interest—filled with triumphs of observation, generalization and fertile imagination. It is filled with sorrows, too. He was born in Paris and attended a classical school at Vauves. His father persuaded him to study law and he was actually called to the bar. However, his desire to study medicine was unabated and he turned to this calling with both enthusiasm and a broad preparation. His knowledge of foreign languages, history and art were to mark him out as an exceptional medical student. Charcot came to regard him as his most accomplished disciple.

In temperament precise and exacting—possibly as a result of the military discipline of his early schooling, and of his legal training—Marie was nevertheless a great teacher. He was deaf to the blandishments of Paris society. He lived for his patients and his family. In turn his daughter, his wife and his son died of infections that today would have been curable. Just before the fall of Paris, Marie was operated upon for an abdominal condition by Count Thierry de Martel—the surgeon who was soon to commit suicide rather than make his life a blank cheque, as he said, for the invading Nazis. Marie died on April 13, 1940, at the age of 87, on the Côte d'Azur he loved so well. Endocrinology and neurology had been powerfully influenced by this one-time lawyer and student contributor.

The triumvirate of Langerhans, Sandstrom and Pierre Marie illustrates the opportunities that were exploited by a microscopist, a gross anatomist and a clinical observer, respectively. The field of endocrinology probably offers more scope than any other today for further observations by enquiring medical students.

Herbert McLean Evans (1882-1971)

Evans was born in Modesto, California, and entered the University at Berkeley, graduating with a bachelor of science degree in 1904. His first publication in that year was the result of a field trip with paleontologists through the state of Idaho. The title was "A New Cestraciont Strain from the Lower Triassic of Idaho."

Evans was the gold medalist in his graduating year and gave the valedictory address on the subject of "The Importance of Biological Research for Human Welfare." He had been exposed to the outstanding scientist at Berkeley at that time, Jacques Loeb. Upon graduation Evans set out to investigate eastern medical schools that might allow him to work in anatomy as well as in the curricular regular courses. Professor Minot at Harvard was a possible choice, but finally Evans settled on Johns Hopkins University Medical School in Baltimore where Franklin Paine Mall was the moving force. Some Hopkins graduates have been known to complain that Mall "taught" them no anatomy. Mall, on the other hand, allowed students to "learn" anatomy. So it was with Evans, who learned the curriculum at Hopkins would allow him one-quarter free for research interests.

Therefore after first-year medicine at the University of California Evans went to Hopkins in the class of 1908. One of the inspiring things that Evans found at Hopkins was a speech by Osler on a visit from Oxford. The lecture was on Michael Servetus, who had discovered and announced the lesser circulation, but who was burned at the stake in Geneva by John Calvin. Evans was also enthused by Harvey Cushing, later to become the world's greatest brain surgeon. Cushing at that time was head of the Hunterian Surgical Laboratory.

In the year 1907 Evans published three papers, one of which was with Professor William Stewart Halsted, the professor of surgery. Halsted had found in one patient in whom he was removing the thyroid gland that tetany followed the operation and the professor felt that possibly the blood supply to the small parathyroids had been interfered with. Halsted realized that there was no one more capable than Evans in injecting small blood vessels, and it was he therefore who demonstrated the fact in cadavers that these vessels might well suffer in thyroidectomy.

Evans was kept busy as an undergraduate by his professors, such as Mall, who persuaded him to write book reviews for his *Anatomical Record*. In 1907, still an undergraduate, Evans was called upon by Mall to prepare a chapter in his new celebrated *Manual of Human Embryology*. Evans was able to show by experimental means that in embryos the large vessels actually come from a network of capillaries during development. This was against the views of all the pundits in the field.

By the time of his graduation in 1908 Evans had seven papers published, one of them leading him into the field of cancer and the lymphatics supplying metastases. Immediately upon graduation Evans was sent to study in Germany, with help from the Rockefeller Foundation and the Robert Koch Foundation. Paul Ehrlich refused to tell Evans the composition of the intra-vital dyes that interested him, so Evans walked out. Eventually one of these dyes, number T-1824, was named "Evans blue." This was used later, in both animals and patients in studying blood volume.

By the age of 84 Evans had produced 600 papers and books by which time he had become the acknowledged head of the scientific community working on the endocrine glands and their function.

As an undergraduate at Berkeley, Amos Christie, later professor of pediatrics at Vanderbilt University, did research with Evans on intra-vital blue dyes.

James Bumgardner Murphy (1884-1950)

After receiving his bachelor's degree at the University of North Carolina Murphy entered Johns Hopkins Medical School in 1905. His anatomical dissection attracted a man who Murphy thought was a senior student. The junior professor was interested in Murphy's excellent drawings of the nerves of the nasal system, so much so that he placed them on the department's bulletin board. He asked Murphy if he would like to come to tea for conversation, but Murphy replied that he was awfully busy. The rejected host was the youthful brain surgeon Harvey Cushing. They later became good friends.

As an undergraduate Murphy published, with William G. MacCallum, another student discoverer, an important paper on "Tetany after parathyroidectomy in herbivora." With his reputation for hard and creative work, Murphy was invited to join Peyton Rous at the Rockefeller Institute for Medical Research on the transmissibility of the chicken cancer found on the leg of a bird brought in by a New Jersey farmer and plunked down on Rous's desk. This led to a lifetime of studies on tissue resistance to grafting and similar interests.

Murphy exhibits a common condition among medical students then and now. He had come upon tough times when he was two years into his medical course, when his father died. Murphy had therefore to leave Johns Hopkins Hospital and was on his way out the door when he ran into the director, Dr. Henry Hurd. On hearing the situation Hurd immediately arranged for the funds needed to keep Murphy, this brilliant student, in medical school until he graduated.

Charles Herbert Best (1899-1978)

Best was born of Canadian parents who lived in the state of Maine. He was a student at the University of Toronto beginning in 1917 and served in the Canadian Army. At the age of 19 he transferred to the honours course in physiology and biochemistry, graduating with his bachelor of arts degree in 1921. Immediately thereafter he took a postgraduate year in chemical pathology, biochemistry and physiology with Professor J.J.R. Macleod, and investigated the pathway of nerve impulses from the medulla oblongata, which influence the liberation of glucose from the liver producing a temporary glycosuria. He began his work with Banting on insulin in 1921 and in the sweltering climate of that summer in Toronto helped Banting to produce the first crude insulin. Best achieved his M.D. degree in Toronto in 1925 and thereafter pursued a very intensive research life, some of it with Sir Henry Dale in London, and much of it with the Royal Canadian Navy in World War II. He headed the department of physiology at the University of Toronto and lived to see the opening of the Charles Best Institute next door to the Banting Institute.

James Bertram Collip (1892-1965)

Collip was born in Ontario and worked with Professor A.B. Macallum at the University of Toronto. Macallum was a close friend of Sir Charles Sherrington at Oxford and the father of the National Research Council of Canada.

Collip graduated with his bachelor of arts degree in 1912 at the University of Toronto and took his master of arts degree the following year. In 1916 he graduated with his Ph.D. and proceeded to a Doctor of Science degree at the University of Alberta in Edmonton, in 1924. Prior to that, however, he received a Rockefeller travelling fellowship that promised six months with J.J.R. Mcleod, six months with Donald Van Slyke at the Rockefeller Institute in New York, and four months with Henry Dale in London. However, he was never able to study with the latter two scientists because insulin was discovered at the University of Toronto in 1921 and he stayed to purify it for human injection. Fortunately for humanity, the first insulin produced by Banting and Best was effective though known to be impure. There was later to be a striking parallel when Florey and Chain's penicillin was found to be active clinically despite the fact that at first it was only one per cent pure.

By the time Collip had graduated in medicine his published papers numbered 58. He went on to great triumphs in the detection and purification of hormones, especially the pituitary and parathyroid, among others. During World War II he succeeded Sir Frederick Banting as chairman of the Medical Research Committee of Canada's National Research Council after Banting was killed while flying to Britain in a Hudson bomber on war work.

Joshua Harold Burn (1892-1981)

Burn was a human dynamo. At the age of 17 he entered Emmanuel College at Cambridge and had Frederick Gowland Hopkins as his tutor. He achieved his bachelor of arts degree with first-class standing in 1912 and then spent 18 months of research with Joseph Barcroft in Hopkins' laboratory. Those were the days when J.N. Langley, A.V. Hill, Keith Lucas, Edgar Adrian, Walter Morley Fletcher and H.K. Anderson were on the physiological side at Cambridge. In 1913 Burn published two papers on measuring the oxygen capacity of the blood. Henry Dale offered him a post at the Wellcome Physiological Research Laboratories, testing the purity of posterior pituitary extracts, ergot extracts, tincture of digitalis and cannabis indica, which was great training for any future professor of pharmacology.

In 1914 Burn was off to the war. He was first offered a corporal's job as motorcyclist dispatch rider. He then joined an infantry brigade as signals officer, and went through the battles of the Somme and Arras. In 1917 he was sent to Guy's Hospital Medical School to complete his medical degree, which he received from Cambridge in 1920.

Burn added to his undergraduate publications in 1915 when with Sir Henry Dale he wrote on "The Action of Certain Quaternary Ammonium Bases." In 1924, again with Henry Dale, he wrote, "On the Location and Nature of the Action of Insulin." In 1937 Burn became the professor of pharmacology at Oxford, and was known as a brilliant lecturer and laboratory demonstrator. He lived to be a great age and was a prolific writer.

Willard Myron Allen (b. 1904)

Allen was born in Macedon in New York State, and attended Hobart College. Prior to his graduation in medicine at the University of Rochester in 1932 he joined in endocrinological research with the distinguished professor of anatomy, George Washington Corner (1889-1981). Their work on ovarian hormones was of primary importance and highly regarded in the field of endocrinology. Their classic paper, "Physiology of the corpus luteum" appeared in the *American Journal of Physiology* in 1929 and was a landmark. In 1940 Allen became professor of obstetrics and gynecology at the University of Washington School of Medicine in St. Louis.

A. McGehee Harvey, as a medical undergraduate at Johns Hopkins published, with E.K. Marshall, Jr., an important paper demonstrating that the loop of Henle in the kidney was the locus of action of the antidiuretic hormone.

Geoffrey Wingfield Harris (1913-1971)

Like J.H. Burn, Geoffrey Harris was a student at Emmanuel College, Cambridge, entering in 1933. There he achieved a first-class in all examinations, graduating with a bachelor of arts degree in 1936. In the same year he published a paper on pseudopregnancy in rats which had received strong electrical stimulation to the head. A year later he began his work on the relationship of the pituitary gland to the brain. He sectioned the pituitary stalk and then stimulated the hypothalamus and recorded his results. He was able to visit the future Nobelist W.R. Hess in Zurich, as well as the prolific John Beattie at the Royal College of Surgeons in London. His research concerned the ovulation produced by the stimulation of both lobes. From 1936 to 1940 Harris completed his medical training at St. Mary's Hospital, London. He contrived to stimulate the posterior lobe of the pituitary by remote control. The release of vasopressin and oxytocin was his objective. Harris displayed great surgical dexterity.

He returned to Cambridge to a lectureship in Adrian's department of physiology, but left in 1952 to develop a laboratory of experimental neuroendocrinology at the Maudsley Hospital, by then the British Institute of Psychiatry. Ten years later he succeeded Professor Le Gros Clark in the blue-ribbon chair of anatomy at Oxford. There his organizational skills were tested to the full as he was able to modify the anatomy course and to bring anatomy, physiology, biochemistry, pathology and pharmacology into a single "Honours School" of physiological sciences. He was ever-mindful of John Fulton's statement that it was easier to move a graveyard than to modify the curriculum of most medical schools. Harris was a pioneer in the relationships between the central nervous system and the endocrine system. He died suddenly of a gastric hemorrhage in 1971.

O.P. Kimball

Two students are often forgotten in discussions of the field of thyroid treatment of goiter. In Akron, Ohio, in 1917 Oliver Perry Kimball, a medical student, explained to the superintendent of schools what was needed to prevent goiter. Kimball knew the relevant literature very well and cited the sporadic cases of goiter described by Captain Cook. He listed the endemic areas for goiter, including the distant Pemberton Meadows of British Columbia where calves, pigs and lambs were affected. He noted that the Greeks had used the ashes of burned sea sponges for treating that illness. He also noted that in Pennsylvania, a small amount of iodine in the water had saved the fishing industry. Kimball's research from 1916 to 1920 was financed by the American Medical Association's Department of Therapeutic Research. Ten thousand school girls in Akron were studied over a three-year period, including those from the fifth to the twelfth grades. Five thousand girls took prophylactic doses of three grains of sodium iodide in water and this group had not a single case of enlarged thyroid gland. An amazingly large fraction of those not treated developed goiters. Under subsequent treatment 60 per cent of these later showed disappearance of the goiter. After being informed of these results Professor Klinger in Zurich, in 1918, began similar research. A stable form of iodine in chocolate was administered.

Kimball's activity was mirrored in that of a Long Island College of Medicine student, Gudernatsch, who described the effect of thyroxin while he was still a medical student.

John Herbert Humphrey (1915-1987)

This medical student researcher was encouraged by Professor C.R. Harrington at University College Hospital (the synthesizer of thyroxine) to find out if it was possible to regulate hormonal action by neutralizing antibodies. Humphrey worked with Neuburger and Pitt-Rivers. The compounds produced were tested in vivo with M. E. Yuil and reported in *The Biochemical Journal* of 1939. Humphrey qualified in medicine in 1940.

Christian René de Duvé

De Duvé was born of refugee Belgian parents near London in 1917. After World War I they returned to Belgium where Christian studied at the Catholic University of Louvain. His medical education was interrupted by World War II. However, he finished his M.D. degree in 1941.

While still a medical student de Duvé worked with Professor J.P. Bouckaert in his laboratory on the action of insulin on glucose uptake. After the war this subject led to a Ph.D. in 1945 by which time he had already published a 400-page book on *Glucose, Insuline, et Diabète*. During the war he had been in a prison camp but managed to escape. He later discovered and named lysosomes and peroxisomes. De Duvé won the Nobel Prize in Medicine in 1974.

Roger Guillemin

Roger was born at Dijon, France, and took his bachelor of arts degree in 1941 and bachelor of science in 1942. He began medical studies in 1943 at the Universities of Dijon and Lyon. However, he spent most of World War II in the French Resistance. During research for his M.D. thesis (1949) he encountered Professor Hans Selye, who invited him to the University of Montreal where he continued his work on steroid-induced hypertension. With Professor Hebbel Hoff he translated the account of the transfusion of blood from animal to man by Jean Baptiste Denis, performed June 15, 1667. Guillemin carried on research at Baylor University in Houston, Texas, at the Salk Institute in California, and with Geoffrey Harris in London. He was awarded the Nobel Prize in 1977.

Daniel Nathans

Nathans was born in Wilmington, Delaware. With his family he suffered greatly in the Depression of the 1930s. Despite their poverty, he was finally able to graduate from the University of Delaware in chemistry in 1950. In the ensuing four years he attended the school of medicine at Washington University, St. Louis, Missouri. There after his first year of medicine he worked summers with Dr. Oliver Lowry on microchemical techniques for the estimation of ascorbic acid and its distribution in the adrenal cortex and the effects of ACTH. Following his graduation in 1954 Nathans was associated with Fritz Lipmann.

At the age of 50 Nathans received the Nobel Prize for his work on cutting the DNA helix using restriction enzymes. He later became a senior investigator at the distinguished Howard Hughes Medical Institute.

A.G.F. Davidson and **W.J. Dubé**

These two medical students at the University of British Columbia in Vancouver, after an all-night session in the laboratory of Dr. D. Harold Copp, carried out the isolation perfusion of the thyroid and parathyroid glands, and were able to demonstrate direct humoral control of parathyroid function in the dog. They carried on their experiment through the night and drew the attention of Dr. Copp next day to the unexpected fall of blood calcium. They first reported their work in the U.B.C. medical undergraduate journal in February 1964 and in the *Canadian Medical Association Journal* in 1968. The basic material was recorded by Dr. Davidson in his M.D. thesis.

R. Neil Schimke

Schimke was born in Kansas and graduated at the State University in chemistry. He was awarded a Fulbright scholarship to the University of Bonn in Germany and returned to complete his medical doctorate in Kansas. His undergraduate work concerned the syndrome that now bears his name: pheochromocytoma and medullary thyroid carcinoma.

[1] One of the best researches done on the posterior pituitary and its function was carried out by the late Alexander M. Fraser as a first-year medical student at McGill University, Montreal, in the summer vacation of 1935. It is a matter for profound regret that following a brilliant wartime career of hazardous investigation into high altitude problems he succumbed to cancer in his early thirties.

CHAPTER NINE

Genetics

Archibald Garrod (1857-1936)

Professor Alex G. Bearn of the Rockefeller University wrote of this student's contributions to science in a masterly 1993 biography, *Archibald Garrod and the Individuality of Man*. If Garrod had a flag or banner it would have read, "One Gene, One Enzyme."

Born in London, at his physician father's house at 84 Harley Street, Garrod had his schooling at Marlborough, where he developed a great interest in spectroscopy, which was to remain with him throughout his chemically-oriented life. At the same school he displayed a penchant for natural history and delivered a paper before the student society devoted to that area of science.

Going up to Christ Church College, Oxford, he had some trouble with the "Holy Scripture" entrance examination that was then obligatory. Once over that antedeluvian hurdle he took a first-class degree in natural science, with a special interest in chemistry. In his final year he won the Johnson Memorial Prize for his essay on "The Nebulae — A Fragment of Astronomical History." He struck a blow for the history of scientific ideas:

> In these days of rapid scientific progress there's a tendency to accept the facts of nature, as at present known, without glancing back at the slow and difficult stages by which the knowledge of these facts has been arrived at. Yet such a retrospect is by no means unprofitable, since it warns us that hasty generalizations upon insufficient data retard rather than advance the progress of knowledge, and that the theories of the day must not be accepted as necessarily expressing absolute truths.

In 1880 he enrolled as a medical student at St. Bartholomew's hospital (founded 1123) and proceeded to win prizes and the coveted Brackenbury Scholarship, giving him sufficient money to visit Norway. While there he visited the leper colony at Bergen, which became the subject, on his return, of a paper to the Abernethian Society that still exists for students interested in research at "Bart's." (Recently they turned out, with their learned librarian-mentor, John Thornton, to hear about their hospital's array of early student contributors.)

Garrod qualified in 1884, as a Member of the Royal College of Surgeons, and a year later took his medical degree from Oxford. Within the unusually short time of three years he was elected to the Fellowship of the Royal College of Physicians. His Oxford M.D. thesis was on the subject of rheumatoid arthritis, as was Charcot's.

After a postgraduate year in Vienna Garrod took up his student interest in spectroscopy again, applying it to "bizarre inherited metabolic disorders," as Bearn describes them. The rest of his life centred around these little understood diseases. His legacy to medicine was composed of two scholarly volumes, *Inborn Errors of Metabolism* (1908) and *The Inborn Factors in Disease*" (1931). Both have become classics.

Garrod succeeded Osler as Regius Professor of Medicine at Oxford in 1920, and retired in 1927. In retirement he kept up his pediatric research and lived long enough to read of Fölling's discovery in Norway of phenylketonuria.

One of Garrod's finest pieces of writing is to be found in his Harveian Oration before the Royal College of Physicians of London on St. Luke's Day, 1924: "The Debt of Science to Medicine."

W.S. Sutton (1877-1916)

Sutton began his work on genetics as a student with the distinguished Clarence Erwin McClung at Philadelphia. McClung was suggesting a relationship of the X chromosome to sex determination in 1901. Sutton became a graduate student of E.B. Wilson at Columbia University in New York and wrote two important papers there in 1902 and 1903. Then for whatever reason Sutton gave up work for his graduate degree and enrolled in medicine and eventually received an M.D. degree, becoming a surgeon.

The next medical student to work in the field of genetics was F. Litz. He worked in the laboratory of Professor A.P. Dustin, Sr., at Brussels and suggested in 1934 the use of colchicine for altering mitosis and in 1937 demonstrated its effect as an agent for inducing polyploidy. Litz, who had been interested in the relationship between colchicine and leukocytosis, went on to write his own "*Contribution à l'étude des réactions cellulaires provoquées par la colchicine.*" This student work first appeared in the *Comptes Rendus de la Soc. de Biol.*, 115: 1421-23, 1933. As Clyde Chandler of the Boyce Thompson Institute for Plant Research has noted, "After the colchicine bandwagon arrived in 1938, numerous publications appeared in various periodicals around the world." In fact a study, "Colchicine—in Agriculture, Medicine, Biology and Chemistry," by Pierre Dustin, Jr., and O.J. Eigsti in 1955 cited 1600 such references.

Robert Gwyn Macfarlane (1907-87)

Early in his medical undergraduate years Macfarlane wrote two arresting papers. He had encountered in the clinic at St. Bartholomew's Hospital a boy who had non-stop bleeding from his chin. So impressed was Macfarlane with this phenomenon that he described it in a paper in the hospital journal soon thereafter. It was entitled "Haemophilia—A Short Survey." As a senior medical student Macfarlane was introduced to laboratory research by Professor C.H. Kettle. He then joined in experimental work with Dr. Burgess Bennett and they produced a paper, "On the Relative Potency of Certain Snake Venoms to Coagulate Haemophilic Blood." This appeared in the proceedings of the Zoological

Society of London in 1934. (Macfarlane was described in the chapter on cardio-vascular contributors.)

As a result of his undergraduate work in medical school Macfarlane devoted his life to research in the field of haematology. He became a well-known writer and produced the excellent volume, *Howard Florey—The Making of a Great Scientist*. In 1984 he wrote *Alexander Fleming—The Man and the Myth*. In turn, the scholarly Alastair Robb-Smith wrote *Life and Achievements of Professor Robert Gwyn Macfarlane*, FRCS: *Pioneer in the Care of Haemophilics* in the Royal Society of Medicine series in 1993.

Francois Jacob (1920-)

In 1965 Jacob was awarded the Nobel Prize "for discoveries concerning the genetic regulation of enzyme and virus synthesis."

In 1938 Jacob completed his baccalaureate studies and entered the medical school of the University of Paris. However, with the outbreak of World War II and the fall of France in June 1940, Jacob went to England to join the Free French. From there he was posted as a medical attendant to North Africa and there saw service in many battles. He was wounded in Tunisia, and later in Normandy. His graduation thesis for the medical degree in 1947 concerned tyrothricin, that important creation of René Dubos. Thereafter he made his home at the Institut Pasteur with Monod, Lwoff and others. Jacob received the Legion of Honour, membership in the Academy of Sciences in France and Fellowship of the Royal Society of London.

Joshua Lederberg (1925-)

At the age of 19 Lederberg completed his bachelor of arts degree in honours zoology at Columbia University in New York. He then entered medical school at Columbia's College of Physicians and Surgeons, and did part-time research with Francis Ryan in the department of zoology. This research he kept up until he completed second-year medicine. Then he took a three-month summer course at Yale University with Edward Tatum on biochemical genetics. In 1958 he shared the Nobel Prize in Medicine with Professor Tatum and with George Wells Beadle for joint discoveries regarding the sexual reproduction and genetic recombination of bacteria.

Karl von Frisch (1886-1982) shared the Nobel Prize in 1973 and, like Lederberg, studied medicine for two years. He then went into the field of entomology where he documented the sensory discrimination and communication skills of bees.

Lederberg served as professor at Wisconsin and then at Stanford and then was named president of the prestigious Rockefeller University in New York City where he built a powerhouse of leading medical researchers and graduate fellows. As a medical student he could hardly have imagined such a future, but he achieved it.

Alan E.H. Emery

After graduating in zoology and botany at the University of Manchester with first- class honours Alan Emery embarked upon three years of research and teaching. At the end of that period he entered the medical course, which he also completed with first-class honours. Later he took his Ph.D. in genetics at the Johns Hopkins University in Baltimore.

Since then he has been professor of genetics at the University of Edinburgh. His early work and his interest in genetics helped him to unravel what is now called the Emery-Dreyfuss form of muscular dystrophy with its slow progression and joint contractures, and its X-linked inheritance.

Hans Renpenning (1929-)

This researcher in genetics was born on a farm in southern Saskatchewan in Canada and took his first degrees in science and engineering before he entered the University Medical School at Saskatoon in 1956. Within two years this medical student undertook genetic research during a university vacation and investigated in the farm population the disorder which now bears his name. He was graduated with the M.D. degree in 1960 and proceeded to the University of Illinois where he undertook specialist training in ophthalmology and otolaryngology. Today he practises in Saskatoon and maintains an interest in medical genetics. Renpenning's Syndrome is an undifferentiated X-linked form of mental retardation.

Lawrie William Powell has been associated most of his life with the Royal Brisbane Hospital in Australia. He is well-known for his work in liver disease. He wrote his M.D. thesis in 1966 on "Human and Experimental Iron Storage and the Liver." There he showed for the first time that so-called idiopathic haemochromatosis was a genetic disorder and quite distinct from alcoholic cirrhosis with iron overload. In 1965 he joined Dame Sheila Sherlock at the Royal Free Hospital in London on a research fellowship and showed that Gilbert's disease covered a heterogenous group of disorders with an important genetic background. He is a member of the Royal Australian College of Physicians and the Royal College of Physicians of London.

In 1986 **Jeremy Nathans**, as a medical student at Stanford University, helped to discover the genes for colour vision and colour blindness with professors Hogness, Vollrath and Davis. Thereafter, he was associated with the Howard Hughes Medical Institute, carrying on research at Johns Hopkins.

CHAPTER TEN

Lymphatics

Basic discoveries in the anatomy of the lymph circulation of the body were made by three medical students, Pecquet, Rudbeck and Joyliffe, independently and almost simultaneously. This fact has been regrettably obscured by squabbles over priority between one of the students, Rudbeck the Swede, and Professor Thomas Bartholin of Copenhagen. For the purposes of this book, the priority issue is of little importance. One could scarcely wish for a better demonstration of student originality and independence of thought than that demonstrated by the following young pioneers.

Jean Pecquet (1622-1674)

Jean Pecquet of Dieppe and Paris studied medicine at Montpellier. He came under the influence of Vesling, the anatomist, who, like Aselli of Cremona, had already seen the lacteals, or lymph-bearing vessels, of the intestine. In 1647 or 1648 Pecquet left what he called "that mute and frigid science"—anatomy—and in the Vesalian temper set about the study of living animals. On removing the heart of a dog he noticed some whitish fluid in the pericardium and thought it must be pus. On further investigation, however, he found that it issued from the superior vena cava and that abdominal pressure increased its flow. This observation led to two momentous discoveries. The first was that contrary to the teachings of Aselli the lacteals, in ascending from the intestine, did not enter the liver at all. The second was that the flow was to the receptaculum chyli and through the thoracic duct into the venous system at the junction of the left jugular and the subclavian veins. His systematic method of working out his problem was in the tradition of William Harvey—whose discovery of the circulation of the blood in 1628 had set the stage for just such studies as Pecquet was now making.

Pecquet's findings were independently confirmed by the Dutch anatomist Van Horne in his *Nova ductus chyliferus* (1652). Pecquet's discoveries were published in his *Experimenta nova anatomica* (Paris, 1651). William Harvey, in a letter to Morison in Paris, in 1652, credits Pecquet with the first demonstration of the thoracic duct and receptaculum chyli. Harvey wrote concerning the lymphatics in general, "I am prepared to award the highest praise to Pecquet and others for their singular industry in searching for the truth. It needs good eyes and a mind free from anxieties to come to any definite conclusion about these extremely minute vessels."

Harvey's views on the centrifugal nature of the arterial blood flow found a supporter in Pecquet who wrote, of a later set of experiments: "I tied the crural artery of the dog, avoiding the vein, and amputating the member a little beyond the ligature. Only a few drops of blood escaped from the divided veins, but there was no haemorrhage."

Pecquet's discoveries were the beginning of the end of Galen's view that the blood was formed in the liver. The fact that the lacteals were now shown to circumvent the liver was something which could be reconciled with Harvey's views on the circulation of the blood. Thomas Bartholin finally accepted Pecquet's views concerning the by-passing of the liver, in his *Vasa lymphatica in humane nuper inventa* (1654).

Olof Rudbeck (1630-1702)

While Pecquet was completing his works for the press, the Swedish medical student Olof Rudbeck in Uppsala was watching the butchering of a calf. He saw a "whey-like fluid" exuding from the supra-clavicular notch, and being an inquisitive student, of 20 years of age, he sought its source. He found what is now known as the thoracic duct, and traced it back to a swollen segment full of a milk-like fluid. His formal medical studies prevented him from further investigating this field until a year later when, in a cat, he was able to demonstrate the flow from the lacteals to the "vesicula chyli" as he called the pooling point, and thence through the thoracic duct into the venous system.

By April 1652, Rudbeck had made observations on various phases of this problem in 400 animals, including cats, dogs, sheep, calves, goats and wolves. The movement of fluid away from the liver, rather than to it, was soon established by his use of ligatures. Rudbeck pressed on to investigate the lymph vessels of the rectum, following them to the cysterna chyli; he later traced lymphatics to an oesophageal gland, to the abdominal wall, to glands between the lung and heart, and to the dorsal side of the sternum.

In April 1652, Rudbeck gave a demonstration of the lymphatics of the liver to Queen Christina of Sweden, before the court and a large assembly of Swedish and foreign university professors. So interested did the Queen become in Rudbeck's work that she later sent him abroad to study. At the royal demonstration Rudbeck learned for the first time of Pecquet's work, and in June 1652 one of the court physicians showed him a copy of Pecquet's publication of 1651. Rudbeck then realized how completely he had confirmed Pecquet's work, even to the discarding of the liver as a blood-forming organ.

In May 1652, Rudbeck defended his graduation thesis at Uppsala, "*De circulatione sanguinis*," in which the Harveian interpretation of the blood's circulation was introduced to Sweden.

In the summer of 1653 Rudbeck's extended observations on the lymphatics were published in his home town of Vesteras, near Uppsala, as "*Nova excercitatio anatomica, exhibens ductus hepaticos aquosos et vasa glandularum serosa*."

In rejecting the liver as a blood-forming organ of the body, Rudbeck substituted a cleansing or purifying role for it. He wrote:

> Even as ordinary cooking requires not only fire but also kettles, skillets, etc., through which that which is being cooked is purified and freed from scum, so in nature the heart is not alone to be considered. It requires help of other organs; e.g. the spleen for fermentation, the kidneys for freeing from watery parts, and the liver for freeing from bile and the new fluid (lymph). Only after this is complete is the blood serviceable for the nourishment of the body.

While passing through Hamburg on his way to Holland, on August 16, 1653, Rudbeck first saw Thomas Bartholin's work on the lymphatics, published in May of that year. When he reached Leyden, on his post-graduate journey under Queen Christina's patronage, he arranged to have his book republished by the physician-publisher Hemsterhugs. This publisher was also bringing out a new edition of Thomas Bartholin's Copenhagen paper, "*De Lacteis thoracicis in homine brutisque nuperrime observatis*," and for some reason produced the two works, bound together, under the title, *The Golden Harvest of the Last Three Years*. The volume contained the seeds of a future controversy in the form of a letter by Rudbeck suggesting that Bartholin had pre-dated his work falsely. Such polemical arguments as developed were relished by supporters on both sides, and brought the much neglected lymphatic circulation into immediate prominence.

Larsell feels that Hammarsten's summary of the controversy is apt:

> The chief honour due Rudbeck is that he, a young student, completed a work which by wealth of observation, better prepared drawings, a deeper insight into and nearer approach of results, together with great independence in interpretation, and clearer grasp of the meaning of his observations, is thus entitled to greater scientific credit than the same work which under similar circumstances would be done by the learned professor, one of the foremost anatomists of the time.

In Holland Rudbeck succumbed to the attractions of botany, returning after a year's absence to teach botany and medicine at Uppsala. The wheel had come full circle—for botany, as well as anatomy and physiology, had been taught by Rudbeck's father in Sweden. The father had originally been a bishop and a professor of theology.

In retrospect Olof Rudbeck's childhood is unusual. He was born tenth in a family of 11 children. At the age of 10 he made a clock out of handcarved wooden parts. A year later he made an abortive attempt to enter the University of Uppsala. However, when he did finally enter he became a real observer, and according to Larsell questioned and tested everything—a trait happily found still in some students despite the lock-step educational systems through which many of them pass.

Rudbeck was made Chancellor of the University of Uppsala at the age of 31. Fortunately for science he did not give up his active investigative career, but ventured into astronomy, architecture, the construction of marine compasses and the furtherance of technical education. He built a botanical garden second only to that of Paris, and founded many new laboratories at Uppsala. When hard times came upon the university he was blamed, as presidents are today, for enlarging the university at the expense of the professors' salaries.

His activity was prodigious in the field of botany alone. In 1666 the entire herbarium of Copenhagen, which had been captured by the Swedes, was taken to Uppsala, and there was catalogued by Rudbeck in 12 volumes containing 7000 plates. Linnaeus named the genus "Rudbeckia" in his honour.

Rudbeck was the scourge of the old scholasticism and poked fun at its devotees in the following manner:

> However primitive was the natural philosophy of the time, yet there were few who would depart from it. . . . With a word it resolved many difficulties without blackening the hands with charcoal in chemistry, neither did one get backache from inquiring into the nature of earths, metals and minerals, nor did the stomach become weak from dissecting, nor the eyes from staying awake nights to observe the peculiarities of the stars, etc., but in a warm house by fictitious words and distinctions, men became learned and he was held most learned who could think in the most subtle manner.

George Joyliffe (1621-1658)

The third member of this triumvirate of student discoverers was George Joyliffe, called by Evelyn in his famous diary (January 10, 1657) the "first detector of the lymphatic veins."

Joyliffe was born in 1621 of an old Oxford family then residing in East Stower, Dorset. At the age of 16 George followed his brother Richard to Wadham College, Oxford. During his three years up at Oxford Joyliffe moved across to Pembroke College, doubtless under the influence of Pembroke's master, Thomas Clayton, who was also Regius Professor of medicine. It is recorded in the diary of Thomas à Wood that Joyliffe gave up the Civil War to return to his studies and "entered on the physic line, and exercising himself in anatomy, with the help of Dr. Clayton, Master of his College and the King's Professor of Physic, he made some discovery of that fourth sort of Vessels, plainly differing from veins, arteries and nerves, now called Lympheducts."

Joyliffe, already a B.A. and M.A. of Oxford, in 1650 entered Clare Hall, Cambridge, as a fellow commoner studying for the M.D. degree. This he received in 1652, having studied under Francis Glisson, then Regius Professor of Physic at Cambridge. In his famous book *Anatomia hepatis* (Amsterdam, 1659), Glisson recalls the history of Joyliffe's earlier observations on the lymphatics:

> I first came upon a notice of them at the instance of Dr. Joyliffe, and that in the year 1652, at the beginning of June; at what time this man who was graduating as a doctor had come to me at Cambridge for that end. He asserted that a fourth kind of vessel was provided, clearly distinct from veins, arteries, and nerves; and that these were distributed to all or at any rate most parts of the body and contained aqueous humours within them. He added further that he had investigated the duct of these same vessels in several animals; in the joints, testicles, uterus and even in other parts; and

> that he was certainly convinced that the fluid in them made its way inwards towards the mesentery, and especially to its origin or root. I thought it better then to leave the whole of this matter to the first Discoverer for further elucidation.

Joyliffe went to London in 1653 where, according to Wood, "he made a full and open discovery of the said Vasa lymphatica in Anatomy lectures at the College of Physicians." He practised in Garlick Hythe where he numbered Pepys among his patients. He died in 1658.

Charles Darwin (1758-1778)

The first Charles Darwin, uncle of Charles Robert Darwin (1809-1882) the author of *The Origin of Species*, was also a student investigator in the field of the lymphatic system. In a short life of 19 years and seven months he accomplished a phenomenal amount of well planned investigation before he died of a dissection wound.

Charles was the eldest son of the physician-scholar Erasmus Darwin (1731-1802) of Lichfield, Shropshire. Erasmus' description of his distinguished son follows:

> [He was] accustomed to examine all natural objects with more attention than is usual: first by his senses simply; then by tools, which were his play-things—by this early use of his hands he gained accurate ideas of many of the qualities of bodies; and was thence afterwards enabled to acquire the knowledge of mechanics with ease and with accuracy; and the invention and improvement of machines was one of the first efforts of his ingenuity, and one of the first sources of his amusement.

He had frequent opportunities in his early years of observing the various fossil productions in their native beds; and descended the mines of Derbyshire, and of some other county, with uncommon pleasure and observation. He collected with care the products of these counties; and examined them by such experiments, as he had been taught, or had discovered; hence he obtained not only distinct but indelible ideas of the properties of bodies, at the very time when he learnt the names of them; and thus the complicated science of chemistry became not only easy, but delightful to him.

After matriculation at Christ Church College, Oxford, in 1775 and spending a year there, he "sighed to be removed to the robuster exercises of the Medical School of Edinburgh." In the early part of the year 1776 Darwin vigorously engaged upon his medical studies under such professors as Robert Whytt in physiology, William Cullen, James Gregory, and Alexander Monro secundus, all referred to elsewhere in this book. The professor of the theory of medicine, Andrew Duncan, invited Charles Darwin to live in his home in Edinburgh and opened his wards at the Royal Infirmary to this comparatively young student soon after his arrival in Edinburgh. Charles Darwin's letters of this date foreshadow the discoveries to be made by this eager mind, and they radiate enthusiasm and high intellectual curiosity. Before graduating Darwin won the Gold Medal presented annually by the Aesculapian Society of Edinburgh[1] for a dissertation on the characteristics of pus as distinct from mucus. His graduating essay or thesis was actually concerned with the lymphatics: "An Account of the Retrograde Motion from the Absorbent Vessels of Animal Bodies in Some Diseases." As his biographer, John Fulton, has said, "This was a more remarkable piece of work than the dissertation on pus and mucus, and it reflects the current teachings of Edinburgh concerning the relations of the lymphatics to dropsical conditions, and it also illustrates a very considerable independence of mind and a capacity to obtain evidence from well-conceived experiments." In addition Darwin wrote a 67-page essay on "What are the Established Varieties of the Pulse, their Causes and Uses in Medicine." This was never published but was discovered by Fulton in the records of the Medical Society of London. This is one of his earliest pieces of work and showed that he knew a great deal about the background literature on studies of the heart and circulation. Among other things he describes the normal variation in the pulse that one finds in aging people, at rest, during exercise, eating and sleeping. Thus, in three important fields, those of the body defences against infection, the lymphatic system, and the pulse, Darwin made notable investigations.

It was during such an investigation into hydrocephalus or "water on the brain" that the boy incurred a dissection wound that proved fatal in about two weeks' time. He developed a high fever with many haemorrhages into the tissues. So great was Dr. Andrew Duncan's affection for this student that he had him buried in the family vault in the Chapel of Ease of St. Cuthbert's at Edinburgh.

Darwin's diversified background learning was such that he would undoubtedly have been a great success in any calling. He has been overshadowed, of course, by his namesake Charles Robert Darwin but the combined roles of nature and nurture would seem to have lost none of their potency as one surveys the various members of this family. Darwin's father, Erasmus, was considered by some to be irascible, but at least he was energetic and saw to it that his son received a good general education. Erasmus waxed eloquent on some traditional methods in education when he wrote: "Ye classic schools! ye not only overcome the struggling efforts of genius and bind his Proteus-forms, till he speaks the language you require; but you then divert his attention from the nice comparison of things with each, and from associating the ideas of causes and their effects, and amuse him with the looser analogies, the vain verbal allusions which constitute the ornaments of poetry and of oratory!" The little-known Charles Darwin was indeed an exemplar of brilliant enquiry and insatiable curiosity flowering before the age of 20.

[1] The Gold Medal of the Aesculapian Society was awarded, one year later, to Edward Stevens of the Island of St. Croix, for his essay: "An Experimental Inquiry Cncerning the Red Colour of the Blood." As President of the Royal Medical Society he had read a paper in 1778, "What is the Cause of the Increase of Weight which Metals Acquire during their Calcination?"

CHAPTER ELEVEN

Muscles

Walter Morley Fletcher (1873-1933)

Fletcher was one of the most experienced and highly regarded administrators ever to enter the medical research field. He graduated in medicine from St. Bartholomew's Hospital Medical School, London, in 1900, having already conducted considerable research at Cambridge on sympathetic nerves and especially on muscle. He set out to determine the time relations of the appearance of carbon dioxide and lactic acid as related to muscle contraction and the supply of oxygen.

Some would wonder why Fletcher should press on to a medical qualification when he was already successfully launched on a research trajectory. It is fortunate for the world that he did qualify in medicine. In 1914, the Medical Research Council was first created in Britain. As its permanent Secretary, Fletcher became the guiding force in much of its development right up to the time of his death in 1933. A nonconformist in religion, with a nature sloping towards the sunny side, as Osler used to say, Fletcher took seriously the role of medical research in modern society. As his research associate of college days, T.R. Elliott, put it:

> From Cambridge, where the looms for every pattern of web in biological knowledge were all in such busy activity . . . he looked out over England and saw how little her people were receiving in bodily welfare from all the newly woven science.

From his bedrock apprenticeship in research, Fletcher was able to cut through the mists of a hobby type of medical investigation that hung over the Thames, even after the First World War. It has been said of him, "There were times when his grasp exceeded human reach and his criticisms of medical practice made him appear unduly intolerant of those in Harley Street." However, his advice was wisely sought by the Rockefeller Foundation in its programme for medical education and research in the United Kingdom, and by the trustees of the late Sir William Dunn. Oxford medical students were raised on the story that Sir William, a wealthy stockbroker, had left his fortune "to the glory of God," and that Sir Walter Fletcher had been quick to act as interpreter for the courts, with the result that Cambridge secured the Sir William Dunn School of Biochemistry and Oxford, the Sir William Dunn School of Pathology.

Cyril N. Hugh Long (1901-1970)

Long was born in Wiltshire and studied in the Honours School of Chemistry at Manchester University where A.V. Hill was the professor of physiology in the medical school. He moved with Hill to University College, London, and by 1925 Long had published eight papers with Hill and his group on lactic acid in muscular exercise.

In 1925 Professor Jonathan Meakins invited Long to come to McGill University in Montreal in the department of biochemistry, to work on diabetes, and endocrine metabolism. He completed his M.D. degree at McGill in 1928. By that time he had published yet another nine papers. Long's further research was recognized by his alma mater, the University of Manchester, which, in 1932, awarded him the D.Sc. degree. In 1936 he succeeded Lafayette B. Mendel as professor of biochemistry at Yale, where he served for 33 years.

Frank Horsfall, Jr. (1906-1971)

Born in Seattle, the son of a surgeon, Frank Horsfall Jr. hoped to be an engineer. However, after two years at the University of Washington, where he became an expert rower, he decided on a medical career and proceeded to McGill University in Montreal. Before graduating there in 1932 he began an anatomical research on muscle with the meteoric John Beattie from the Royal College of Surgeons of England, who energized the teaching of anatomy at McGill. It was providential that Beattie did that in spades, for the languid professor, Samuel Whitnall, with his Oxford gown of silk and his monocle, barely deigned to notice his students. To an enthusiastic freshman who called out to him that he had discovered something remarkable in the dissecting room, "Adolf Menjou"—as the professor was described—put his monocle in place and expatiated: "I am the Robert Reford Professor of Anatomy, and not to be hailed as one does a taxi."

Horsfall carried on further research with C.N.H. Long, and published his major undergraduate contribution, on the recovery process after exercise in the mammal. Their paper, which appeared in the *Journal of Biochemistry*, was 18 pages long, contained 25 references, and reported their work on "the conversion of infused d-lactic acid into muscle glycogen." Horsfall was financed through a grant from the Banting Research Foundation, which Sir Frederick had set up for just this purpose—to get young researchers started.

Horsfall graduated with McGill's M.D.C.M. degree in 1932 having achieved the highest marks ever recorded in the five-year course.

The paper concluded that "the recovery process in the intact mammal is a function of the organism as a whole rather than one affected by the muscles only."

In preparing for a career in surgery Horsfall was studying pathology when it became clear that he had a serious sensitivity to formaldehyde, and he gave up his training at the Brigham in Boston. In 1934 he joined the researchers at the Rockefeller Institute in New York and began his researches on the treatment of lobar pneumonia using type-specific serum. He succeeded Tom Rivers at the Hospital of the Institute. After 25 years with the Institute, Horsfall succeeded Cornelius Rhoads as head of the Sloan-Kettering Institute. His services to medical science and its application to the public's health were of a high order. He died of cancer in 1971.

Ann Michelson

Ann Michelson, a Harvard medical student working at Bar Harbour, Maine in 1955, discovered the mutant mouse, which became an important laboratory animal in many subsequent studies in the field of muscular dystrophy.

Arthur J.L. Strauss

Arthur Straus, a medical student at Columbia University's College of Physicians and Surgeons, published the results of his work on myasthenia gravis in 1960. To quote Lewis Rowland, the professor of neurology there, Straus "found the antistriation antibodies in patients with myasthenia gravis. This was the first solid evidence that there were humoral antibodies. His observation that antistriation antibodies were almost invariably present in patients with thymoma has stood the test of time." After graduation Strauss specialized in psychiatry, which he carried on with the Louisiana Department of Mental Health in New Orleans.

CHAPTER TWELVE

Nervous System

The brain has known many kinds of investigators in its long history, isolated as it is in its bony enclosure, and insensitive itself to pain. The Edwin Smith papyrus (circa 1600 B.C.), the oldest scientific document the medical profession has, shows that the Egyptians knew that an injury to one side of the brain affected the opposite side of the body. Gradually the idea evolved that there were localized areas on the surface of the brain controlling specific parts of the body. This chapter will discuss the discoveries by medical students in the field of neurology, from the earliest attempts at cerebral localization to their contributions to the anatomy of the nerves, the pathological changes in the brain, the clinical diseases of humans, the physiology or functioning of the nervous system, and finally the student works of some pioneers in psychiatry.

CEREBRAL LOCALIZATION

Francesco Gennari (1750-1797)

Francesco Gennari was born in 1750 in the village of Mataleto de Langhirano, near Parma, Italy. He studied medicine at Parma with the help of an annual bursary. His biographer, Marimo, states that Gennari was very open-handed with even this small subsidy and shared it with the indigent and his gambling companions.

At the medical school in Parma, Gennari studied under Michele Girardi, a most able teacher of pathology, and a pupil of Morgagni, the father of modern pathology. Girardi is known to medical historians as the editor of Santorini's works and a pioneer in inoculation.

Girardi was himself possessed of an active mind and encouraged students to work independently. He provided a large number of cadavers for Gennari who was interested in the structure of the brain, and must have felt it worthwhile when this undergraduate student discovered the white line in the visual area of the human brain.

To some this may seem an insignificant contribution to medical science, but its importance lies in the fact that it was the first discovery of that structural specialization of the cortex of the brain that today so occupies physiologists in search of functional correlates.

Gennari's book, published in 1782, was dedicated to Count Giuseppe Camuti, rector of the University of Parma, court physician and professor of chemistry. Its title was: *De peculiari Structura cerebri nonnullisque eius morbis*. It contained four copper plates, and was printed in Parma, probably by Bodoni. In it Gennari relates that on cutting the brain of a frozen cadaver, on February 2, 1776, he saw for the first time the line of white matter, or medulla, interposed between two layers of grey matter, or cortex, in the visual or occipital pole of the brain, posteriorly. A translation of his description follows:

> None of the anatomists I have come upon in reading have taught that, besides the cortical substance and the medulla, there exists in the brain another substance which I shall call the third substance of this viscus. If anyone has looked at the horizontal strata of the cortex of a brain dissected at the point where it conjoins with the medulla, he will have found a certain whitish substance ('subalbida'). This does not always present itself in exactly the same spot, appearing a little farther from or a little nearer to the medulla; it is however always observed with the same extension, with the same colour, sometimes more abundant and sometimes more obscure; sometimes subtle, sometimes clearer; at points, difficult, at others it is easy to demonstrate. In a defect of a section especially if it is transected obliquely, this substance disappears; not only in single brains, but also in diverse parts of the same brain I have observed such variations, as if many times it reappeared in such points, *afterwards with a duplicate line* (italics ours). Especially in the anterior parts or solely 'subobscure', it is possible to retrace it, but since it becomes denser to the posterior, I have come to the conclusion that its appearance can be more certainly obtained. In the internal part of the posterior lobe of the brain not far from the point in which it extends itself into the tentorium was where the substance of which I am speaking stretched in a line even whiter, but I have not observed it in any other place to be so evident.
>
> This line I first saw the 2nd February 1776 and having often followed it, it seemed to run finally to the ultimate substance of the hippocampus. For the rest I am ignorant to what purpose that substance may be formed, like so many others of which the use is still hidden, at any rate some of those who combat by the animal spirits, may perhaps draw such an argument for their existence, which in every time, even the hour in which I write, is much disputed. I exhort the anatomists in every way to enquire into this substance.

Originality can show itself in the discovery of unsuspected relationships and of more accurate causes for conditions for which wrong explanations are current and generally accepted. Your own opportunities will lie in those directions.
Sir Geoffrey Jefferson (1951)

Little is known of the later life of Gennari, save that he published a case report on one of the hospital attendants and a medical work long since lost. It is known, however, from Verga's work on the brains of mental patients, published in Milan in 1896-97, that Gennari was greatly interested in the icicles that he found in the hollows or ventricles of the brain in frozen cadavers. He surmised, correctly, that since the frozen fluid was also interposed between the brain and its coverings, it served to cushion the brain against blows or sudden movements of the unyielding skull.

The exact date of Gennari's death is not known, but it occurred some time before 1797, the year in which his teacher Girardi died. To

Girardi, more than to anyone else, Gennari owed his fame, and he gracefully refers to his teacher in the preface to his book: "No one was superior to him and few have been his equal."

Fifty years after Gennari's discovery, a medical student in France, L.F. Bravais, was writing his thesis, *Recherches sur les symptômes et le traitment de l'épilepsie hémiplégique* in Paris. In this, for the first time, there was described a case with convulsions localized to a part only of the body. The French still refer to such a fit as a "*crise Bravais-Jacksonienne.*"

Marc Dax

Nine years later, in 1836, another French student, Marc Dax, wrote a thesis on his research on the brains of patients dying after the loss of speech (aphasia). He found that in right-handed aphasic patients the left hemisphere was selectively involved. Though he searched for a right-handed patient with a right cerebral lesion he never found one. This student investigator wrote with a firm grip on the truth concerning aphasia. His thesis was never published, though copies of it existed in the faculty of medicine in Montpellier where he graduated, and where he had actually communicated the substance of his research to a medical congress in July 1836. As Sir Geoffrey Jefferson said, neurologists must give "full credit to the prior observations of Marc Dax, who, before anyone else, observed that it was the left hemisphere that was usually found damaged in aphasics, a fact that did not dawn on Broca until he had seen Dax's posthumous but unpublished thesis."

Sir Henry Head (1861-1940)

So far-reaching were his studies, that Sir Henry Head must be mentioned wherever aphasia and brain damage are discussed. He came to this work well prepared, with a scholarly Quaker background, an honours B.A. degree in natural science from Cambridge, and two years of study in Prague and Halle before doing the clinical or hospital years of the medical course. In Prague he reputedly introduced soccer, while in Hering's laboratory in Halle he published two papers-one on the action potential of nerve and the second, in 1889, on the role of the vagus nerve in respiration. This was such a competent study that Head became widely known as an investigator. Upon qualifying with the M.B. degree in medicine at University College, London, Head wrote his M.D. thesis, "On Disturbance of Sensation, with Special Reference to the Pain of Visceral Disease," and this was of such high calibre that Hitzig insisted on its translation into German.

Head experimented on himself, cutting branches of the radial nerve in the arm to study changes in feeling in the skin affected. His work on changes in sensation from brain injuries preceded World War I, and was greatly added to during that conflict. The speech difficulties associated with penetrating wounds of the head were studied in minutest detail and much of the descriptive terminology in this field today stems from Henry Head. As well as his medical works his verse was widely read. He died in 1940 after suffering, without complaint, from paralysis agitans for 20 years.

One of the keenest minds in the field of cerebral localization was the great French neurologist, **Jean Martin Charcot** (1825-1893). As a student, he contributed to the knowledge of arthritis and joint diseases.

At the height of his powers Charcot was such a physician, teacher and artist that some would see him as the dividing line between the old neurology and the modern. This son of a carriage-builder shot like a comet across the sky, scattering light in such diverse fields as poliomyelitis, hysteria, epilepsy, cerebral function, multiple sclerosis, locomotor ataxia and the insensitive swollen joints, now called "Charcot joints." Charcot's graduation thesis in medicine in 1848 was entitled, "The Affection Described Under the Names of Primary Asthenic Gout, Nodosities of the Joints, and the Primary Form of Chronic Articular Rheumatism." It was in this student work that he sorted out for the first time the wastebasket classification of joint disease. It reflects his systematic approach to the mélange of arthritic problems that he saw lumped together in the wards of the Salpêtrière. This sense of discernment is to be seen over and over again in the work of French physicians, whose clinical observations set off a chain-reaction in basic research—Charcot, Claude Bernard, and Broca being pre-eminent in this regard.

When it became possible to speak of specific areas of the brain being connected with definite functions of the human body, neurologists began to wonder if special microscopic structures were involved. For instance, were motor areas on the surface of the brain similar in composition to sensory areas?

Constantin von Economo (1876-1931)

One of the first to provide answers to this problem was Constantin von Economo, a restless son of aristocratic Greek parents. He first studied engineering, to please his father, and was, after two years, allowed to proceed to medicine upon which his mind had been set since the age of 14 when he had read Lombroso's book *Genius and Insanity*. Baron von Economo graduated in medicine in Vienna after writing an undergraduate paper on the pituitary gland in birds. His early endocrinological interests gave way to those for which he is famous today—the parcelation of the surface of the human brain according to its microscopic structure. He pursued this interest from 1912 until his death in 1931, with frequent interruptions, usually concerned with aeronautics. In 1908 he gave up hot-air balloons and learned to fly airplanes. He fought as a pilot in the First World War and became prominent in an early movement to get airports built in major cities. His life was certainly varied.

Important as it was to appreciate the relation between structure and function in the cerebral cortex, it was still more important to develop the technical methods for showing up the precise microscopic anatomy of the various brain areas. **Rudolph Berlin**, as a 25-year-old medical student at Erlangen, in 1858, reported on his researches in this field in his 27-page graduation dissertation. He illustrated his work with two plates, and his designation of the cells which he stained, as pyramidal, spindle and granular, is still used daily.

Related to the subject of localization of function in the brain, is the pioneering work done by Niclas and Spurzheim as student assistants to the father of phrenology, **Franz Joseph Gall** (1757-1828). Though Gall operated on fantastic assumptions at times, his labours in Paris undoubtedly advanced the problems to the stage where Bravais, Charcot, Dax and Broca could help to solve them.

NEUROANATOMISTS

Johann Friedrich Meckel (1724-1774)

The work of gross anatomists has been covered generally in Chapter II. However, there remain for brief consideration here some student contributors whose work lay largely in the nervous system, such as the Meckels. Johann Friedrich Meckel established a line of Prussian anatomists—father, son and two grandsons. He was born at Wetzlar and graduated in medicine in 1748 with a dissertation on the anatomy and physiology of the "Fifth Pair of Nerves from the Brain." In this he described for the first time the spheno-palatine ganglion, since called Meckel's ganglion, lodged, as the name implies, in the bony cavities above the palate and below the base of the skull.

In the same year Meckel described the submaxillary ganglion, which lies at the angle of the human jawbone and is protected by it. These studies were soon extended to the innervation of the face. Three years after graduation he was made a professor in Berlin where he taught botany, anatomy and obstetrics. In fact he was the first physician to give instruction in midwifery at La Charité Hospital there.

When J.F. Meckel's son, **Phillip Friedrich Theodor Meckel** (1756-1803) graduated in medicine in Strasbourg in 1777 he wrote an important dissertation on the labyrinth of the internal ear. He became professor of anatomy at Halle two years later, and was eventually obstetrician to the Russian court. His two sons were also distinguished anatomists, particularly Johann Friedrich (1781-1833) who has been called "the German Cuvier," so eminent was he in the fields of comparative anatomy and pathology. From 1821 to 1830 he wrote his system of comparative anatomy, which demonstrated the recapitulation of earlier attributes at some stage of the development of higher animals.

Alexander Monro, Secundus (1733-1817)

One of Meckel's most distinguished pupils was Alexander Monro, Secundus, son of the professor of anatomy at Edinburgh, and father of Alexander Monro, Tertius, who completed the 128-year dynasty in which the three Monros occupied the chair of anatomy at Edinburgh. Monro, Secundus, studied in London under William Hunter, the distinguished older brother of John and the brilliant teacher of the Great Windmill Street School of anatomy in London. Of this period Monro has written:

> So far back as 1753, soon after I began the study of Anatomy, I discovered that the Lateral Ventricles of the Human Brain communicated with each other, and, at the same place with the Middle or Third Ventricle of the Brain: And, as a passage from the Third Ventricle to the Fourth is universally known, it followed, that.what are called the Four Ventricles of the Brain, are in reality different parts of one cavity.

The Foramen of Monro, thus described, has since become familiar to all medical students. Monro himself lectured to 40,000 of them in his 50 years as professor at Edinburgh—a post that he assumed at the age of 25. He was a brilliant teacher of anatomy and the leading physician of his time in Edinburgh. He was a fearless controversialist and as a young man crossed swords with William Hunter over priority in discovery of the function of the lymphatics. Monro had done considerable undergraduate work on these vessels and actually wrote his thesis on them, *De Venis Lymphaticus Valvulosis*, in Berlin, at the age of 24. A letter written by Joseph Black, the chemist, mentions that Monro had been working on the vessels at the age of 22, and had, by a very ingenious method, shown that the lymphatics "are a distinct system of vessels, having no immediate connection with the arteries and veins, but arising, in small branches from all the cavities and cells in the body, into which fluids are thrown; and that their use is to absorb the whole, or the thinner parts of these fluids, and restore them to the mass of circulating humours." By injecting fluids into arteries against the direction of the stream of blood he was able to show, in the lungs, that the foreign matter thus injected was taken up by the thin lymphatic vessels and transported away by them.

Monro's other original contributions were concerned with the little cushions or bursae underlying some muscles, the seat of the common disease bursitis, and with the comparative anatomy and physiology of fish.

Domenico Cotugno (1736-1822)

Any biographical note on this student might be entitled "The Father of Sciatica" or "From Radishes to Rectorship." Thanks to the diligent researches of Dr. Henry Viets, the Boston historian and neurologist, Cotugno's fascinating life has been rescued from oblivion, and to him all students of history are indebted.

Cotugno was born on the southern Adriatic coast of Italy and grew up with his brothers in humble circumstances. The feudal lord in this part of Italy, the Duca d'Andria, sponsored his entrance into the University of Naples. There Cotugno encountered a wise professor of philosophy, Antonio Genovesi, who told him: "If you have an original idea write it down and put it among your papers; after some time read it, and perhaps a second idea will come to mind in a similar manner to the first. Add this to the original thought and later re-read them both. A third and fourth idea may be created and perhaps a complete work will be the result of the first idea." The student took this advice so literally that he wrote three medical books by the time he was 32.

Cotugno began his medical training at 17 and within his first year began to study sciatica and its causes. His financial situation was pitiful. He asked for and was given some sort of work in the Ospedali degli Incurabili; he was classed there at age 19 as "resident physician." This more fittingly described his duties than his rewards, and he lived on radishes and bread until he suffered an haemoptysis, possibly tuberculous in origin. The hospital authorities thereupon provided him with a better room and a much better diet.

Before long he was tutoring surgical students in anatomy, a subject he liked so much that he made independent dissections on hundreds of dogs, rabbits, birds, rats and humans. He became interested in the secrets locked securely in the petrous portion of the temporal bone of the skull. Subsequent generations have probably wished that Cotugno had never uncovered the series of traps that this intricate area holds for the student being examined in anatomy. However, Cotugno was not being examined, he was examining, and he found a veritable gold mine. He found that there were two nerves to the ear, one for hearing and one for balance. He found the semi-circular canals, connected with the latter, to contain a clear liquid, the better to remind humans of their position in space. He thought that the spiral cochlea, or shell-like organ of hearing, had represented on its two-and-one-half turns the necessary structures for recording and distinguishing pitch. This was a century before Helmholtz proved it so in detail. This investigation that he began as a third-year student was published in Naples in 1761 as *De aquaeductibus auris internae-anatomica dissertatio*.

His research on sciatica and the cerebrospinal fluid was continued for 10 years before he published on it at the age 28. The treatise is a masterpiece of exposition. He begins by differentiating from sciatica all those afflictions that superficially may resemble it, such as arthritis, sacroiliac disease and tuberculous affections of the spine.

In describing the origin of the sciatic nerve from the lower segments of the spinal cord he introduces the subject of the clear liquid that surrounds the cord and is contained by the meninges. He notes that it resembles the fluid found in the pericardial sac about the heart, or that found in the hollows of the brain and the semicircular canals of the ear, and "in other cavities of the body impervious to the air."

Occasionally, he says, the fluid is yellow, but it is invariably red and opaque in the case of a foetus strangled in a difficult labour. He thinks the liquid is manufactured by the choroid plexus in the hollows of the brain and re-absorbed over the surface of the brain, as is thought today. He thought the liquid "to be in a continual state of renovation," which view is borne out by modern studies using radioactive isotopes.

The causes of sciatica were difficult to ascertain but, in cadavers, he forced air and quicksilver along the sciatic nerve elements peripherally in search of blocks, compressions and other affections. He knew that the lifting of heavy weights could lead to sciatica. His general conclusion was that the cerebrospinal fluid itself caused the pain, and in support of this he was able to demonstrate "dropsy of the nerve" in known cases.

Valsalva is said to have mentioned the spinal fluid in 1692, noting that it resembled the fluid within the joints of the limbs. In order to be sure that the fluid did not arise post-mortem, Cotugno experimented on sea tortoises and found it present during life. He showed that there were times when the fluid was coagulated. Cotugno was the first to show that albumen in the urine could be coagulated by heat. His other discoveries include the nasopalatine nerve, according to Castiglioni, and it is recorded that in 1783 "while dissecting a mouse, he observed, imperfectly, animal electricity."

Cotugno became professor of anatomy at Naples, and was known to the pathologist Morgagni of Padua. As the wheel came full circle the erstwhile resident physician, aged 19, became the leading physician of Naples, chief of service at the "Incurabili," dean of medicine of the University, and finally Rector. Before he died he headed the Royal Academy of Sciences. He started the preventive movement in the field of tuberculosis in Naples.

Throughout his long and constructive professional life he maintained a dispensary for poor patients in his home. In gratitude for shelter when he most needed it, and for the opportunity to study, he left his fortune to the Hospital for Incurables. His life was determined in large measure by the hospital to which he turned as a penniless youth, in a manner reminiscent of John Shaw Billings' life. Small hospitals will probably always have souls, and the educational opportunity that they present to the enquiring mind is as limitless as it is unique. If the walls of such hospitals could speak they would tell of a camaraderie, unknown to oft-vacant lecture halls, but regnant in the wards and corridors where human beings are born, cared for and die—where from midnight to midnight, century after century, a living river flows. Perhaps the incurable patients in the wards of his hospital were in Cotugno's mind when he wrote: "Medicine does not have masters; it has but one teacher, Nature."

Rudolf Albert von Kölliker (1817-1905)

Rudolf Albert von Kölliker's lifespan covered almost a century—a century in which the microscope came to displace the scalpel in laboratories dedicated to research. He was one of the truly noble creations of nature—a Swiss mountaineer with the presence and resourcefulness of a guide—approachable, the friend of young men struggling uphill, and a trusted teacher.

As a medical student in Bonn and Berlin, he spent his summers in Heligoland in zoological investigations. They culminated, two years before he graduated in medicine, in a publication on the sexual physiology of the invertebrates. From 1847 to 1902—a period of 55 years—he served as head of the Institute of Comparative Anatomy, Microscopy and Embryology at Wurzburg—retiring at age 85. Gerhardt von Bonin relates that Kölliker in the last eight years of his life published 20 papers.

Kölliker was one of the important forerunners of "the neurone theory" and years before it was popularized wrote: "All nerve cells must have essentially the same function and their functional dignity depends solely upon the different extraneous stimuli which might impinge upon them or upon the many possibilities of answers to a stimulus" (von Bonin). He championed the work of the unknown stranger from Spain—Ramón y Cajal—at a meeting of the German Anatomical Society held under his chairmanship in Berlin in 1889.

He stands as one of the most benevolent and human figures in the history of neurology. His contributions were great, his meticulous textbooks milestones in themselves, and his encouragement of young scientists a monument to his memory.

Benjamin Archer Kent (1808-1864) and **William D. Carpenter** (1813-1885)

The study of ganglia appears to have taken hold with other young researchers. In July 1831, for instance, "An Inaugural Dissertation on the Composition, Functions, and Diseases of the Sympathetic Ganglia" was presented for the M.D. degree at the University of Edinburgh by Benjamin Archer Kent. He had been born in Abingdon outside Oxford in 1808 and at the age of 16 began an apprenticeship that lasted four years in Oxford, followed by his entry into the University of Edinburgh Medical School. There Kent blossomed and became a Fellow of the Plinian Society with interests in natural history and in the Royal Medical Society, that ancient association to which so many important papers have been delivered in its history. Kent's dissertation was well received and was published in Edinburgh in 1831 with excellent illustrations. More than a century after Kent's death in 1864 P.H. Schurr, F.R.C.S., in London published a biography of him entitled *Benjamin's Son*. Kent's thesis is notable for the background of historical information that he furnished. He began with Galen (131-201 A.D.). His bibliography in the thesis incorporated more than 20 references to ancient writers. Vesalius and Thomas Willis and their views are brought into the discussion by Kent. The conclusion to his thesis was sweeping in its outlook: "Let each man for himself, with his own eyes, study the changes caused by diseases; let him trace the various interlacings and harmonies between each part of the body. Then at last he can bring succour to failing health at its very origin, and he might hope to drive the very dangerous enemy from its deepest hiding places."

William D. Carpenter also submitted a thesis for his graduation from the University of Edinburgh in 1839 on the function of the ventral cord ganglia of the arthropoda, all done in 83 pages. One year later, in 1840, Johannes Müller translated it into German.

Charles Hastings (b.1794)

Hastings was born in Worcestershire, England and was apprenticed to two surgeons. They wisely advised him to add to his armamentarium a session in London where he could attend lectures in the existing medical schools. Those that he chose had memorable names, such as Blenheim St. School of Joshua Brookes, Dr. John Taunton's Private School, and lectures on medicine by Dr. Hooper in Savile Row.

Late in 1812 Hastings returned to Worcester and at age 18 competed for the post of house surgeon in the infirmary, a competition he won by a vote of 134 to 133. For an 18-year-old that was a remarkable result, given that his opponent was older and better qualified. However, one factor which seems to have been important in Hastings' case was the fact that he had been working on a research with Dr. A.T. Wilson Philip "On the Functions of Spinal Ganglionic and Cerebral Nerves." This work must have been of some merit, for it was communicated to the Royal Society of London by Dr. Philip and published in the *Philosophical Transactions*.

It is likely that Hastings' personal interest in research was responsible for placing it in the objects of the British Medical Association. This eventually-powerful group he organized, with the help of physicians from other parts of England, on July 19, 1832, at the Worcester Infirmary. One of the researches which the BMA financed early in its career was that by Dr. Richard Caton in Liverpool in the year 1874. Caton was the first to show that electrical activity could be recorded from the surface of the brain in rabbits and monkeys.

Robert Remak (1815-1865)

Polish patriots living within the borders of Germany have never led an easy life. Robert Remak was born in Posen soon after its incorporation into Prussia following Napoleon's defeat. Remak was the son of a local merchant and attended the Gymnasium in Posen. On his graduation there his schoolmaster wrote of him: "Diligence, attendance and conduct must be regarded as exemplary. Progress in all subjects was excellent so that I am able to certify with good conscience I never before had such an excellent pupil in my class." At the age of 18 he earned a place in the medical faculty of the University of Berlin where he soon came under the influence of the outstanding German physiologist of the century, Johannes Müller. With Müller's personal microscope Remak embarked on a study of the finest nerve fibres in the body, a study which he published three years later, and incorporated in his graduation thesis in 1838. Such was the worth of his contribution to knowledge that these nerve fibres are still referred to as "Remak's fibres."

His investigation showed that the principal structure in any nerve fibre was the central core of conducting material known as the axis cylinder, and that this material was continuous with the interior of the single nerve cell from which it originated. He showed, moreover, that there was a preponderance of those non-medullated or non-insulated fibres in what he called the organic nervous system, which today is called the autonomic nervous system because it regulates digestion, blood pressure and many vital functions occurring even during sleep. Remak's vertebrate conclusions were confirmed in the invertebrate nervous system five years later by another medical student, Helmholtz.

Remak's 42-page thesis was entitled "*Observationes anatomicae et microscopicae de systematis nervosi structura*," and began with a quotation from Francis Bacon, "Neither manual work alone nor imagination unchecked by facts is worth very much." His text and drawings attracted the favourable notice of Alexander von Humboldt, the naturalist and explorer.

From his graduation in 1838 to his death 27 years later Remak's contributions to knowledge poured out as if from an inexhaustible fountain. His interests ranged from retinal physiology to the nervous structures of the tongue, the larynx, pharynx, bronchi and lungs, to the liver and its nerve supply, to red blood cells, ossification, involuntary muscle, the secretion of glands and to localization in the brain of visceral functions of the body.

After lecturing in his apartment for 20 years he was invited to lecture in the University of Berlin. His importance in the development of the cell theory is still poorly recognized. Like John Hunter, he worked on inflammation and the blocking of blood vessels, and extended his researches to: the stimulation of blood regeneration by the bleeding of horses, the absorbing structures of the intestine, the inflammation of the lining membrane of the lungs in pneumonia, and the single muscle cell, which he showed to be the unit of all muscles. He first described the disorder known as pulsus paradoxus in 1844. He pioneered in the field of the development of the embryo and wrote of the germinal layers from which the tissues of the body are selectively developed. His student researches, however, proved to be the central core around which his other fundamental contributions to neurology were grouped. His stature in the history of this subject is likely to grow larger as time goes on.

Theodore Billroth (1829-1894)

Theodore Billroth is well-known as one of Germany's greatest 19th-century surgeons. As an undergraduate he and Meissner assisted Professor Wagner in physiological research and accompanied him to Trieste in 1851 where they did a microscopic study of the nerves of the electric ray. It was as a result of this apprenticeship at the microscope, similar to that of the young Joseph Lister, that Billroth turned to experimental pathology and wrote his graduation thesis in 1852 on "The Nature and Cause of a Pulmonary Affection which Arises from Cutting the Vagus Nerve," at the age of 23. His first teaching post was in pathological anatomy and from a sound background in the post-mortem and microscopic observation of diseased tissues he went on to surgery. He was a teacher who trained teachers, among them the brilliant abdominal surgeon, Mikulicz, and the versatile Kocher of Switzerland. During his lifetime his textbooks passed through eight editions and his name is still a household word in surgery. In the field of music he was well-known, as a close friend of Brahms who dedicated various works to him, and as the author of a most interesting study, "Psycho-Physiological Aphorisms on Music."

Ernst Philipp Eduard Bischoff (1807-1882) published his graduation thesis in 1865 on the subject: "Microscopic Analysis of the Anastomoses Between the Cranial Nerves."

Victor Horsley (1857-1916)

On to that enigmatic dynamo, Sir Victor Horsley—an anatomist as an undergraduate. The third child born to John Callcott Horsley, R.A., and his wife was named Victor at the request of Queen Victoria. He was born in Kensington into a family of unusual gifts. His mother was descended from a long line of artists and surgeons, and was herself raised in France. His father came of a family of musicians and artists. He combined a hot temper with generosity and, above all, activity. On occasion he found it necessary to write to *The Times* cautioning against the dangers of modernity.

It is necessary for physicians to study the healed cases of supposedly incurable disease.
Wagner Jaurreg, quoting Bacon

A year after Victor's birth the family moved to Cranbrook in Kent, and the formative 15 years of his life were spent in this country setting. He became an observer of everything in nature, and his childhood letters are remarkable for the detail with which he describes the birds' nests, silkworms, boats and people he encountered. At the age of 15 he decided that he would study medicine, and at once began to dissect birds, and to work with the microscope. Like Osler, he ground his own sections of bone for observation.

In January 1874 he matriculated at the University of London. He attended lectures at University College and was tutored by Philip Magnus. In July 1875 he passed his preliminary science examinations and was awarded the Gold Medal in Anatomy. From this time until July 1878 he concentrated on physiology under Burdon Sanderson and Schäfer. His classmates numbered among them C.E. Beevor, Francis Gotch, F.W. Mott and Dudley Buxton.

Horsley's biographer, Stephen Paget, relates that as an undergraduate Horsley gave two papers that embodied his own researches to the Students' Medical Society of University College. The first, given during the session of 1875-76, was entitled, "On the Endings of the Tendons in the Rat's Tail." The other, presented a year later, was, "On the Terminations of Muscular Fibres; and a Note on the Structure of Intervertebral Discs." This long and painstaking paper, based upon excellent microscopic work, was awarded a prize by the students' society, which also elected him president for the year.

After completing the 1876-77 term with further distinctions and medals, Horsley travelled in Germany for four weeks. His diary for the month covers 120 pages. He carried a letter of introduction from Burdon Sanderson and visited a number of laboratories. His criticisms of some laboratories were cryptic. He saw, however, in Strasbourg, some of the dogs on whose brains Professor Goltz had operated, and this made a lasting impression on him.

At The Club in University College, Horsley gave a well illustrated lecture on "Reformed Dress for Women." He favoured "trousers to the ankle" and a "very full frock-coat buttoned up to the throat." He also took up the anti-alcohol, anti-tobacco crusade, which was later to waste so much of his energy in fruitless political struggles.

As Horsley progressed into the clinical part of his course, his interests turned to pathological anatomy, in which he won the Filliter Exhibition. His regular attendance at operations soon overcame his fainting tendencies. His artistic abilities were often called upon by his Chiefs, and in 1879 he was drawing the relations of the spinal nerves to the vertebral column for a lecture by Gowers. While clerking for Bastian, Horsley drew two plates for his book, *The Brain as an Organ of the Mind*. In the April issue of *Brain* in 1880, Horsley published, with Bastian, an important paper, "Arrest of Development in the Left Upper Limb in Association with an Extremely Small Right Ascending Parietal Convolution." The drawings were done by Horsley.

It was clear in what direction he was heading, as his association with the neurologists Gowers and Bastian developed. Another of his teachers was Rickman Godlee, who was the first surgeon in Britain to remove a brain tumour that had been localized pre-operatively through a study of the attendant clinical signs and symptoms. While a student, Horsley also carried on bacteriological work with F.W. Mott, although their paper was not published until 1882.

In November 1880, Horsley took his M.R.C.S., which allowed him to practice, and in 1881 he completed his University of London M.B., B.S., winning the Gold Medal in Surgery. He lost no time in taking off to Europe for a breathing spell, and visited the laboratory of the noted pathologist Cohnheim in Leipzig. On his return to London, Horsley once more took up bacteriology, and was interested in the demonstration of the tubercle bacillus under the microscope. He worked on the transplanting of tumours from man to cats, and from rats to rabbits. His clinical observation of a sick mouse, which he encountered in a railway cut at Wimbledon, led him to examine its blood, which he found to be alive with trypanosomes.

The incessant activity inherited from his father was manifest at all times, but between drawing illustrations for the ninth edition of Quain's *Anatomy* and reading a paper on December 13, 1883, to the Physiological Society, "On Four Cases of Injury to the Brain; Illustrating the Position of the Motor Centres," Horsley found time to take his F.R.C.S. John Marshall prevailed on him to illustrate the Bradshaw Lecture for him, "On the Operation of Nerve Stretching for the Relief or Cure of Pain."

From 1884 to 1890, Horsley served as Professor Superintendent of the Brown Institution, that singular research centre that can boast among its one-time chiefs, Burdon Sanderson, Greenfield, Roy, Sherrington, Rose Bradford and Brodie. It was established in 1871 by the will of Mr. Thomas Brown of Dublin, "for the founding, establishing and upholding of an Institution for investigating, studying, and without charge beyond immediate expenses, endeavouring to cure maladies, distempers, and injuries, [which] any quadrupeds or birds useful to man may be found subject to." The University of London was "to control the number and cases of diseased or injured animals to be taken charge of, and to decide about the purchase of diseased or injured animals or their carcases for the promotion of science."

Horsley's work at the Brown Institution proceed along three main lines. First was his study of the localization of function in the brains of animals, with related studies on the pathology of epilepsy and of chorea in dogs. Second was his pioneer work on thyroid gland deficiencies as related to myxedema and cretinism. The third segment of his investigations was on means of protection against rabies.

As neurosurgical practice and political campaigning came to absorb more of Horsley's time and energy, so did his scientific publications decrease in frequency. In 1908, he presented to the Royal Society a report on the brain of Mr. Charles Babbage, F.R.S., who invented intricate mechanical calculators a century ago, and who proposed, in vain, a design for a reflecting ophthalmoscope to Wharton Jones in 1845. Also in 1908, Horsley and R.H. Clarke published an account of their now-famous stereotaxic apparatus for the exact placing of electrodes at predetermined points within the brain.

In 1911, Horsley received a prize from the Société de Chirurgie of Paris for having made the greatest contribution to the advancement of surgery in the preceding 10 years. He also received a white kangaroo from a grateful patient in Australia.

Horsley, the father of neurosurgery, had opened the door on the most difficult of all surgical specialties. He had shown that it was possible to learn something about the human brain while attempting surgically to cure some of its grosser maladies. While he did this, and made his own artistic drawings, and laboured too in opening the field of endocrinology, a younger man across the Atlantic—Harvey Cushing—persevered, refined neurosurgical techniques, transfused his cases with blood, skilfully sketched his operative fields and, not least of all, broke down the barriers of ignorance that surrounded the functions of the pituitary gland. Both men soon became enmeshed in the World War I, Cushing first having to fight a political battle on Boston Common, and Horsley first having to condemn the rotten heart of Europe. On August 25, 1914, Horsley wrote to a colleague: "The situation is exactly what you would expect from the aristocrats who rule Europe. Austria trying to smash Servia; Germany coolly smashing Belgium. Burglary and murder arranged in the name of God by rulers and nobles. And all the while the people who are starved, tortured and killed have not had a single voice in the matter."

Horsley was among the first to volunteer for service and was eventually dispatched to Egypt. He then served in Gallipoli, India and finally in Mesopotamia. His letters were full of delightful sketches of people and scenes encountered. His student interest in archaeology was revived. But he was restless and heedless of danger. He succumbed to heat stroke on July 16, 1916, after walking miles at midday to attend an ailing colleague.

Horsley willed his skull and brain to the Neurological Society of London, and the rest of his body to University College, London, for the preparation of anatomical specimens for the museum. This was typical of his complex, inflexible and generous nature.

In a busy lifetime with many peripheral interests Horsley managed to contribute 125 papers to the medical literature. He worked all his life for medicine as a student, researcher, teacher, surgeon and finally, a soldier. At age 58 he said goodbye to his wife in Egypt: "Don't worry about me; I don't matter; I can't live forever; it's the young that matter."

Camillo Golgi (1844-1926)

Golgi was to become one of the basic contributors to the study of the structure of the nervous system through use of silver staining of the constituents in their finer detail. He was born in the Lombardy town of Corteno, which is today called Corteno Golgi. He was the son of a physician trained at Pavia and in 1865 Camillo received his degree from the same institution.

It has been said many a time that the problem of Spain is a problem of culture. It is necessary in fact, if we would enroll ourselves with the civilized peoples, that we must cultivate intensively the desert of our land and brain, thus rescuing by prosperity and mental vigour all those national riches that have been lost in the sea, and all those talents which have been lost in ignorance.

Ramón y Cajal

Golgi's thesis for graduation in 1865 was a critical review on the need for a classification of mental diseases according to microscopic structural changes in the brain, and causal factors. Golgi was a pioneer in intravital staining of nervous tissue, and an early researcher on malaria, which was endemic in his native area. The plan of much-needed research set out by Golgi in his thesis was to occupy him for the rest of his life. His great technical contribution, the sliver chromate staining method, was produced in his kitchen where he was isolated from his scientific contemporaries as he struggled to make a living as physician to the hospital at Abbiategrasso. With osmic acid and with silver chromate he probed the secrets of the terra incognita of the nervous system. He was a determined man with a tough mind that carried him through to the Nobel Prize in 1906, which he shared with his rival Santiago Ramón y Cajal. This meant that Golgi's techniques for the microscopic study of the nervous system were, in the hands of others rather than his own, the key which opened many neurological secrets. Unfortunately, Golgi mistakenly held all his life that the nervous system was made up of endless interconnecting networks rather than discrete pathways. As well, his bitter denunciation of Ramón y Cajal and other supporters of the theory of the nervous system made up of discrete nerve cells upset the Nobel ceremonies at Stockholm. From his student thesis at Pavia to his death in the same city in 1926, however, Golgi remained an unremitting researcher, always with the big picture in mind of delineating the structures and underlying conditions in the brain that produced mental illness.

The contributions of Ramón y Cajal were described in the chapter on anatomy earlier in this work. In conclusion, Cajal left an extensive school extending throughout Europe, Britain, Latin America and Canada. Within Spain Cajal's best-known pupils were Nicolas Achúcarro, Pío del Rio-Hortega and Fernando de Castro.

One student, R.B. Hirsch, in his graduation thesis in Vienna in 1765, memorialized his teacher Johann Ludwig Gasser in naming the great sensory ganglion that supplies the face, the Gasserian ganglion. One is re-

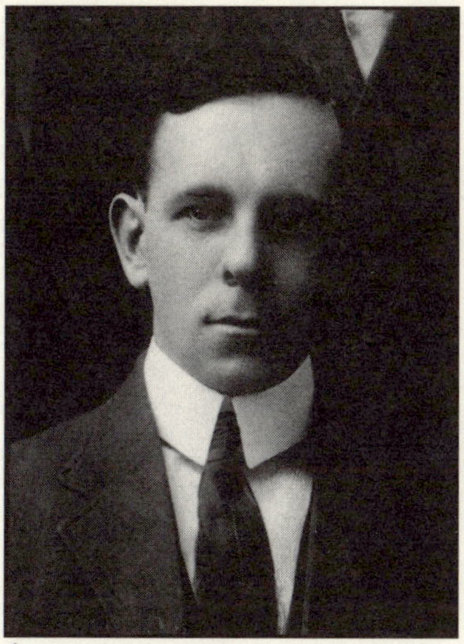

1

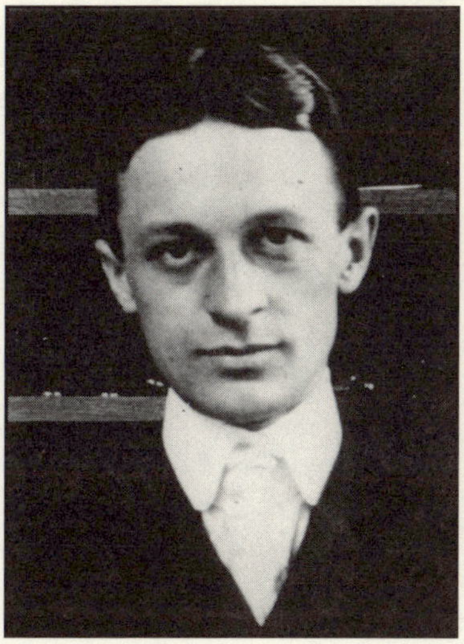

2

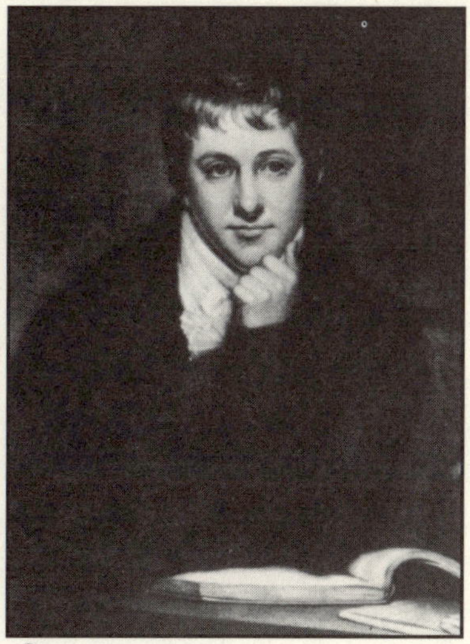

3

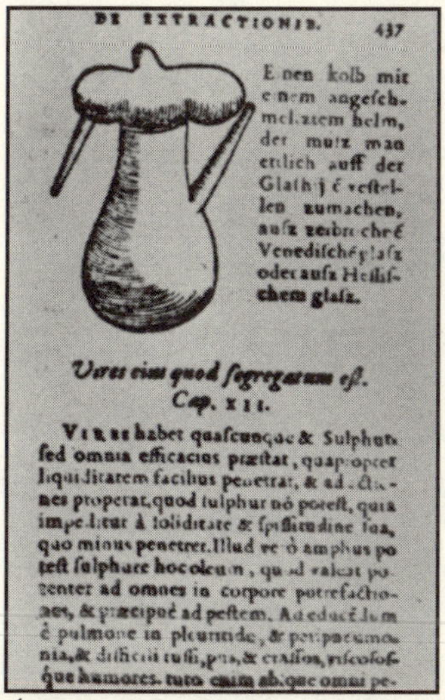

DE EXTRACTIONIB. 437

Einen kolb mit einem angeschmelztem helm, der mutz man etlich auff der Glath j ċ vestellen zumachen, ausz zerbrochnē Venedischē glasz oder ausz Heilischem glasz.

Vires eius quod segregatum est. Cap. XII.

VIR habet quascunque & Sulphuris sed omnia efficacius præstat, quapropter liquiditatem facilius penetrat, & ad actiones properat, quod sulphur nō potest, quia impeditur à soliditate & spissitudine sua, quo minus penetret. Illud verò amplius potest sulphure hoc oleum, quod valeat potenter ad omnes in corpore putrefactiones, & præcipuè ad pestem. Ad educēdum è pulmone in pleuritide, & peripneumonia, & difficili tussi, pus, & crassos, viscososque humores. tuto enim absque omni pe-

4

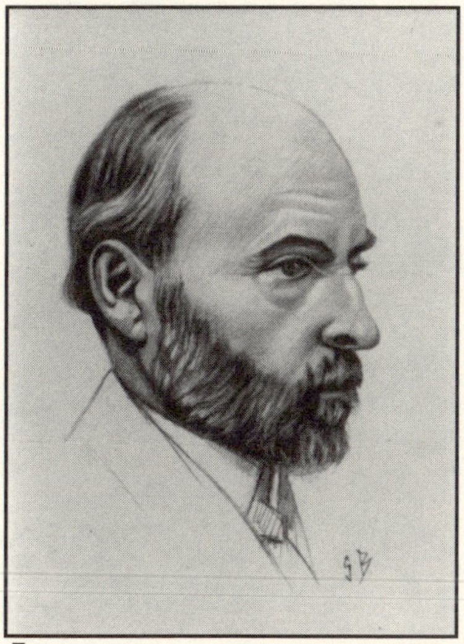

5

1. H. Thoms (Ch. 1)
2. Harvey Cushing (Ch. 1)
3. Humphrey Davy (Ch. 1)
4. Valerius Cordus (Ch. 1)
5. Ramon Y. Cajal (Ch. 2)
6. Lister's drawing (Ch. 2)
7. Vesalius in Medical Historical Library, Yale (Ch. 2)

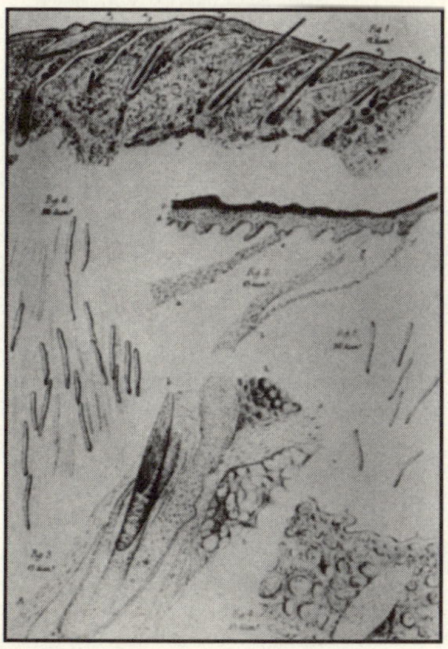

6

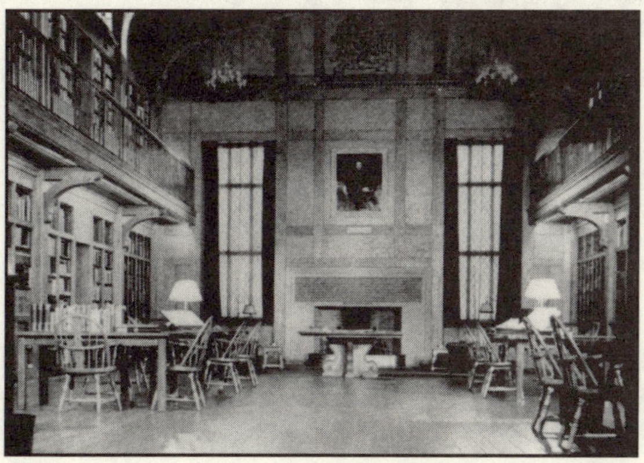

7

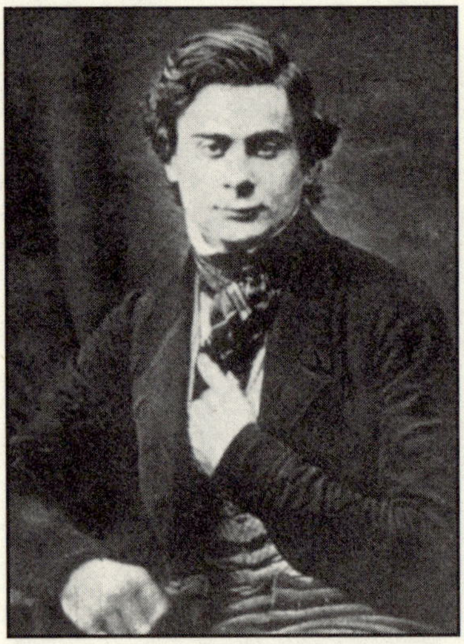

1

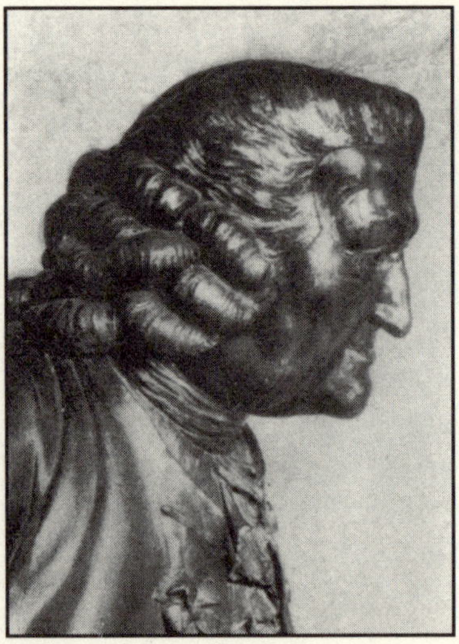

2

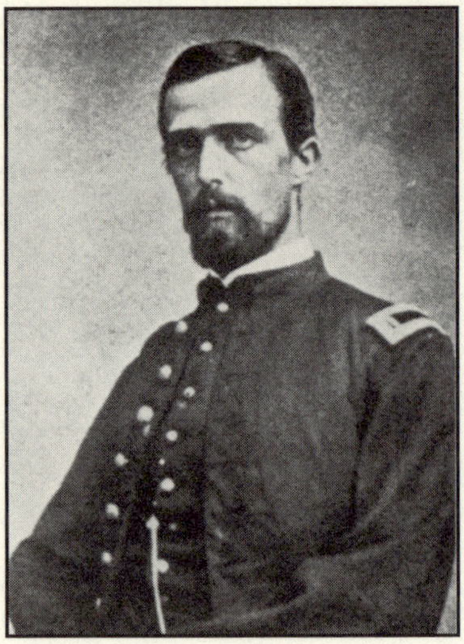

3

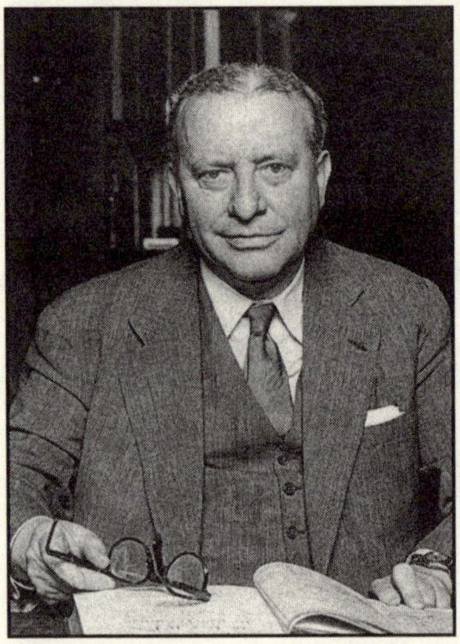

4

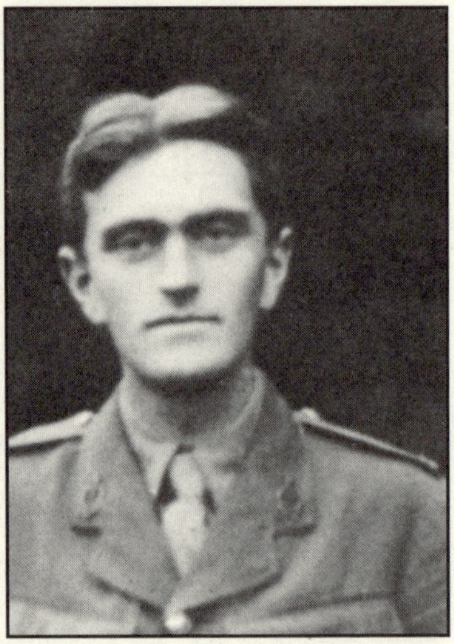

5

1. T.H. Huxley (Ch. 2)
2. A. Von Haller (Ch. 3)
3. Billings (Ch. 3)
4. John F. Fulton (Ch. 3)
5. Geoffrey Keynes (Ch. 3)
6. Robert Thornton (Ch. 4)
7. Linnaeus (Ch. 4)

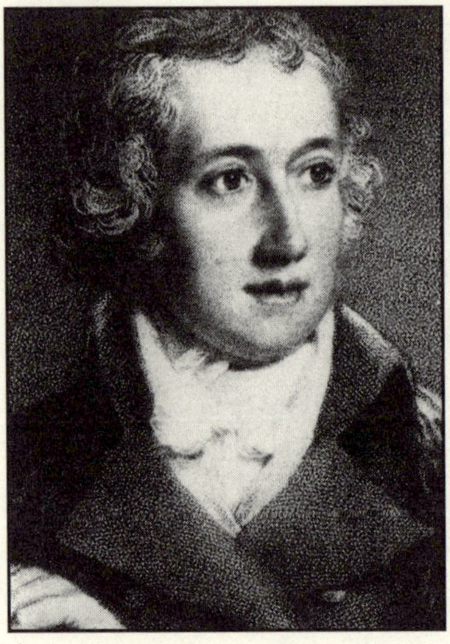

6

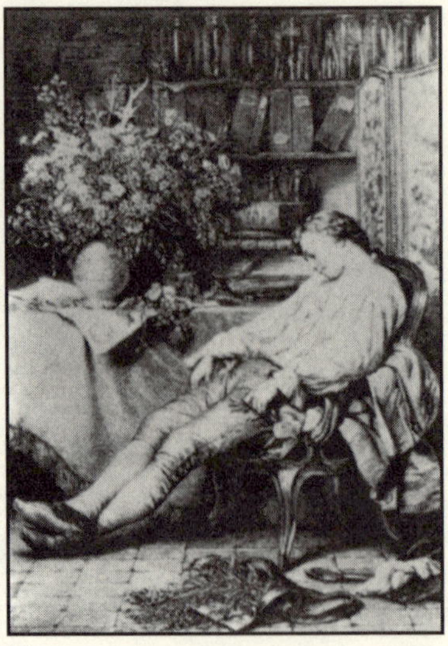

7

8

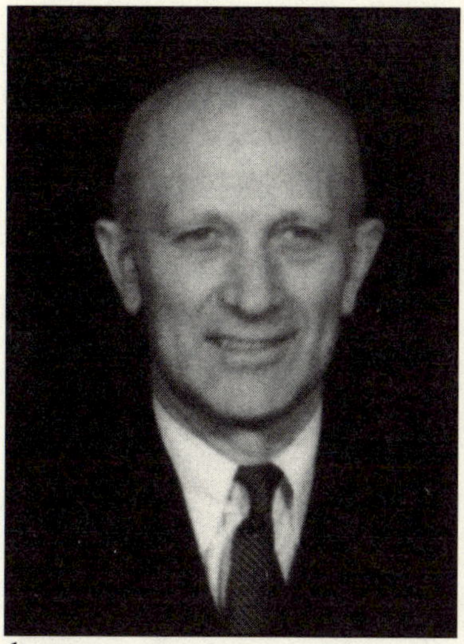

1

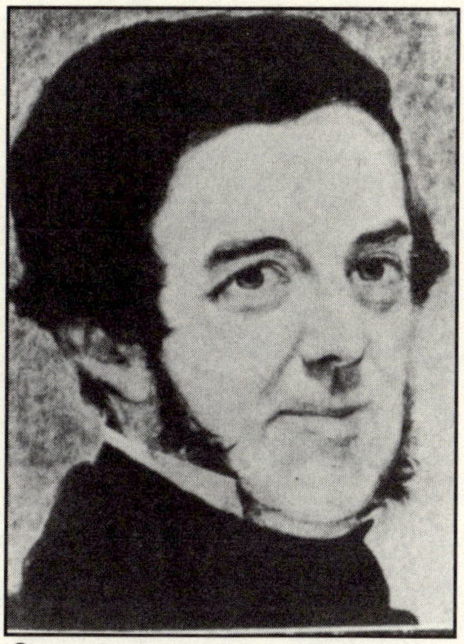

2

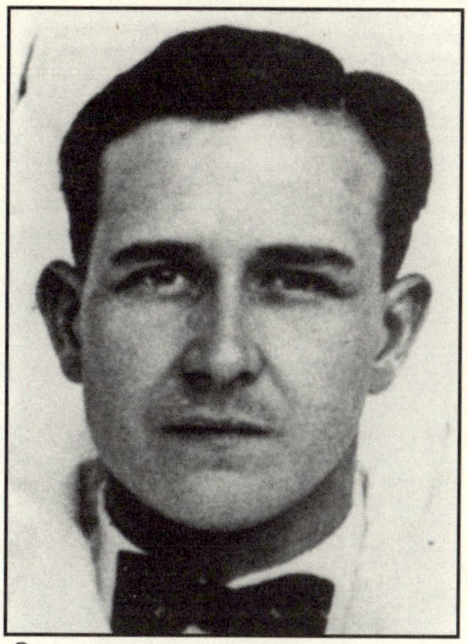

3

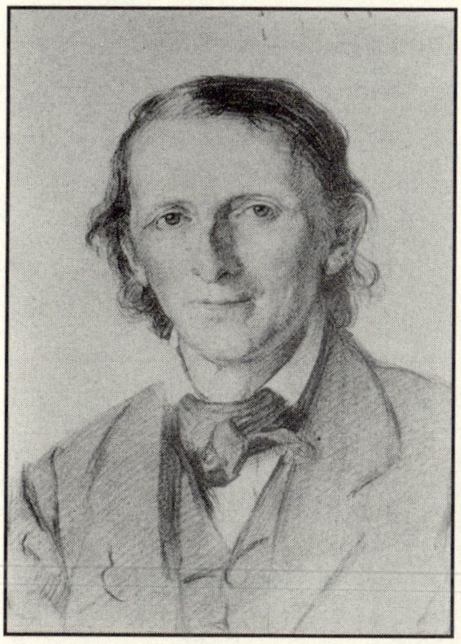

4

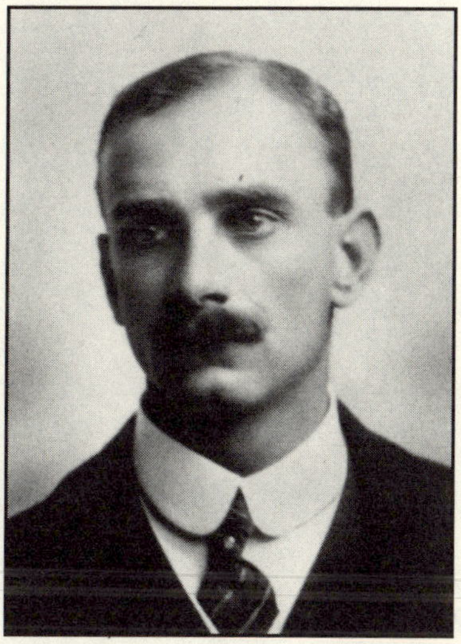

5

1. W. Penfield (Ch.5)
2. O.W. Holmes (Ch.5)
3. Jay McLean (Ch.5)
4. Carl Ludwig (Ch.5)
5. Thomas Lewis (Ch.5)
6. Raynaud (Ch.5)
7. A.V. Waller (Ch.5)
8. Sir Astley Cooper (Ch.5)

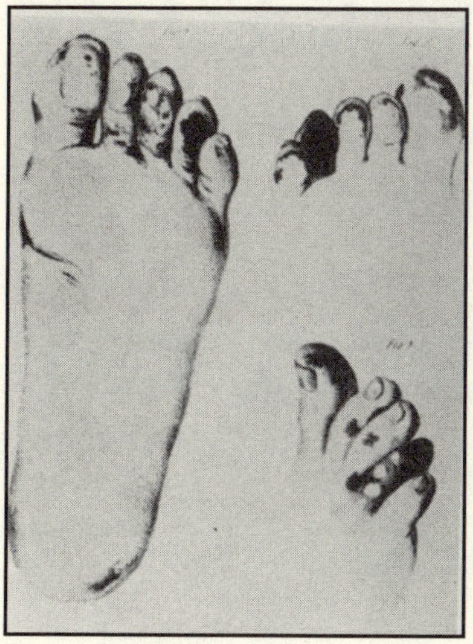

6

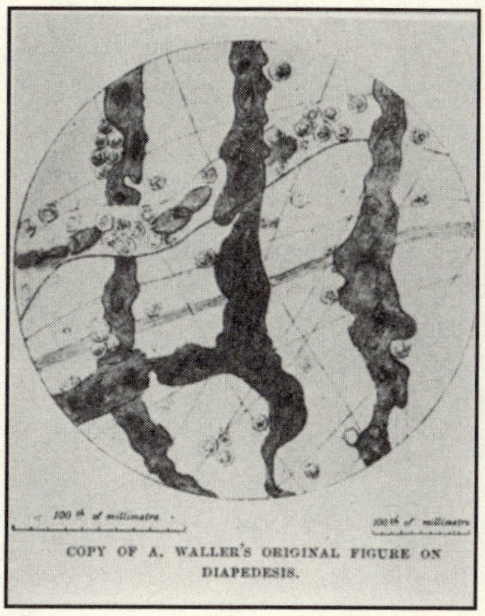

7

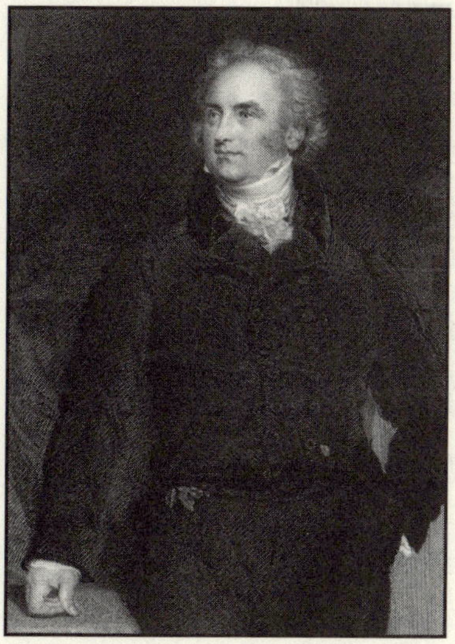

8

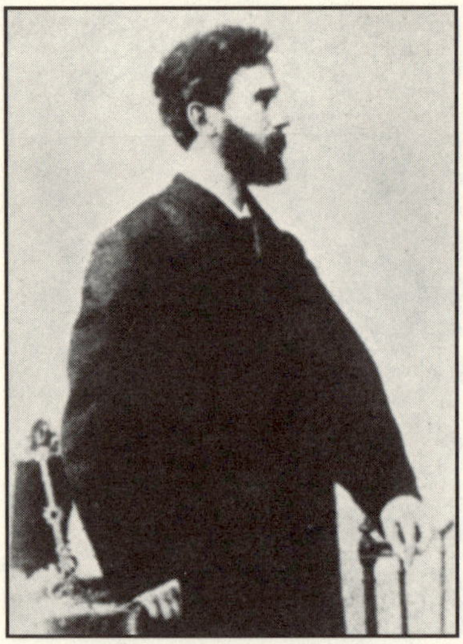

1

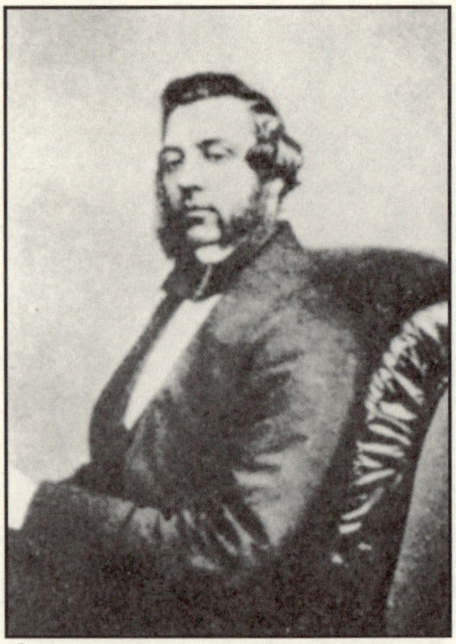

2

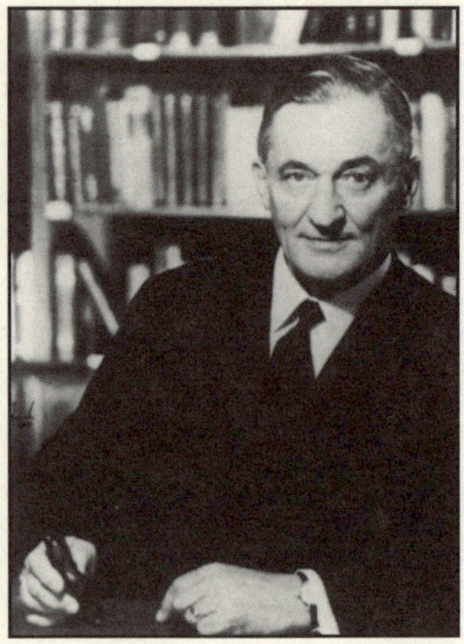

3

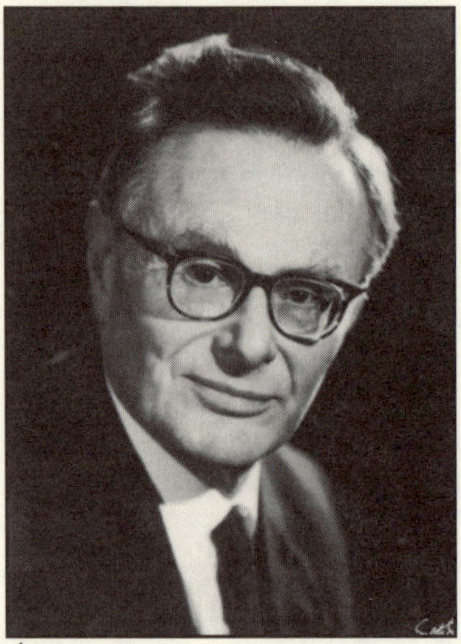

4

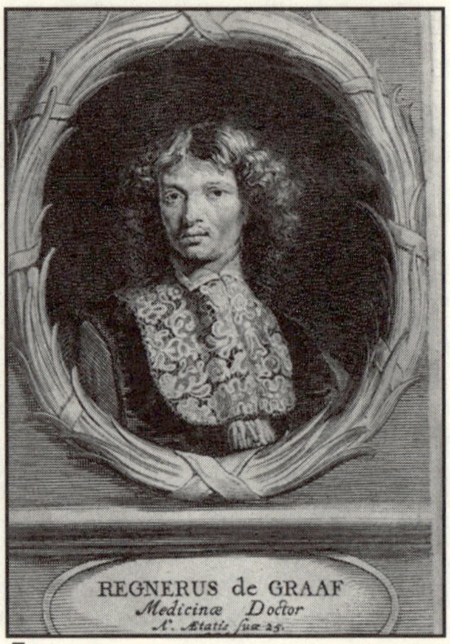

5

1. Ehrlich (Ch.6)
2. Thudichum (Ch.6)
3. Theorell (Ch.6)
4. Hans Krebs (Ch.6)
5. de Graaf (Ch.7)
6. Pavlov (Ch.7)
7. Stensen (Ch.7)
8. Benjamin Rush (Ch.7)

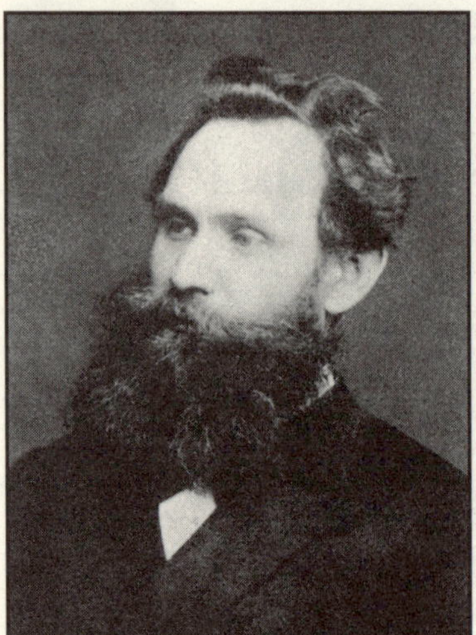

6

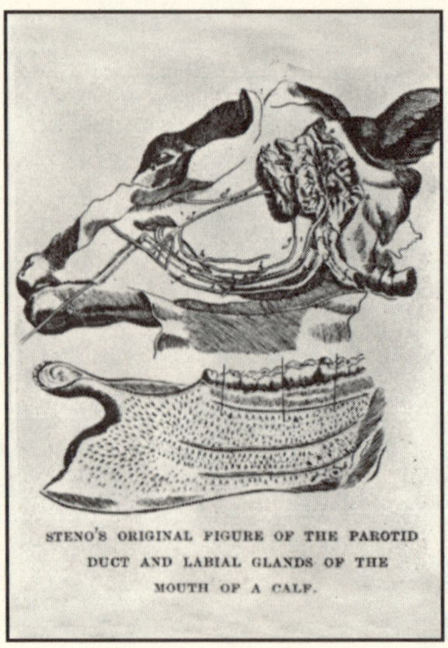

STENO'S ORIGINAL FIGURE OF THE PAROTID DUCT AND LABIAL GLANDS OF THE MOUTH OF A CALF.

7

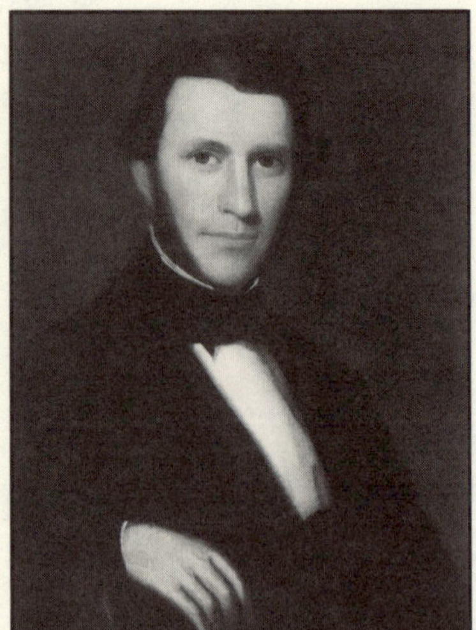

8

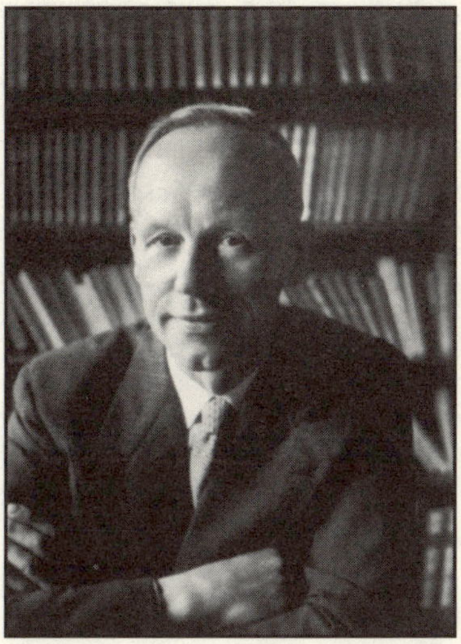

1

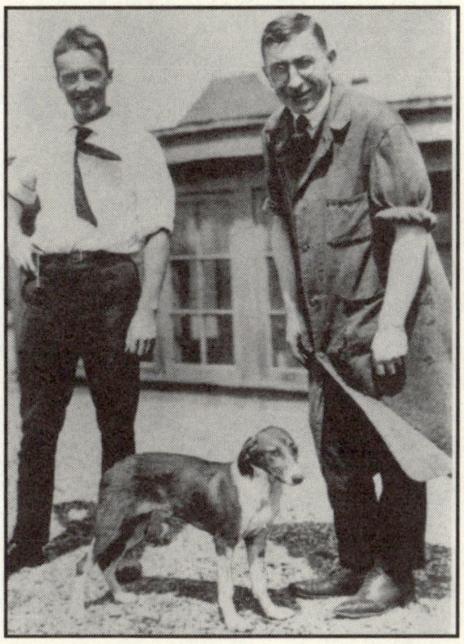

2

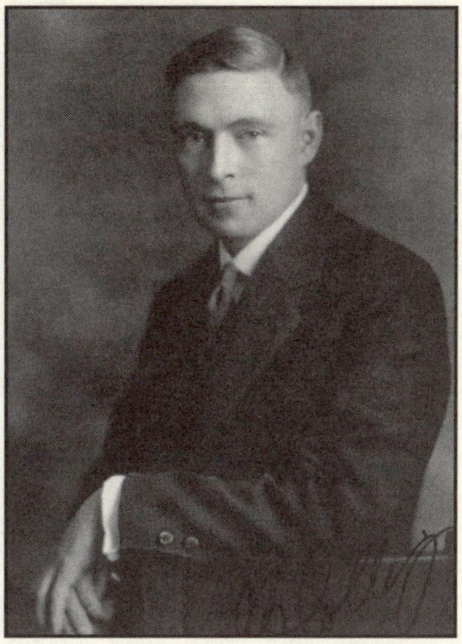

3

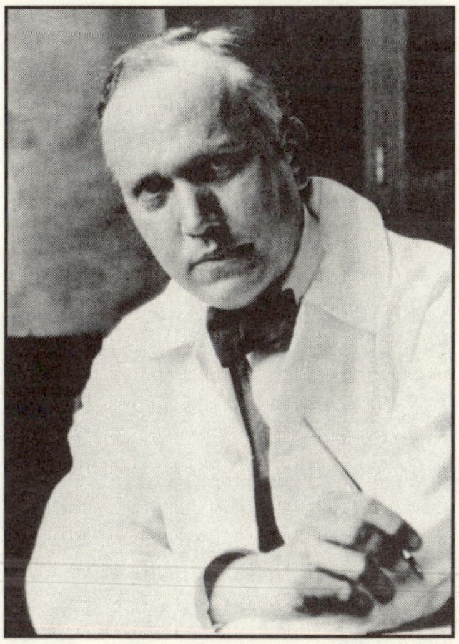

4

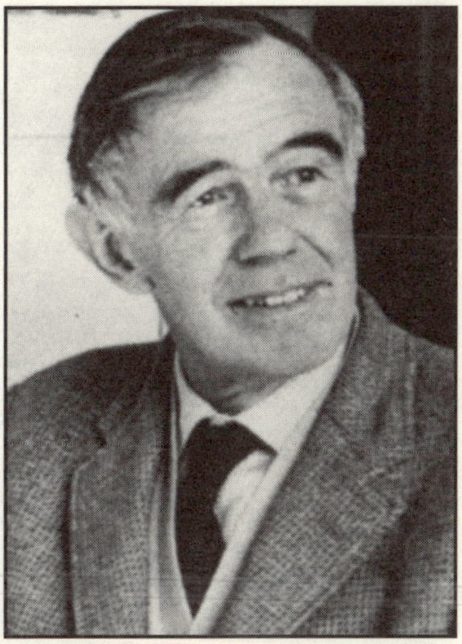

5

1. J.H. Burn (Ch.8)
2. Best and Bauting (Ch.8)
3. J.B. Collip (Ch.8)
4. Herbert Evans (Ch.8)
5. Gwyn Macfarlane (Ch.9)
6. Dr. Archibald Garrod from Green College (Ch.9)
7. Rudbeck (Ch.10)
8. Pecquet's figure of the thoracic duct in the dog (Ch.10)

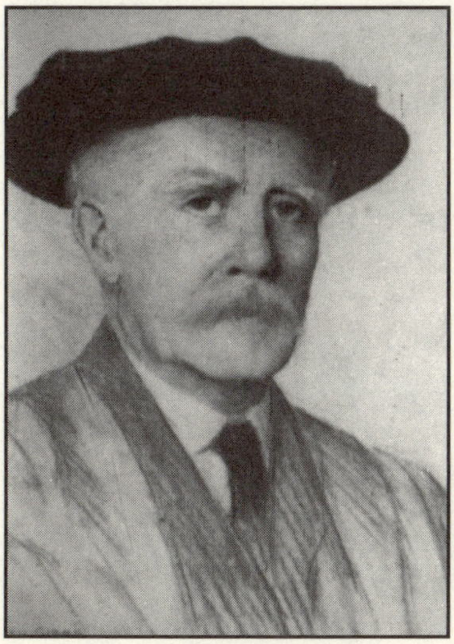

6

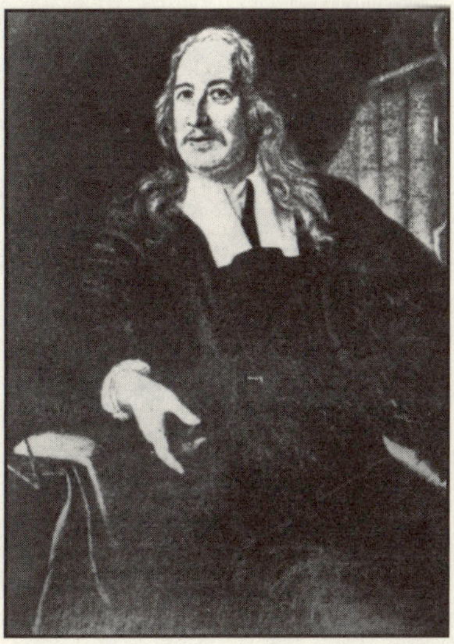

7

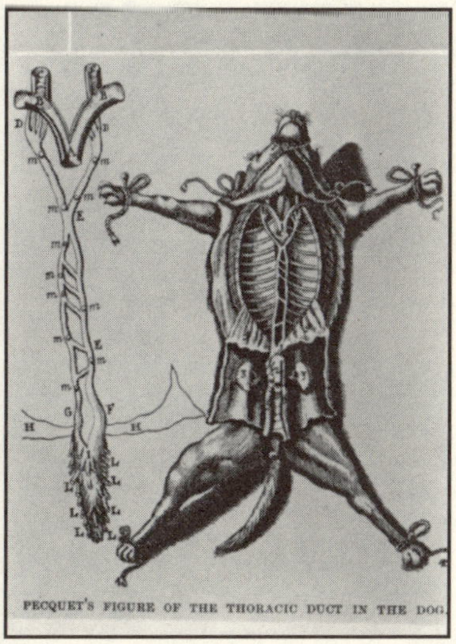

8

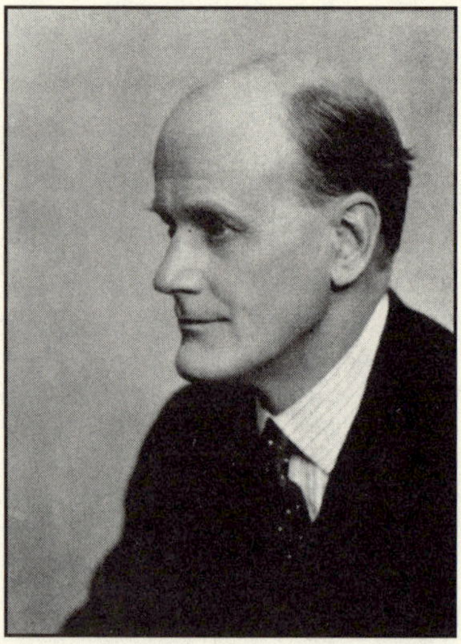

1

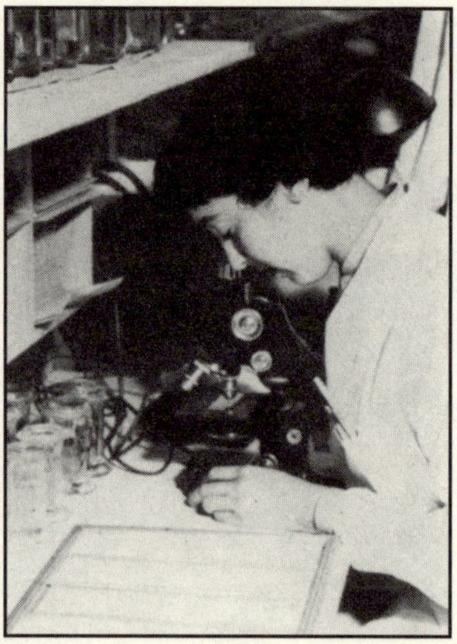

2

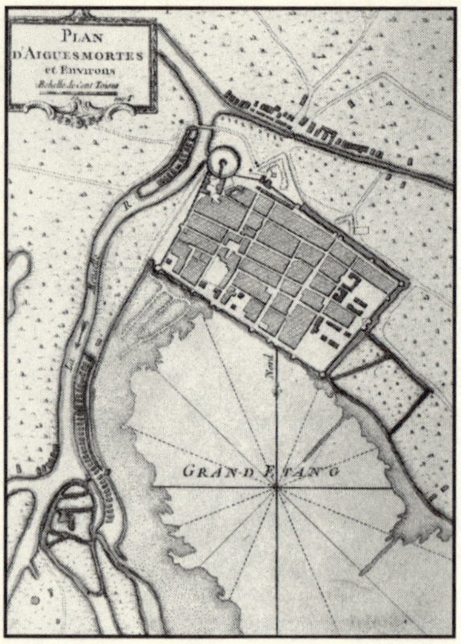

3

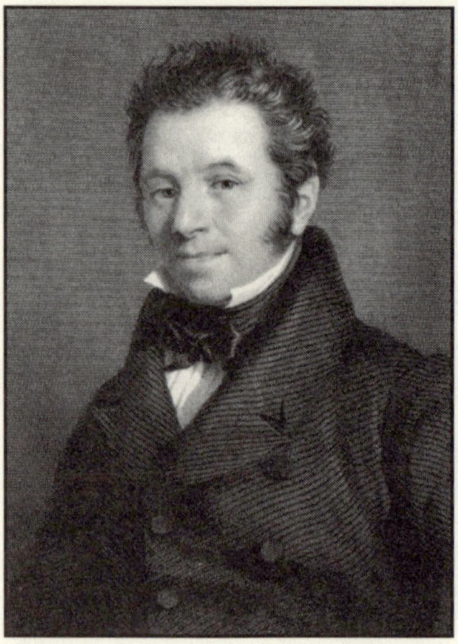

4

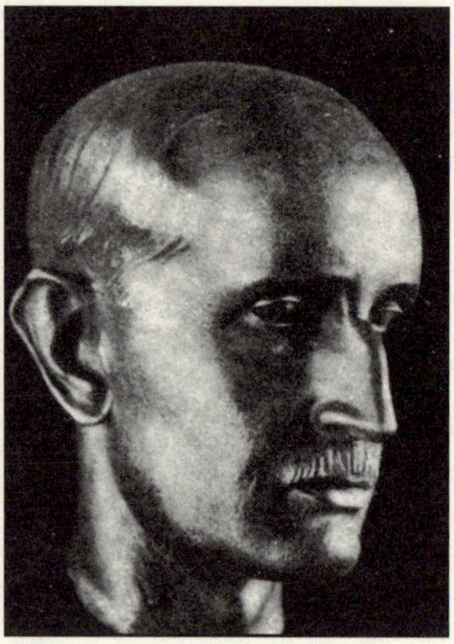

5

1. W.M. Fletcher (Ch.11)
2. Ann Michelson (Ch.11)
3. Marc Dax "Aignes Mortes" (Ch.12)
4. Marshall Hall (Ch.12)
5. Pio del Rio-Hortega, bronze by Juan Cristobal (Ch.12)
6. Alan Gregg "Difficult Art of Giving" (Ch.12)
7. W.M. James (Ch.12)
8. U.S. Von Euler (Ch.12)

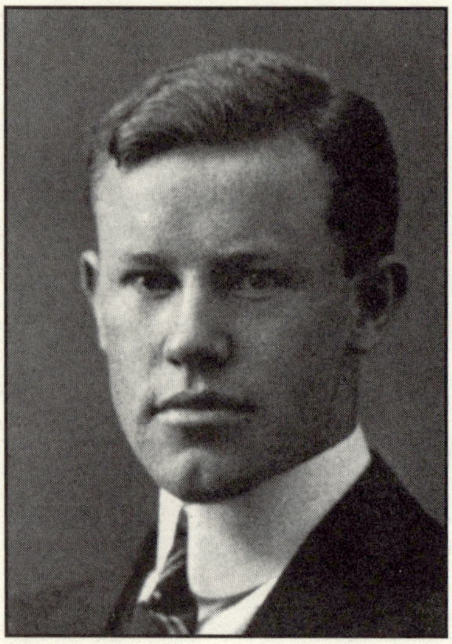

6

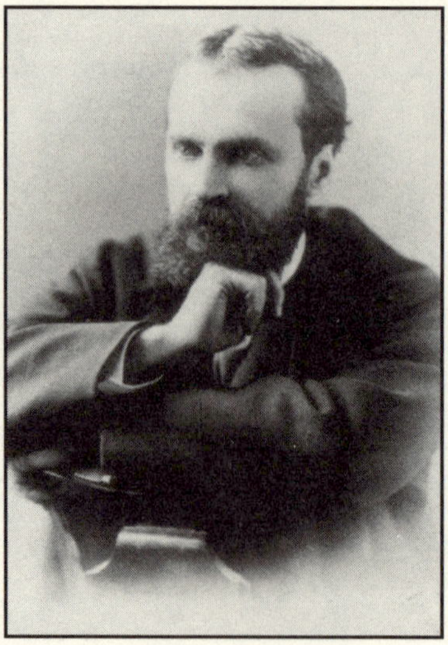

7

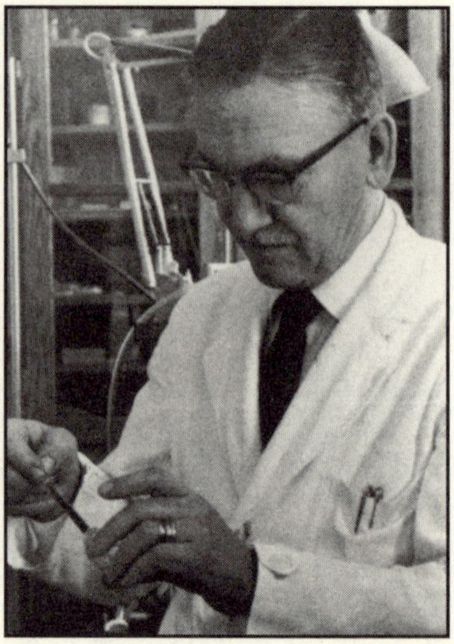

8

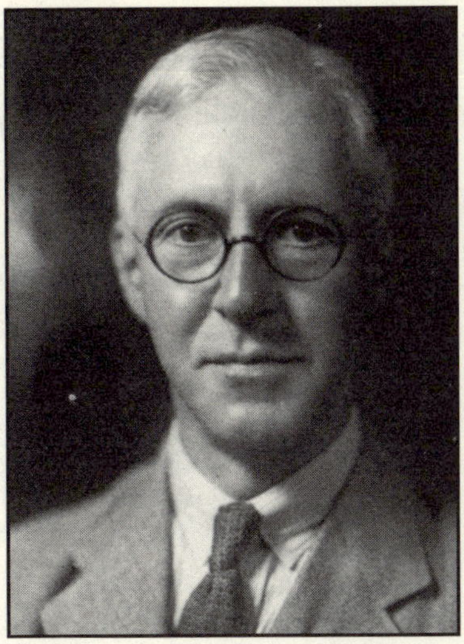

1

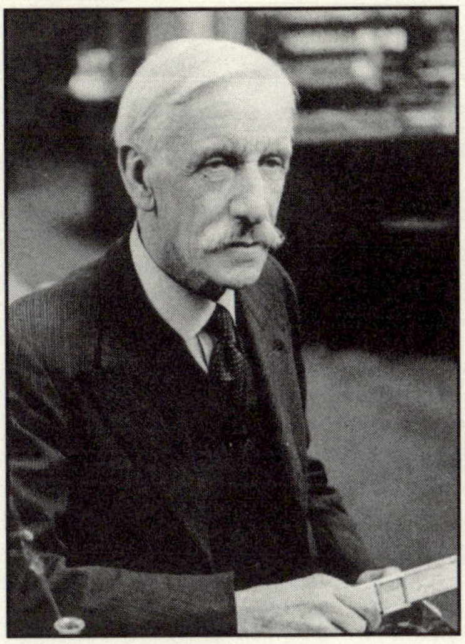

2

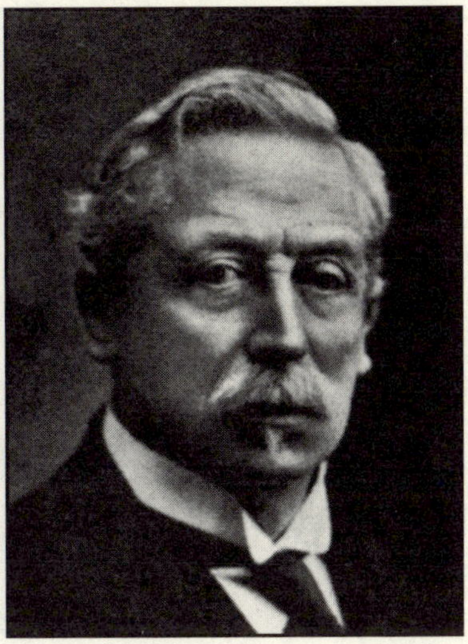

3

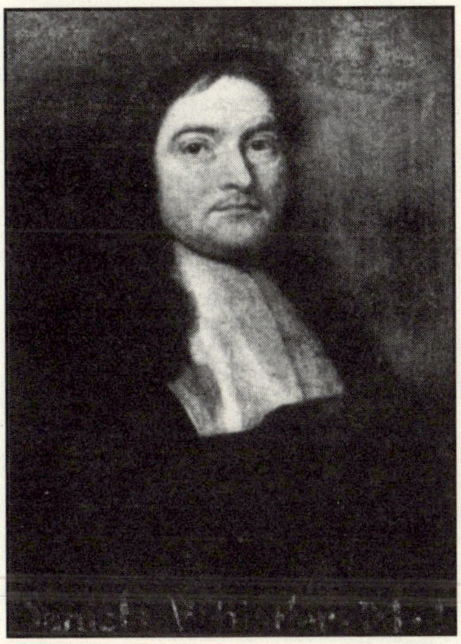

4

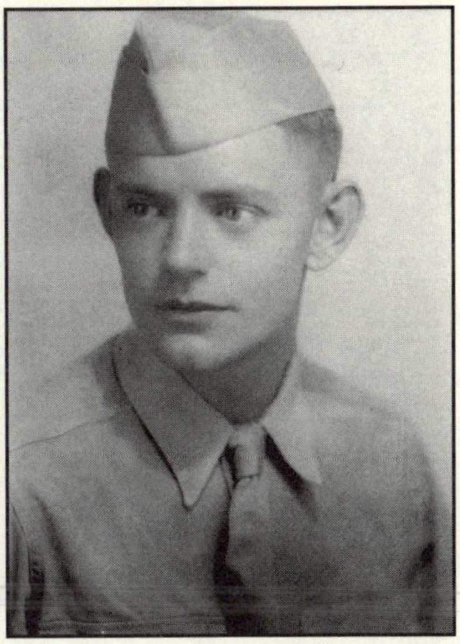

5

1. H.H. Dale (Ch.12)
2. F. Gowland Hopkins (Ch.13)
3. Eijkman (Ch.13)
4. Daniel Whistler "Classic Descriptions of Disease" (Ch.13)
5. John P. McGovern (Ch.14)
6. De Graaf (Ch.13)
7. Florence Sabin (Ch.14)

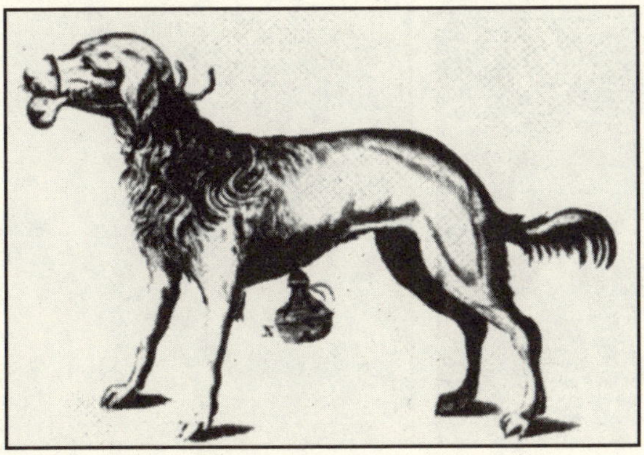

6

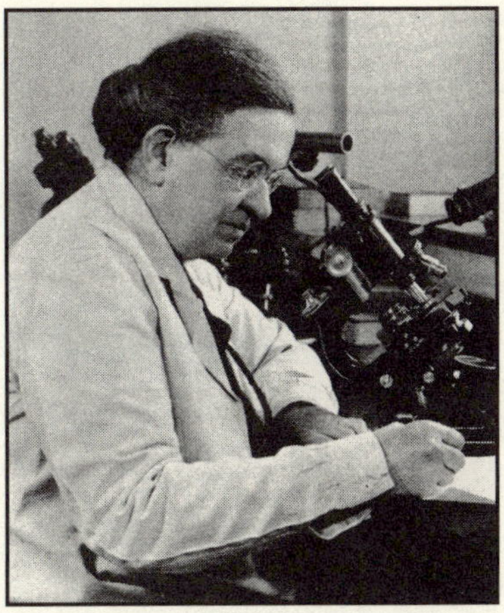

7

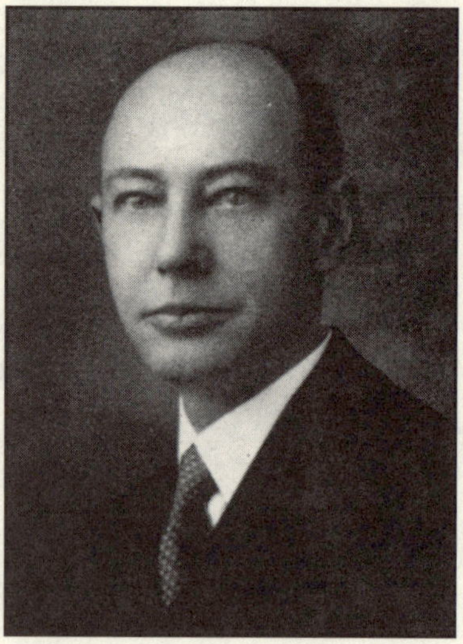

1

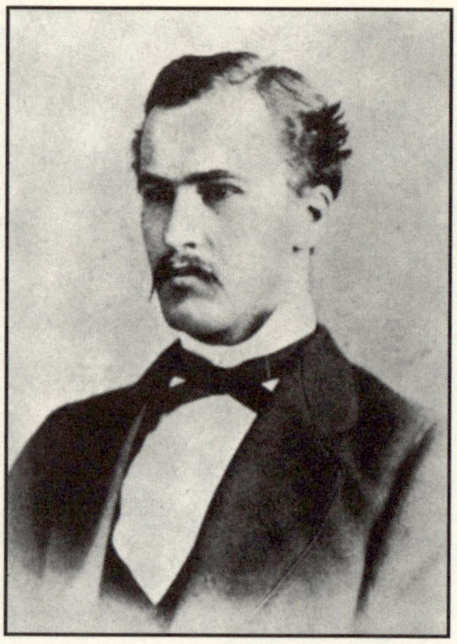

2

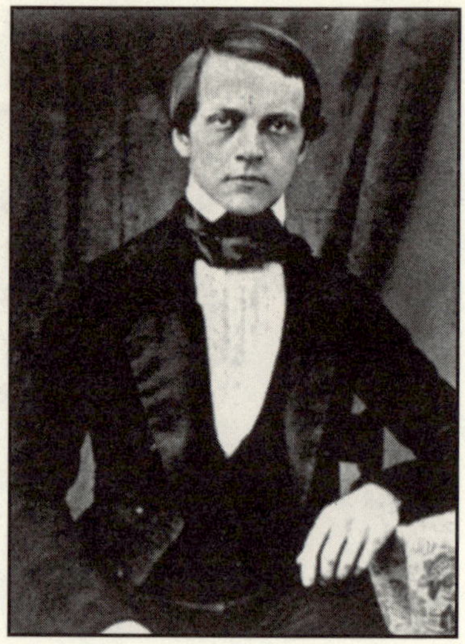

3

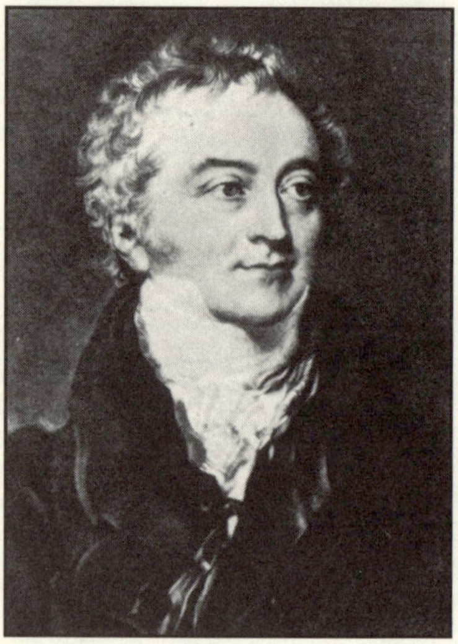

4

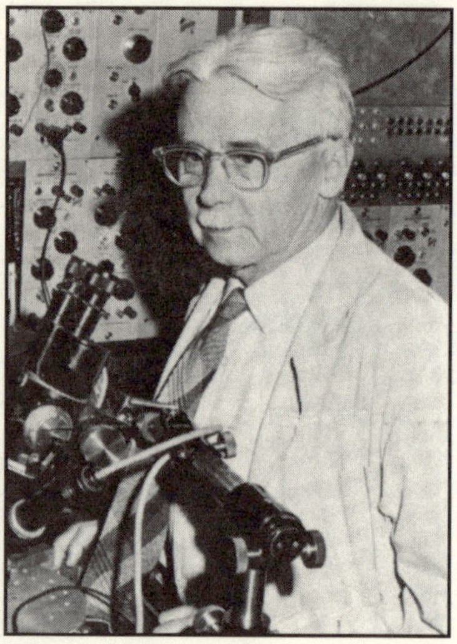

5

1. George Richards Minot (Ch.14)
2. W. Osler (Ch.14)
3. Helmholtz (Ch.15)
4. T. Young (Ch.15)
5. H.K. Hartline (Ch.15)
6. Galileo "Diagrams of the Pulsilogia" (Ch.15)
7. Swammerdam (Ch.16)
8. Johannes Muller (Ch.16)

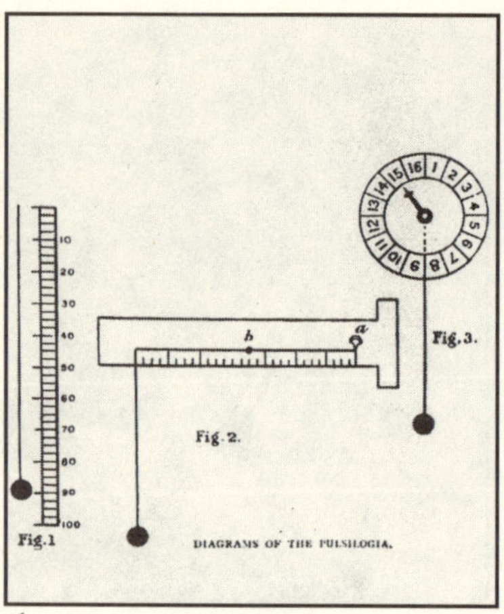

6

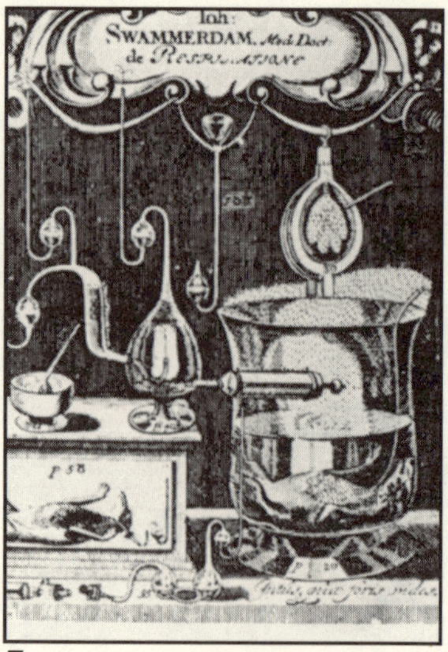

7

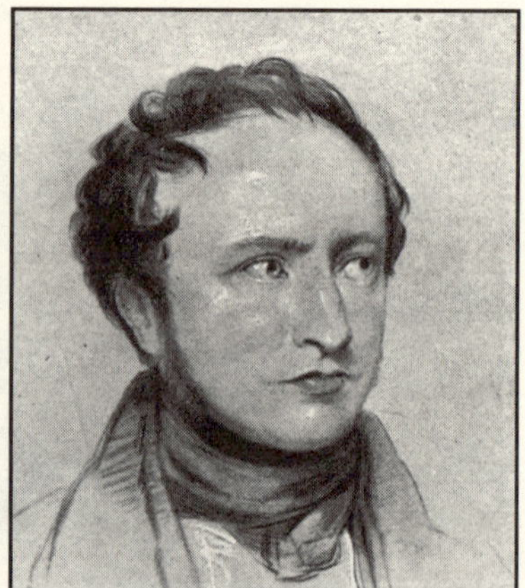

8

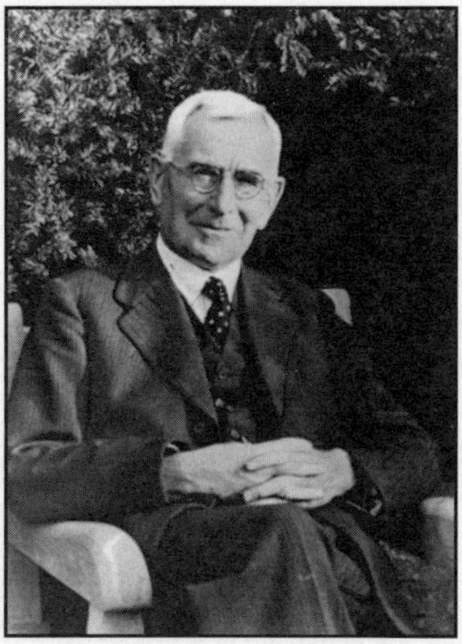

1

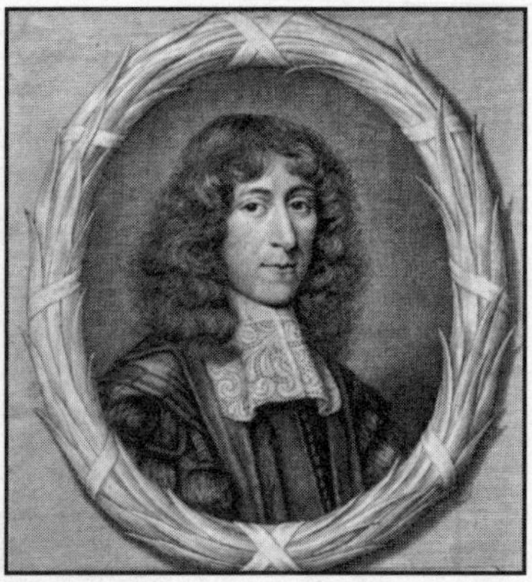

2

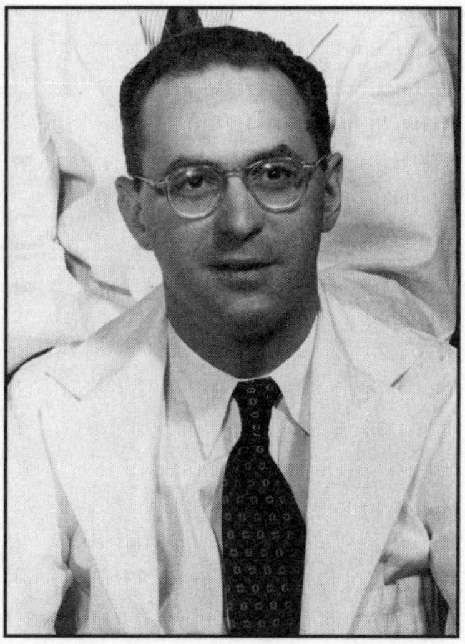

3

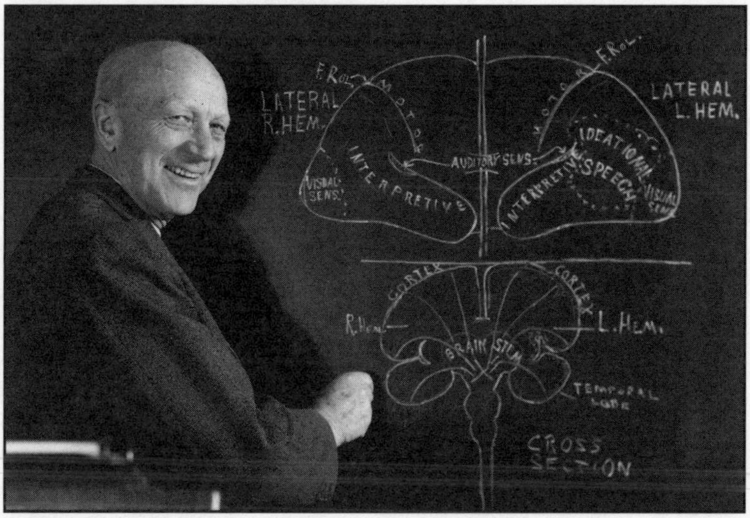

4

1. C.G. Douglas (Ch.16)
2. John Mayow (Ch.16)
3. Dr. William Feindel (Ch..17)
4. Wilder Penfield (Ch.17)
5. From Keats Notebook (Ch.18)
6. Robert Bridges (Ch.18)

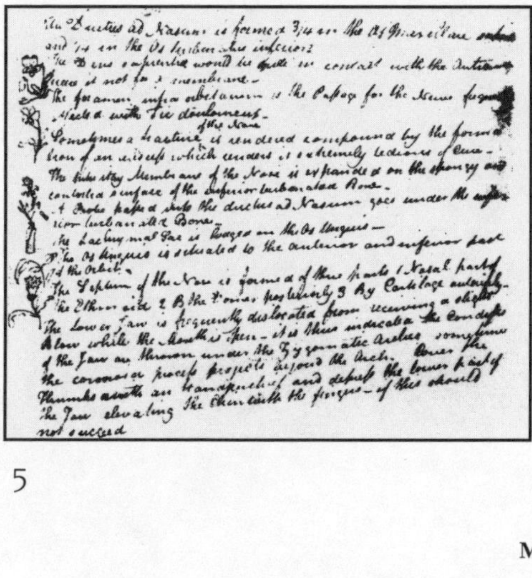

The Ductus ad Nasum is formed 3/4 on the Os Maxillare [illegible]
and 1/4 in the Os turbinatus inferior
The Bone [illegible] would be [illegible] in contact with the Antrum
[illegible] it not for a membrane.
The foramen infra orbitarum is the Passage for the Nerve [illegible]
[illegible] with the [illegible]
Sometimes a fracture of the Nose is rendered compound by the forma-
tion of an abscess which renders it extremely tedious of cure.
The [illegible] Membrane of the Nose is expanded on the spongy and
convoluted surface of the inferior turbinated Bone.
A Probe passed into the ductus ad Nasum goes under the infe-
rior turbinated Bone.
The Lachrymal Sac is lodged on the Os Unguis.
The Os Unguis is situated to the anterior and inferior part
of the Orbit.
The Septum of the Nose is formed of three parts 1 Nasal part of
the Ethmoid 2 By the Vomer posteriorly 3 By Cartilage anteriorly.
The Lower Jaw is frequently dislocated from receiving a slight
blow while the Mouth is open — it is thus indicated [illegible] the Condyle
of the Jaw are thrown under the Zygomatic arches sometimes
the coronoid process projects beyond the Arch. Cover the
Thumbs with an handkerchief and depress the lower part of
the Jaw elevating the Chin with the fingers — if this should
not succeed

5

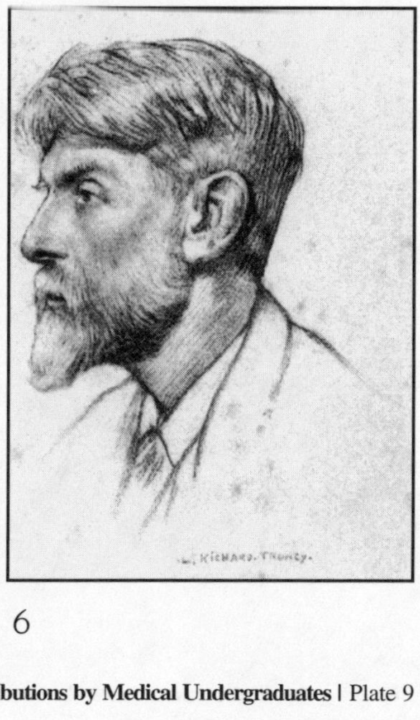

6

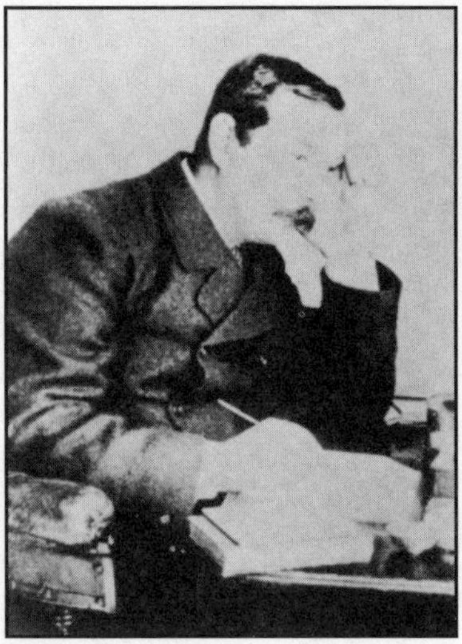

1

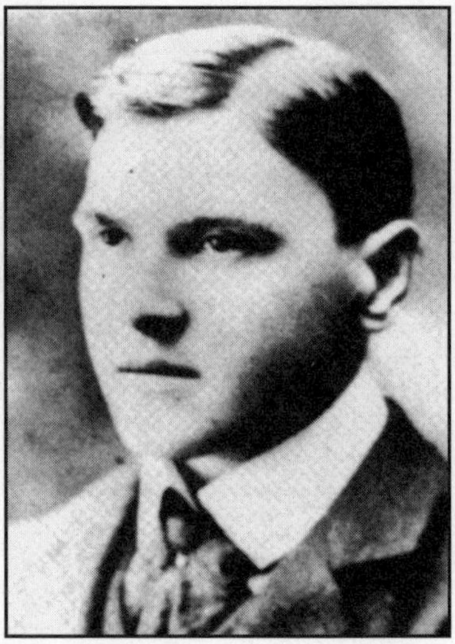

2

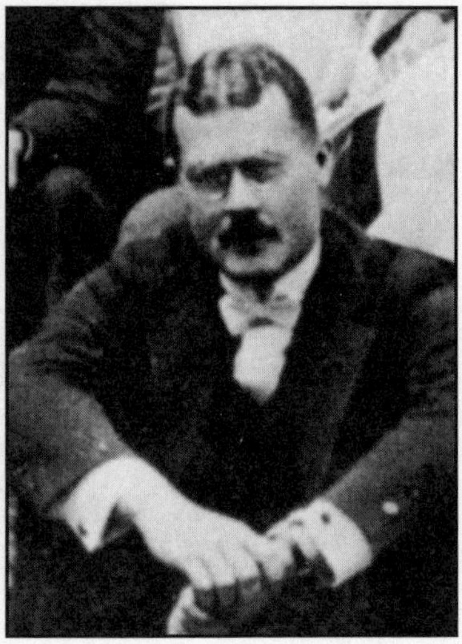

3

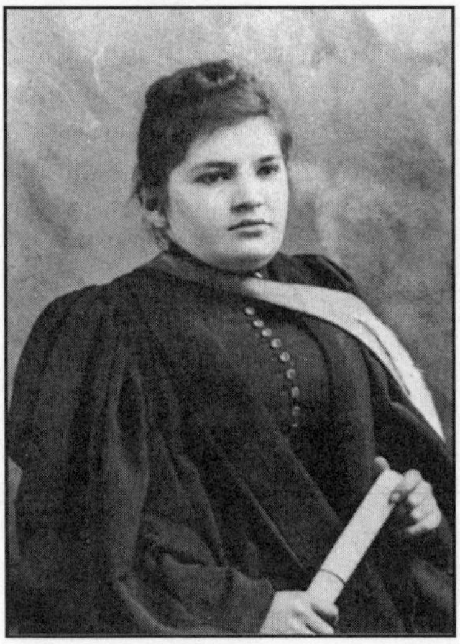

4

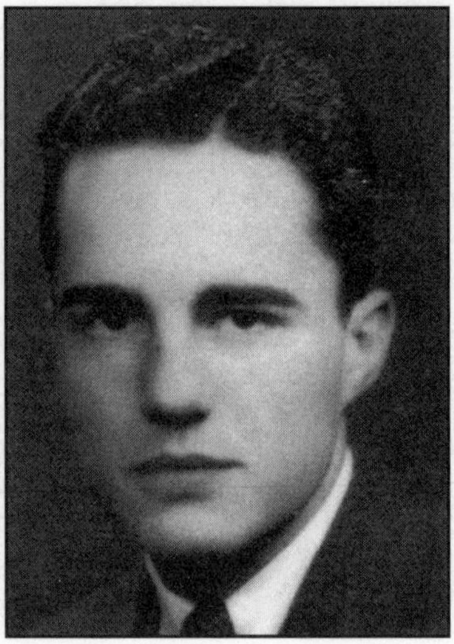

5

1. A. Conan Doyle (Ch.18)
2. W. Somerset Maugham (Ch.18)
3. Wilbert Davison at Oxford, 1916. (Ch.19)
4. Maude Abbott (Ch.19)
5. Grey Dimond (Ch.19)
6. Virchow (Ch.19)

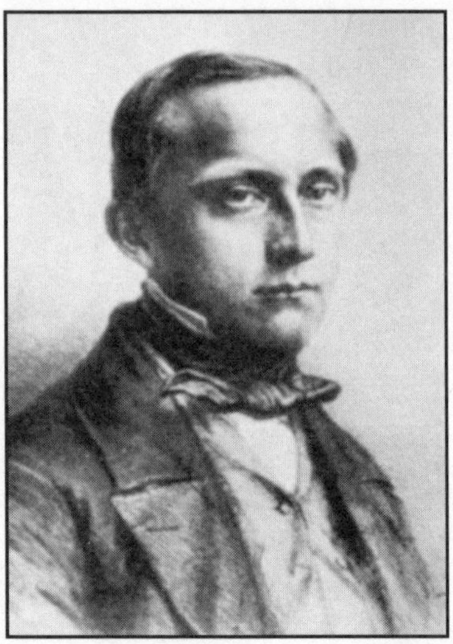

6

minded of Christopher Wren's famous drawing of the arterial circle at the base of the brain which, it is said, he named "the circle of Willis," after his teacher at Oxford. The method of naming and numbering the cranial nerves—those to the eyes, ears, tongue and so on, which Willis devised, was eventually replaced by an improved system that originated with a German medical student. In 1778 Samuel Thomas von Soemmering presented this new classification of the cranial nerves in his graduation thesis. He became a physician, a disciple of Jenner, a contributor to physics and to the early work that preceded the electric telegraph. Independently he described the "white line of Gennari" in the grey matter of the human brain. He wrote on sunspots and on fossils. Thirteen years after graduation he described the disease of developing structures known as achondroplasia. The classical description of this condition, however, was to await the medical student, M.H. Romberg (1795-1873), whose graduation thesis, "On Congenital Rickets," in Berlin in 1817 embodied a most thorough study. Every medical student knows Romberg's name in connection with the loss of the erect posture with the eyes closed in certain ataxic disorders.

August Forel (1848-1931)

The versatile August Forel is remembered the world over for his studies on ants and their social behaviour. Like so many Swiss physicians he was a biologist with a broad base of experience and manifold interests. At the age of seven, on the shores of Lake Geneva, he became enamoured of ants, and wherever he went, in his schooling, he kept learning their lore. When he entered medical school in Zurich in 1866 he was already writing papers on ants, and when, 32 years later, he retired from his chair of psychiatry there, he was still writing about them.

As a medical student Forel met the gifted von Gudden—a pioneer in neuroanatomy and psychiatry, later to be drowned by his patient, Ludwig II, the mad king of Bavaria. Forel's doctoral thesis was begun in 1871 under the anatomist, Meynert. It was a contribution to the structure of the mammalian thalamus and its role in vision. Meynert disagreed with some of his student's conclusions, but he had the grace, nevertheless, to have it published in the *Proceedings of the Vienna Academy of Sciences*.

Fortunately for science Forel failed in a competition for a local health officer's appointment, though he bitterly resented the petty medical politics which entered into the selection. Within eight years he was made professor of psychiatry at Zurich succeeding that pioneer in electrical stimulation of the brain, Eduard Hitzig. Forel was also made director of the Burgholzi Asylum. He clearly and independently enunciated the neurone theory in 1887. With Oskar Vogt he founded the *Journal für Psychologie und Neurologie*. His crusading pen was stilled temporarily by a stroke at the age of 64, but he learned to write with his left hand and continued on until his death at age of 83.

Sigmund Freud (1857-1939)

One of the most controversial figures in the history of medicine and thought, Sigmund Freud, was a student investigator in anatomy. Freud did not emerge from some sort of penny-in-the-slot-machine with psychoanalysis on his lips, at the turn of the century. Rather he came from the exacting discipline of the neuro-anatomical laboratory and from the hard realities of speech disorders and cerebral palsy in the neurological clinic.

Freud was born in Freiberg, Moravia, and from the age of four lived in Vienna. In grammar school he was a consistently good student and developed broad cultural interests. He was early conscious of the Darwinian theories that were then breaking on the world.

Despite the fact that his family lived in straitened circumstances, Freud began to study medicine, although he was at one time on the verge of studying law. However, his reading of Goethe's essay *Die Nature* determined him on a medical career.

Freud entered the University of Vienna in 1873. In 1876 he commenced to work, as a student, in Ernst Brucke's laboratory of physiology, and continued almost uninterruptedly until 1882. He graduated with his M.D. degree in 1881, aged 25. The first undergraduate study set him by Brucke concerned a larval form of the early vertebrate, petromyzon. This may have been the beginning of Freud's thinking concerning phylogeny and levels of development and of function within the nervous system.

On January 4, 1877, Brucke communicated Freud's first paper to the Vienna Academy of Science. It was entitled "Spinal Ganglia and the Spinal Cord of Petromyzon," and was later printed, being 12 pages long and accompanied by a colour plate. In 1878 the study was elaborated into one of 80 pages and four plates. He clearly showed the derivation of unipolar posterior root ganglion cells from bipolar sensory cells in this species. Freud was no newcomer to the field of comparative neurology, having spent the summer of 1876 with Professor Clause, of the Institute of Comparative Anatomy in Vienna, at the Zoological Station at Trieste.

Freud was one of the lesser forerunners of the neurone theory, as it came to be called in Germany. In the summers of 1879 and 1880 he worked on the nervous system of the fresh water crab and emphasized the finely neurofibrillar structure of its axones. He was also impressed by the similarity of the pattern of the nervous system in invertebrates and vertebrates.

Also from Brucke's laboratory Freud published his papers on the tracts and nuclei within the medulla oblongata. At about the same period (1880) he translated into German John Stuart Mill's book, *The Emancipation of Women*. Freud's co-workers in Brucke's laboratory had equally broad interests and published on such subjects as collateral innervation, the origin of cell nuclei, corneal innervation, the conception of movement and space, and "the nature of the psychical process."

Freud graduated in 1881, and in 1882, on Brucke's advice, embarked on a clinical training as his only hope of earning a living. While on the neurological service of the Allgemeines Krankenhaus in Vienna, Freud found time to carry on some neuropathological studies in Meynert's laboratory. One of these was on the use of gold salts in the staining of the axons of nerve cells as a means of tracing fibre tracts in the nervous system.

His papers thereafter show an increasing preoccupation with clinical neuropathological matters, such as cerebral and basal ganglion lesions in a case of scurvy, muscular atrophy associated with syringomyelia, and acute multiple neuritis. With Meynert he wrote a paper on the acoustic nucleus and the interolivary tract.

In 1884 Freud received a supply of cocaine from the Merck Company and carried on many experiments with it. These are detailed in a small book which he produced on the subject. He told his ophthalmological colleagues Konigstein and Carl Koller of its potential value in anaesthetizing the eye. Returning from a vacation he found that Koller had publicly demonstrated this effect in animals. Freud tested the effect of cocaine on human endurance, and with a dynamometer was able to show that the effect was not subjective only.

In 1885 Freud was awarded a travelling fellowship in neuropathology that took him to Paris. There he worked with Darkschewitsch on the connections of the inferior peduncle of the cerebellum with the posterior columns of the spinal cord, which had not been understood previously. Freud's apprenticeship in comparative neurology came to his assistance when he developed the thesis of the homology of the sensory nuclei in the medulla oblongata with the posterior roots of the spinal cord at a lower level.

Despite all this, however, Charcot's clinic became the outstanding interest of Freud in Paris. At the Salpêtrière he heard the great clinician say that he wished his lectures might be translated into German. Freud offered to carry out this onerous work and was soon admitted to the inner circle. The chief interests of Charcot at that moment were hypnosis, suggestion and hysterical paralyses and contractures. Freud suggested that study might be made of organic paralyses as compared with those of an hysterical nature, which always conformed to the patient's view of such phenomena. However, as Freud remarks in his autobiography, Charcot "took no special interest in penetrating more deeply into the psychology of the neuroses."

Returning from Paris in 1886, Freud spent some time in Berlin at paediatric clinics, with a view to future collaboration with Kassowitz in Vienna. Actually, some of Freud's best clinical studies came out of Kassowitz's institute, on "The Cerebral Palsies of Children."

On returning to Vienna, Freud gave to the Society of Medicine an account of his tenure of the travelling fellowship in neuropathology. As he recounted the things that he had seen and learned in Paris he was given the prophet-without-honour reception reserved for returning postgraduate fellows in the medical profession. His attempts to get access to patients to prove what he was talking about were as ineffectual as those of Semmelweis, 40 years earlier, in the same hospital, who had been denied access even to his own clinical records. The laboratory of anatomy was closed to Freud, and he was allowed no place in which to lecture.

Locked out, therefore, Freud began medical practice with what he called "the crowds of neurotics whose number seemed further multiplied by the manner in which they hurried, with their troubles unsolved, from one physician to another." Using electrical machines and hypnotism he waded into the totally uncharted sea of psychotherapy. He soon gave up electrotherapy and began to move towards the use of suggestion in therapy. As he later wrote: "Psychoanalysis is the administrator of the estate left by hypnotism."

He travelled to Nancy to observe Liébault and Bernheim, as he says, "working among the poor women and children of the labouring classes,

... . and I received the profoundest impression of the possibility that there could be powerful mental processes which nevertheless remained hidden from the consciousness of men."

In 1891 Freud published his work on "Aphasia" and showed that he had grasped the significance of the great generalizations being propounded in England by Hughlings Jackson in this field, such as "the dissolution of function." This was followed, in 1893, by a monograph of 168 pages on cerebral diplegia, a work that drew the praise of Pierre Marie. In the same year Freud, in company with his old colleague from Brucke's laboratory, Josef Breuer, wrote, "On the Psychic Mechanisms of Hysterical Phenomena."

With this publication and with his translation of Bernheim's 414-page book on suggestion, Freud started out upon his second writing career, though this one completely overshadowed his first in terms of volume. As if Freud had not written enough on psychoanalysis, a band of interpreters has arisen, and at the hands of some of these Freud has suffered. The importance of what he had to say is too great to allow it to be drowned in the currently fashionable semantic torrent, and for that reason a brief and clear summary by Franz Alexander is quoted in part:

> Freud's main accomplishments were to demonstrate that man's personality, normal or morbid, is shaped by life experiences; that among these experiences early childhood experiences are of overwhelming significance and, above all, that behind a layer of civilized veneer man harbours in his unconscious mind an asocial nucleus with destructive impulses directed against others and himself. He discovered a method by which this asocial core of the personality can be explored in spite of man's natural tendency to hide it from himself and others. Freud called this tendency repression, and the method by which repressed unconscious impulses can be made conscious, psychoanalysis.

According to Freud, psychoneuroses and many psychoses are the result of this inability of the patient to face the entirety of his emotional situation. This inability Freud considered as a failure in the highest integrative functions of the personality or, in terms of neurophysiology, of the highest integrating centres of the brain.

Freud's phylogenetic thinking never left him, and it may have been one of the most useful things that he carried with him from his undergraduate medical education. Certainly his early practice in drawing generalizations from his observations stood him well in later life. From petromyzon to psychoanalysis was a long journey, but as Brill concluded, in his excellent biographical study: "Freud had, as it were, started from the ranks, as a private, yet from the beginning he carried the commander's staff in his knapsack."

A prophet without honour in 1886, Freud has nevertheless become a prophet to many, and with reason, as the following extract from his address to the International Psychoanalytic Congress in 1918 suggests:

> But one day the conscience of society will awaken, and we shall realize that... man has the same claim to mental treatment that he now has to surgical aid. And we shall also come to see that the

> neuroses menace the health of the people no less than does tuberculosis, and that, like tuberculosis, the neuroses cannot be left to the ineffectual care of the individual himself. When that time comes, institutes and consultation centres will be established, and staffed with trained physicians, so that men who would otherwise give way to drink, women who would break down as a result of overwhelming deprivations, and children whose choice would be limited to delinquency or neurosis, may be strengthened to resist such unhealthy tendencies and become capable of social achievements.

Ross Granville Harrison (1870-1959)

While histology, pathology and physiology were coming to the support of the neurone theory, one of America's most original minds was finishing up his postgraduate studies at the University of Bonn in Germany. Ross Granville Harrison was a Ph.D. graduate of Johns Hopkins University (1894), and an M.D. graduate of Bonn (1899), who set out to elucidate embryological development in the nervous system. He did this against a background of three existing developmental theories that can be quickly summarized. He knew his history well, as his papers and discoveries show. The first theory was the "cell chain theory," which Schwann enunciated in 1839, one year after his great generalization, "the cell theory." Schwann thought that the nerve fibres were formed by the same chain of cells that gave rise to the neurilemmal or Schwann sheath. The second theory was the "outgrowth theory," which was put forward, in rudimentary form, by Bidder and Kupfer in 1857, but was much more firmly established by His (1886-1890) and by Ramón y Cajal (1890). This stated that the nerve fibre was an outgrowth of a single cell or neuroblast. Finally, the third was the "plasmoderm" theory of Hensen (1864). He believed that nerve fibres were produced *in situ* by differentiation of a pre-formed set of protoplasmic bridges.

Writing of his own research Harrison said:

> The decision between neuroblast and sheath cells was reached by removing the source of each element in turn, and finding that neurones with naked axis cylinders developed when the ganglion crest, the source of the sheath cells, was removed and the neuroblasts were left intact, while no nerve fibres developed at all when only sheath cells remained.

Harrison continued:

> The nerve cells send out protoplasmic processes which gradually expand to nerve fibres... The ends of these developing nerve fibres consist of a thickening with finely-branched pseudopodia. These are precisely the structures that later make contact,. as synapses, with other nerve cells. Harrison saw the whole problem as revolving around a special application of the general proposition, the cell theory.

To answer the protoplasmic bridges problem posed by the third theory mentioned above, Harrison, in 1907, working at Yale University made one of the greatest advances in the study of living matter. He states it simply: "The next and final step was to remove the embryonic nervous tissue from the organ entirely by means of the explantation experiment, the method now known as tissue culture." There is no need here to expand on the scientific value of the tissue culture technique and of the great benefits to mankind that have flowed from its use, as in the field of anti-poliomyelitis vaccine. Suffice it to say that it was the product of a well trained and inventive mind.

Harrison concluded as a result of his study of embryonic nervous tissue removed entirely from the body, and cultured in a drop of lymph on a special microscopic slide, that, "The substance of the axone originates in the neuroblast and is spun out by means of the amoeboid activity of the end, without material contribution from the surrounding protoplasmic bridges, which may serve however as a framework to support and guide the fibres. The outgrowth of the nerve fibre is, therefore, a mode of protoplasmic movement and not a progressive differentiation *in situ*."

Cajal regarded the work of Ross Harrison as giving the neurone theory some of its most powerful support. He turned to tissue culture work in Spain and eventually handed it over to his adept pupil Pio del Rió-Hortega, director of the Cancer Institute in Madrid.

As he proceeded further with studies on degeneration in the nervous system Cajal laid the foundation for a great many modern neuroanatomical studies that stain, with silver, degenerating fibre tracts that have been interrupted experimentally in order that they may be traced to their eventual termination on the dendrite or cell body next in the circuit. The reactivation of this method of tracing bouton terminal degeneration in Sherrington's laboratory at Oxford by Ebbe Curtis Hoff, an American medical student, set off a chain-reaction that is still going. For more than 20 years students have been immersed in this subject, applying Rió-Hortega's beautiful double impregnation technique, among others, to the spinal cord, sympathetic nervous system, cerebellum and finally to human brains in which frontal lobotomy or other tract-cutting operations have taken place.

The list of active workers in this field would today run into several dozens, which precludes individual mention of them here. The most recent work on the numbers of boutons terminaux to be found on the surface of large anterior horn cells in the spinal cord deserves special notice. There is a beautiful reconstruction on a three-dimensional basis by Professor Murray Barr of the University of Western Ontario, of the bouton endings on anterior horn cells. There is also the superb work of Professor J.Z. Young of University College, London, who with his group has pioneered a post-chroming type of staining that suggests nerve cells probably have not too few, but probably too many, bouton terminals on their surface to be counted.

Harrison's announcement about his revolutionary technique of tissue culture was greeted with derision by some classical anatomists. However, his techniques were used at the Rockefeller Institute by Montrose Burrow, Warren Lewis and Alexis Carrel. Many scholars find it inconceivable that Harrison was passed over by the Nobel advisory committees in the field of medicine or physiology.

In 1907 Yale asked Harrison to head up the department of zoology which, in 1913, occupied the new Osborn Laboratories. After retiring from Yale, at age 68, Harrison took on the chairmanship of the National Research Council for the tumultuous war years 1938-1946. Harrison was one of the truly great scholars who made Yale University a good centre for learning and research. One of his biographers, Dorothea Rudnick, wrote of him: "He quite obviously enjoyed the racy talk of young people in the laboratory; perhaps the most telling commentary on his character is that, once the ice of shyness was broken, the students saved their best stories for him." He must have quietly enjoyed the transformation of his original home on York Street, New Haven, to become the famous club "Mory's," where the irrepressible Cole Porter's music was performed by generations of songsters, including the Whiffenpoofs. "The tables down at Mory's" have as many students' initials carved in them as those in Heidelberg or at Harrison's medical alma mater, Bonn University.

Florence Sabin (1871-1953)

Florence Sabin was born in a mining camp in Colorado, the daughter of a mining engineer. After a busy life in medical research she retired to Colorado and there drafted many public health measures for that state.

After graduating at Smith College, Florence Sabin taught school and biology at her alma mater. She was admitted to Johns Hopkins University medical faculty in 1896 where she did student work with Professor Franklin Paine Mall in anatomy. She prepared a wax model of the brain stem of a newborn child. It aided students in the teaching of this difficult area of the nervous system and was copied in Germany. She became the first woman to be a full-time professor at Johns Hopkins Medical School, and her portrait bust is in the Statuary Hall in the Capitol in Washington, D.C.

It is amazing to learn of her output in her studies of the chromaffin glands, and in the vascular system her staining, supravitally, of white blood cells and of the maturation of cells in leukaemia. She also studied the origin of the lymphatics and of red blood cells. Antibody formation was another of her areas of interest.

Joseph Erlanger (1874-1965)

Erlanger was born in San Francisco and took his bachelor of science at the University of California at Berkeley. He was in the top dozen students in the graduating class in Johns Hopkins in medicine in 1899. The first of his many student papers dealt with the developing eggs of the newt. He spent a summer with the Canadian-born Lewellys Barker in the histology laboratory at Hopkins, because he could not afford the fare home to San Francisco for the summer. He removed the soleus muscle from the leg of a rabbit and studied subsequent changes in the cells of the spinal cord. He thus found which cells in the cord innervated which muscles. When Barker came to write his classic work, "The Nervous System and its Constituent Neurones" in 1909, he cited Erlanger's research six times and reproduced three of his histological preparations.

Erlanger's second student paper was published in 1901 with another student contributor, Albion Walter Hewlett. (Hewlett became the revered professor of medicine at Stanford University but died at the age of 50 of three separate and malignant brain tumours.).The Erlanger-

Hewlett paper studied how much of the intestine could be removed at operation without interfering with digestion. Professor William Howell at Hopkins was so impressed with Erlanger's work that he later offered him the assistant professorship in his department. After graduating at Hopkins in 1899, Erlanger took up his interest in cardiovascular disease, on the use of intravenous solutions in shock and eventually shared the Nobel Prize with Herbert Gasser in 1944. Their work concerned signals in nerves of varying diameters, their excitability and the propagation of the transmitted information.

Two pupils of Sir Victor Horsley, **Frederick Mott** (1853-1926) and **Arthur MacNalty** carried on student research in London. In 1905 Mott was anticipated by Schaudinn's discovery of the *treponema pallida* by a few months. MacNalty had been helping Dr. Gustav Mann with his researches in Oxford on the histology of the optic thalamus. Francis Gotch, professor of physiology at Oxford, told his brother-in-law Victor Horsley that this bright student was en route to University College Hospital, London, for his clinical work and soon MacNalty was invited by Horsley to work in his laboratory from October 1904 to December 1909 on the cervico-spinal-bulbar and the spino-cerebellar tracts, as well as on the question of topographical representation in the cerebellum. For the rest of his life Mott was immersed in the fields of neuropathology, and.psychiatry, and gave the Harveian oration before the Royal College of Physicians of London in 1925. McNalty went on to become Britain's outstanding public health campaigner and administrator.

Henry Hallett Dale (1875-1968)

As a Cambridge undergraduate Dale worked with Professor J.N. Langley on nerve fibre counts. With that genius W.H. Gaskell, Dale studied the origin and conduction of the heart rhythm and the relationship of the autonomic nervous system to the central nervous system. After two years at St. Bartholomew's Hospital, Dale qualified in medicine in 1902. He became director of research for the Wellcome Group and for his work on the chemical transmission of impulses at the synapse shared the Nobel Prize in Medicine in 1936 with his old friend Otto Loewi. When the Nazis refused to let Otto Loewi leave Germany until his half of the Nobel Prize was transferred from a Swedish bank to a bank in Germany, Sir Henry Dale shared his part of the prize with his old friend. Though he never occupied a university chair, Dale published 295 papers, and was the heart and soul of the early years of the Medical Research Council of Great Britain. When he became chairman of the Wellcome Trust his influence on the development of medical research and on medical history became enormous. Henry Dale in his long life did much for medical research and medical education. He was the most approachable man in the world of foundations, so powerful in fact that he was called by his juniors, "The Pope." His ever-present help for young writers was manifest in the foreword that he wrote to *Young Endeavour*.

NEUROPATHOLOGY

Robert Carswell (1793-1857)

Robert Carswell, born in Paisley, Scotland, was drawing pictures of multiple sclerosis lesions when he was a student. He graduated at Aberdeen in 1826 and he became, two years later, the first professor of pathology at University College Hospital, London. In his long and productive life he prepared, from pathological specimens, 2000 water colours, which he painted and lithographed by himself. These have never been improved upon. It is sometimes forgotten that he studied morbid anatomy under P.C.A. Louis in Paris. It was also in Paris that he completed the great collection of pathological drawings which had been commissioned by U.C.H., London, where they are still preserved. It took three years of constant work to prepare these illustrations. Because of poor health Carswell became physician to the King of the Belgians. He died in 1857.

Antoine Bayle (1799-1858)

On November 21, 1822 Bayle presented his thesis for graduation in Paris. It was entitled *Traité des maladies du cerveau et de ses membranes*. In this he first described general paresis of the insane as one disease. It had previously been known as several diseases. The 109-page student discourse was published under the title *Research on Mental Illnesses*.

William Wood Gerhard (1809-1872)

At the age of 25 Gerhard presented the first clinical study of tuberculous meningitis with adequate backup in a paper of 46 pages. The following year he followed this with a paper of 12 pages. He is credited by Osler with having given an early differentiation between typhus fever and typhoid fever from cases seen in the epidemic of 1836 in Philadelphia. Gerhard was said to be one of the most brilliant American pupils of Louis in Paris and as early as 1830, at the age of 21 was writing on the endermic application of medicines. He was in Paris during the cholera epidemic of 1832 and has written concerning that, as well as smallpox that year, and pneumonia in children in 1834. He later wrote on acute rheumatism and on the pathological anatomy of phthisis. He was a classmate, from Paris days, of Oliver Wendell Holmes.

Constantin von Monakow (1853-1930)

The Russian-born Constantin von Monakow, who was to become a leader in the field of neurology, and whose life has been so gracefully chronicled by Colin Russel, was a student who fled from the wax models of neuroanatomy after attending only three lectures, to be caught in the mesmerizing web of neuropathology. As a psychiatric student on Hitzig's wards at Zurich, he was allowed to work over the neurological specimens from the autopsy room. It was in his sixth semester that von Monakow started on histological studies on the brain in dementia. He investigated damage to the cerebral blood vessels, the brain cells and liver in experimental chloroform poisoning. Hitzig, who had discovered the electrical excitability of parts of the cerebral cortex, was so impressed with von Monakow's organizing ability, as a student, that he sent him on a tour of investigation and study of mental institutions. In Munich, von Monakow saw von Gudden's anatomical methods, his microtome, and his set of serial sections of the human brain. This fired his imagination, and took him out of the field of neuropathology and into that of cortical localization of function, his greatest work. His discoveries bear out the thesis that, given the means, a student can be stimulated to do original research.

Von Monakow's life illustrates the value to a researcher of sufficient isolation from the busy world to enable him to concentrate on tough problems for long periods at a time. The seven most productive years of von Monakow's life were spent in an old Benedictine monastery that had become a mental hospital, in St. Gaul in Switzerland. For his microscopic studies he sectioned brains that had been hardened in formaldehyde and fixed in chromic acid. These were held firmly in a mixture of pig's fat and suet, within a metal cylinder, while the very thin sections were cut with a two-handled draw-knife under water. It was with such primitive equipment and far away from any cultural centres that this dynamic man demonstrated some of the cardinal truths of modern neurology. His life illustrates the fact that many first-class discoveries have been made by physicians isolated in rural mental institutions. In such surroundings A.W. Campbell, the Australian, spent 13 years as resident medical officer and pathologist in an asylum in the Liverpool area and, with Sherrington's support, produced his classic atlas on the microscopic structure of the brain's surface. His maps are used today wherever the brain is studied.

J.F.F. Babinski (1857-1932)

The French interest in multiple sclerosis stems also from J.F.F. Babinski. Every student knows that if a patient's great toe goes up when the sole of his foot is stroked he is said to have Babinski's sign. Few realize that Babinski was once a student too—and that he wrote his graduation thesis for the University of Paris on multiple sclerosis. He had already written a paper on typhoid fever two years previously. At the age of 39 he reported on his "cutaneous plantar reflex," now called Babinsky's sign. This milestone in neurological diagnosis was presented in a communication of only 28 lines. Dozens of papers and even books have since been written about it by others.

George Huntington (1850—1956)

George Huntington was born in East Hampton, Long Island, New York, on April 9, 1850. His father and grandfather had, in succession, practised medicine in East Hampton for over 50 years. The unique contribution that George Huntington made to medical knowledge is the description of the chorea, now known by his name. His was not the first description of the disease, but as Osler put it, "In the history of medicine there are few instances in which a disease has been more accurately, or graphically, or more briefly described."

Although it was not until a few months after graduation from the College of Physicians and Surgeons, New York, in 1871, that George Huntington's work appeared in print, he had been a student of chorea since his boyhood. Huntington's own description of how he became interested in the disease and made a study of it throughout his student years cannot be improved upon. He told the New York Neurological Society on December 7, 1909:

> Over fifty years ago in riding with my father on his professional rounds, I saw my first case of "that disorder," which was the way in

which the natives always referred to the dreaded disease. I recall it as vividly as though it had occurred but yesterday. It made a most enduring impression upon my boyish mind, an impression every detail of which I recall today, an impression which was the very first impulse to my choosing chorea as my virgin contribution to medical lore. Driving with my father through a wooded road leading from East Hampton to Amagansett, we suddenly came upon two women, mother and daughter, both tall, thin, almost cadaverous, both bowing, twisting, grimacing. I stared in wonderment, almost in fear. What could it mean?.My father paused to speak with them, then we passed on. Then my Gamaliel-like instruction began; my medical instruction had its inception. From this point on, my interest in the disease has never wholly ceased.

Huntington's formal description of this type of chorea was read before a medical society meeting on February 15, 1872, in Middleport, Ohio. He had worked on the manuscript while assisting his father at East Hampton, immediately after graduation. Throughout the manuscript are corrections in his father's handwriting. George Huntington gave much credit to both his grandfather and his father for teaching him what they did, not only about chorea, but about medicine in general. Commenting upon this, George Huntington remarked, "In old Greece the pupil sat at the feet of his teacher; so your essayist sat at the feet of these two, and whatever of honour, whatever of praise, whatever of scientific worth there is, is due much more to them than to him to whom has come the unsought, unlooked-for honour."

As one reads Huntington's paper today one can hardly believe that it was written by a man only 22 years old. It bears the stamp of long experience that Huntington already had with this disease. As Osler remarked, "It is truly a classic and has scarcely been improved upon since it was first set down." The following are brief extracts from Huntington's original paper:

The hereditary chorea, as I shall call it, is confined to certain and fortunately a few families, and has been transmitted to them as an heirloom from generations away back in the dim past. It is spoken of by those in whose veins the seeds of the disease are known to exist, with a kind of horror, and not at all alluded to except through dire necessity, when it is mentioned as "that disorder." It is attended generally by all the symptoms of common chorea, only in an aggravated degree, hardly ever manifesting itself until adult or middle life, and then coming on gradually but surely, increasing by degrees, and often occupying years in its development, until the hapless sufferer is but a quivering wreck of his former self... . There are three marked peculiarities in this disease: 1) Its hereditary nature. 2) A tendency to insanity and suicide. 3) Its manifesting itself as a grave disease only in adult life... .In all the families, or nearly all in which the choreic taint exists, the nervous temperament greatly preponderates, and in my grandfather's and father's experience, which conjointly covered a period of seventy—eight years, nervous excitement in a marked degree almost invariably attends upon every disease these people may suffer from, al-

> though they may not when in health be over nervous... I have never known a recovery or even an amelioration of symptoms in this form of chorea; when once it begins, it clings to the bitter end. No treatment seems to be of any avail, and indeed nowadays its end is so well known to the sufferer and his friends that medical advice is seldom sought. It seems at least to be one of the incurables.

Typical of the thoroughness and penetrating nature of Huntington's observations as a boy and young man, is the fact that he noted in his paper the location of the geographical pockets in which his cases were discovered. The leads that he and others gave in this direction were of the greatest value to Macdonald Critchley when he came to draw together, in skilful fashion, the tangled threads of the story of this hereditary chorea.

Augusta Klumpke (1859-1927)

In 1885 Augusta Klumpke of San Francisco, a student of Dejerine in Paris, first described the paralysis of the arm from a traction injury to the brachial plexus that is still known as "Klumpke's Paralysis." Two years later she became the first woman in France to hold the title "interne des hopitaux"—a matter that raised so much opposition that it was only settled by the Minister of Public Instruction, the physiologist Paul Bert. The following year Klumpke married the neurologist Joseph Jules Dejerine (1849-1917).

Karoly Schaffer (1864-1939) and **Hermann Oppenheim** (1858-1919)

The role of heredity and constitution in diseases of the nervous system continues to attract investigators. Two of these, historically, were student contributors. In the case of Karoly Schaffer, the father of Hungarian neurology, the approach to the nervous system was through an undergraduate study that he made of the mechanism involved in the transmission of the virus disease rabies. This early paper was published in Budapest. He carried on postgraduate study in Germany with the versatile Weigert and there encountered Edinger, a brilliant colleague and researcher.

Schaffer's work is reported in 200 published papers. His triad of criteria for judging a neurological disease hereditary consisted of: a defect in the germ plasm of ectoderm of the developing embryo; localization of symptoms to correspond with the anatomical abnormality; and selectivity of the clinical defect for a specific system or faculty. His last paper was on his hero Semmelweis. He had just put down his pen when the end came, at age 75.

Congenital abnormalities of the nervous system are of the greatest interest today when medical professionals know something of the effects of diseases such as rubella complicating pregnancy. One of the early students of this field was Hermann Oppenheim, who described amyotonia congenita—also called Oppenheim's disease. When a doctor picks up a limp, toneless infant today, he or she thinks back to Oppenheim's original cases of the year 1900. They might think further back to his graduation thesis of 1881 on the metabolism of urea in the body. He had already published three papers on this problem while a student, so keen was he in physiological pursuits.

Franz Nissl (1860-1919)

Franz Nissl, after deserting theology and gaining a medical education after much privation, made his first contribution at the age of 24 in Munich when, in a prize-winning dissertation, he analyzed "The Pathological Changes of the Nerve Cells of the Cerebral Cortex." Using alcohol-fixed brains and by staining with magenta red (a forerunner of the blue dyes now associated with his name) he showed many new details of the finer structure of nerve cells. Such was his student reputation that immediately upon graduation he was taken into von Gudden's Institute and given a laboratory and assistants.

Every medical student learns early in his career about "Nissl granules"—those "spots on the tiger's skin" that so delicately indicate the state of health of a nerve cell. The reactions to injury of the cell or of its conducting process—the axon—are easily-read barometers that have aided in thousands of researches since Nissl's earliest descriptions. It is a shame that all medical students could not have known Franz Nissl as well as his granules, for he was a man full of humour, an excellent pianist and a deflator of his overly serious colleagues. The late A.T. Rasmussen used to tell of Nissl's endless teasing of his friend and colleague Kraepelin—the psychiatrist, full of brilliance but also of distractions. Nissl would arrange an armful of beer bottles outside a suitable laboratory, informing all who passed that there was serious inebriety abroad in the department, headed, of course, by the militant crusader against alcoholism, Kraepelin himself.

Nissl had a technique for winnowing down the number of students who sought interviews. Only the truly serious ones ever met him—for he saw them "at twelve"—meaning midnight, after his patients had been visited, his research concluded for the day, and his favourite sonata played in peace at home. Such was the puckish, human and industrious Franz Nissl. He died at age 58 of a chronic kidney ailment.

Henri Claude (1869-1945)

This neurologist has been inexplicably neglected by historians of medicine. His education was thorough and he came to his chosen work with a brilliant record. On graduation he picked up the threads of his earlier thesis work and pushed ever further into the mysteries of multiple sclerosis and the elimination of salt in kidney diseases. He wrote on epilepsy, tumours of the pineal gland—once alleged to be the seat of the soul—tumours of the third ventricle of the brain, the propagation of tumours, and on encephalitis. The First World War brought him into close touch with peripheral nerve injuries and with hysteria.

The measurement of cerebrospinal fluid pressure was of great interest to Claude and he did pioneer work in graphically recording its changes in various postures, after the administration of drugs, and after the compression of the jugular veins. He was one of the first to develop an interest in the possible role of the thymus gland in muscle diseases. He also surmised that deep in the hypothalmus—that primitive part of the nervous system just above the pituitary gland—there must be some central representation of the autonomic or involuntary nervous system.

Claude occupied Charcot's chair in nervous and mental diseases in Paris from 1921 to 1939. He was a forerunner of much that is thought to be modern or advanced today. He was a psychobiologist, a good psychiatrist, and a pioneer in preventive mental health services, including the use of psychiatric social workers. His work on experimental epilepsy in animals with brain wounds has a modern ring to it.

Pio del Rio-Hortega (1882-1945)

This student contributor was born in the Spanish city of Valladolid, and after training in an art school entered the university of that city. At the medical school, his first contribution was to a student journal where he described, very thoroughly, a carcinoma, which may have been the start of his career in cancer research. His graduation thesis as a doctor of medicine, in 1909, at the same university, was a work of 324 pages with over 100 references to the medical literature. Its title was *Etiology and Pathological Anatomy of Brain Tumours*. It was such a massive thesis that the first half was published in 1911 and the second in 1912. He did his own illustrations, 16 in all, most of them in pen and ink. This was the beginning of his later artistic career as he illustrated the nerve cells and the neuroglia in normal and pathological conditions. He later became famous for his discovery of the microglia, now colloquially called "the garbage collectors of the nervous system." Today they are centre stage in the etiology of Alzheimer's disease. From an early age, Rio-Hortega exhibited an extensive knowledge of clinical neurology.

Paul Schilder (1886-1940)

Paul Schilder made his first contribution in neuropathology while an undergraduate. Two years after graduation he published papers on his research into the anatomical lesions that produce bizarre choreic and athetoid movements. The affliction now called Schilder's Disease—encephalitis periaxialis diffusa—he first described in 1912, three years after graduation.

Though well grounded in structural neuropathology he was also a keen student of philosophy and psychology, probably because of his student association with Laurenz Miller, the philosopher, and Exner, the physiologist, in Vienna. From Freud he learned much, but he was not a strict adherent to his theories.

Schilder's pen was ever-active and his breadth of interest wide. His outstanding contribution, he felt, was his *Das Körperschema*—published in Berlin in 1923, and translated as *The Image and Appearance of the Human Body*, in London, in 1935. He died in 1940, struck down by an automobile in New York City.

Edith Bülbring (1903-1990)

Having learned from the distinguished professor of histology Jan Boeke at the University of Utrecht how to stain neurofibrils, Edith Bülbring applied these methods to staining of pheochromocytomas of the adrenal glands. She presented this work for her M.D. thesis in May 1928 at Bonn University. The work was soon published in Virchow's *Archiv*. Subsequently Dr. Bülbring lived a full and brilliant career as a teacher and researcher in Professor J.H. Burn's department of pharmacology at Oxford University.

NEUROPHYSIOLOGISTS

The physiologists of the nervous system encompass one of the most influential groups in medical history. Though most of them worked in laboratory sciences their contributions have changed much of clinical neurology.

Johannes Evangelista Purkinje (1787-1869)

Johannes Purkinje was born in Libochovice, Bohemia, and received his early education there from the Piarist monks. He became a novitiate and for three years taught in the school, but then decided to study philosophy in Prague. Lacking any support from home—his father died in 1797—Johannes became tutor to the family of Baron Hildprandt. The baron eventually made it possible for Purkinje to take up the study of medicine, and soon he was engrossed in pharmacological studies, in which he himself was the experimental subject. The interest that he showed in intoxications by belladonna, camphor and other substances was maintained throughout his life.

Under the influence of the poet Goethe's *Farbenlehre*, Purkinje became attracted to visual problems, and for his graduation thesis at Prague, in 1819, wrote a dissertation on "The Subjective Features of Vision." This essay was expanded six years later to include an account of his experimental work on "after-images" and on differences in the threshold of vision for various colours.

The following year Purkinje began his work on dizziness and on the jerking motion of the eyes, known as nystagmus, following rotation of the body, as in a swivel chair. In this, as in many other fields, Purkinje anticipated by many years the workers still regarded in the West as the pioneers or discoverers.

Purkinje was a friend of Goethe, the poet, Hegel the philosopher, and the brothers von Humbolt in Berlin. Together they persuaded the German government that their brilliant protégé merited a professorship. Accordingly, Purkinje was installed in the chair of physiology in Breslau, in 1823.[1].Breslau's German University received the young Czech professor in a cold fashion, and when he started elementary laboratory exercises and demonstrations for the medical students, his colleagues urged upon the government his early removal. The ministry of education responded by building him a first-class physiological institute.

Purkinje ranks as one of the fathers of histology—the science of tissues. He was the first to develop a microtome for cutting thin sections of tissues for microscopic study. This led to important studies in embryology. He discovered the sweat glands of the skin in 1833, and kept up a running fire of researches, assisted always by his students.

In 1835 his wife, a daughter of Rudolphi, the Berlin anatomist, died of "the pest," along with their two children. Thereafter Purkinje worked in a small laboratory in his home—much as Ramón y Cajal did in Madrid after a large institute was built in his honour. From Purkinje's home came many important theses by students, reporting, for the first time, their master's discoveries. Thus Adolph Wendt in his Latin graduation dissertation at Breslau in 1833, *De Epidermide Humana*, described in detail the opening of the sweat glands on the surface of the human skin.

In 1837 Purkinje made his broad microscopic survey of the substance of the brain, giving the first accurate account of the billions of nerve cells that make it up, together with their nuclei, their receiving apparatuses "the dendrites," and their transmitting fibres, covered with insulation of "myelin." In the cerebellum he described those "flask-shaped ganglionic bodies," known to this day as "Purkinje cells."

More important, however, were his observations in 1837 on the basic similarity in structure between the cells of plant and animal tissues. He laid the groundwork for that great generalization—the cell theory—in 1838 by Schleiden and Schwann. In 1839 Purkinje introduced the term "protoplasm" to facilitate discussion of animal tissues, since the physician-botanist Schleiden had used chiefly botanical terminology.

The all-important fibres of the heart that are specialized for electrical conduction—known as the Purkinje fibres—were first described in the thesis, *De musculari cordi structura* (1839) by Bogislaus Palicki, one of Purkinje's students, who gave his master full credit for their discovery. Another student dissertation, *De structura fibrosa uteri nongravidi*, by Wilhelm Kasper in 1840, reported the discovery of what are still called the "Purkinje fibres" of the uterus.

Purkinje's interests ranged from the microscopic structure of the teeth, to that of the skin, bones, blood vessels and seminal vesicles. He did the early basic work on the ciliary motion by which particles are carried along moist epithelial surfaces within the body. He showed that deaf mutes could receive and appreciate the vibrations of a tuning fork in contact with the skull.

A significant paper was written by Purkinje, in 1846, on dreams as possible indicators of personality structure. Purkinje had already anticipated Barany on nystagmus, Galton on fingerprints, Schleiden and Schwann on cell structure—why not Freud on dreams?

In 1850, at the age of 63, Purkinje was welcomed home to Prague and was given the chair of physiology and a good laboratory in which to work. He became a great national figure, known not only for his discoveries, but also for the translations of Shakespeare, Schiller and Tasso that he made into Czech. He lived until 1869, greatly beloved by his people.

Purkinje was more than a great discoverer in physiology who started as a student contributor. He stands as an important representative of a culture in the cockpit of Europe that has nurtured great minds amidst religious and political conflict. The subjection of the Czechs did not prevent John Wycliffe in England from proclaiming John Huss as a great leader. This nation, prostrated twice in 10 years by modern police states, should not be forgotten. Purkinje should remain in the minds of freemen of science as a great pioneer and powerful beacon.

Marshall Hall (1790-1857)

The physiology of the nervous system has been well represented by such medical students as Marshall Hall. Hall came from a remarkable family in the cotton-spinning and bleaching industry of Nottingham. They were the first in the United Kingdom to use chlorine for bleaching. It is said that Marshall and his inventor brother, Samuel, were raised on a mixture of religion and chemistry. After a four-year apprenticeship to a pharmacist, Marshall Hall embarked upon medicine at Edinburgh, where he was known as a student who dissected from early till late every day.

As an undergraduate he contributed a paper to *Nicholson's Journal*, on a chemical research. He was popular with his colleagues and elected president of the Royal Medical Society in his third year. While a student at Edinburgh he began work on a manuscript of a book that was to be the turning point of his life, *Diagnosis of Diseases*. He took the uncompleted manuscript with him when he left for London at the age of 24, and it was published three years later. A copy of this book came into the hands of John Hunter's nephew, Matthew Baillie, in London, who was so impressed with its contents that he sent a host of patients to Hall to be studied. Eight years later Hall set up in practice in Keppel Street, in London, near the present site of the School of Tropical Medicine of the University of London. He built a research laboratory in his house and was soon at work on a study of the circulation in animal tissues. His first paper in this field propounded the argument that the capillaries were the all-important structures in accomplishing the true work of the circulation.

One day in his laboratory Hall found that the tail that he had just removed from a salamander jumped when he handled it. With a curette he removed the spinal marrow that remained in this segment of the tail and thereafter found that touching it no longer caused it to move. He carried out the same experiment on a snake, making a transection of the spinal cord just below the head. He then found that even a breath of air would make the tail twitch, whereas if he wrapped it in cotton wool, no movement whatever was induced. He also found that if he cut off the head of a turtle and touched the nose, breathing movements ensued. From these observations he came to generalize that one message sent into the spinal marrow reflected another one along the motor pathways. For his work, on what would today be called "reflex action of the spinal cord," he was awarded his fellowship in the Royal Society. He is also remembered for his pioneer studies on artificial respiration of more than a century ago.

One of Marshall Hall's biographers, Sir Geoffrey Jefferson, concluded his writing about Hall: "His degree of importance was much debated in his own lifetime, and he took an embarrassingly active part in the discussion."

Charles-Edouard Brown-Séquard (1818-1894)

Poets and playwrights are common enough in the annals of French medicine but the playwright Brown-Séquard, successor in the chair of medicine at the Collège de France to the playwright Claude Bernard, was no ordinary Frenchman. In fact he was half American. His father was a Philadelphia sea captain, Charles Edward Brown, who sailed into the island of Mauritius, or the Isle de France, in the Indian Ocean, on his merchant ship. There he married Charlotte Séquard, a vivacious French resident. Their "Paul et Virginie" existence was interrupted by a famine that threatened the island and Captain Brown volunteered to sail a ship to India to collect rice. On the return journey the ship foundered with the loss of all on board.

Charles-Edouard was born then into a fatherless world, and had to make his way by working in a shop, while he wrote his plays and poems. His friends saw in him such promise that they financed his passage to Paris, where, discouraged by the critics, as Claude Bernard had been, he burned his manuscripts and entered medicine. To earn a living he tutored other students in his class, for he was ahead of them in his studies, especially since his gift for writing eased his way at examination time.

Two years before he graduated Brown-Séquard carried on research on the effect of human gastric juice on the food ingested. He swallowed sponges, which, when saturated, were pulled up by a string and the gastric juice collected and tested. His M.D. thesis, presented in 1846, was a preview of his life's work. In his words:

> This work is composed of two distinct parts: the first has for its object the study of reflex movements in batrachians, especially the augmentation of the reflex faculty after section of the cord; the second treats of the properties and functions of the columns of the cord and has for its chief aim the demonstration that the transmission of sensation is by way of the grey substance and not by the dorsal (posterior) columns. In this second part the author remarks that pricking the anterior columns of the cord in frogs, eels, pigeons, rabbits and dogs causes only local contractions, an important fact which shows the inexcitability of the longitudinal fibres of the anterior columns.

Here then, in his student thesis, is the germ of his later generalization that a spinal cord lesion produces a distal sensory loss on the opposite side of the body, and a motor deficit on the side of the lesion—the well-known "Brown-Séquard syndrome."

His American heritage may have taken him to Richmond where he held a chair in the Medical College of Virginia. He oscillated back and forth across the Atlantic, being at one time a professor at Harvard. He finally settled at the Collège de France where his life work was done, on the physiology of the nervous system and on the importance of the adrenal glands to survival of animal life.

Ivan M. Sechenov (1829-1905)

At the age of 22 Sechenov applied to enter the Moscow University Medical School, having already graduated in a military engineering school. He held the rank of lieutenant in an engineering regiment in Kiev. On entering the Moscow University medical faculty, he resigned his commission and studied with I.T. Glebow (1806-84). Glebow's dissertation for graduation in 1834 had been on physiological and pharmacological subjects; he then worked in European laboratories such as those of Bernard and Flourens. Sechenov became interested in reflexes and in psychophysiology. He graduated in Moscow in 1856 with a dissertation on the physiology of alcohol intoxication and concluded that vodka played a great part in Russian life.

Following in Sechenov's footsteps was **Vasili Danilevsky** (1852-1939). He was the son of a Kharkov watchmaker and began his studies at Kazan University (from which Lenin had been expelled as a law student). In 1873 Danilevsky won the Gold Medal for an original work by an undergraduate; in his case, on muscle physiology. This was published in Pflüger's *Archiv*. When at the age of 25 Danilevski graduated, his thesis was on "An Investigation into the Physiology of the Brain." He was one of the group of highly productive neurophysiologists so well chronicled by Dr. Mary Brazier. She reports that all the old buildings of the University of Kharkov were destroyed by the German Army in 1942, including the library with its collection of theses.

Napoleon Nicodemus Cybulski (1854-1919)

This notable student was a Lithuanian who attended the Military Medical Academy in St. Petersburg where he was a student of Tarkhanov, the discoverer of the galvanic skin response. As a second year student in 1878, Cybulski published his first paper, "Concerning the Influence of Body Posture on Blood Pressure, Pulse and Respiration in Animals." In 1880 he graduated with the Gold Medal for his class, for his work on the velocity of the nerve impulse. By the age of 31 he was professor of physiology and histology at Krakow. Citizens of Krakow helped him to equip his laboratory and in order to raise additional funds he gave popular public lectures. In fact, to achieve a decent income he invented a mouthwash.

Sir Charles Sherrington (1857-1952)

The great explorers in history have had rivers, seas and continents named for them. There is probably no single continent in the neurological world large enough to adequately memorialize the name of Charles Scott Sherrington as the explorer of the nervous system. He was a veritable Columbus. His name is associated with so many of the milestones in this sphere that one can appreciate the truth of the statement, "Sherrington did for the nervous system what Harvey did for the circulatory system."

Sherrington, though born in Islington, was associated throughout his life with Ipswich and the cities of Britain's eastern seaboard. His father died at an early age and his mother later married an Ipswich physician and scholar, Dr. Caleb Rose. Under his tutelage Charles was to develop, with his three brothers, into an active lad with artistic and literary interests, and with a flair for athletics—playing rugby for St. Thomas' Hospital and rowing for Caius College, Cambridge.

Throughout his life Sherrington was interested in the works of the physician-poet John Keats, as his own style of writing would suggest. With a classical education and an interest in science Sherrington found himself doubly prepared for a world that was rapidly changing in philosophical and scientific concepts. A colleague might be talking with him about some occult theory of consciousness when he would suddenly say, "Of course Cicero really expressed it better than we can." He maintained this ability to call on classical allusions to the end of his 95 years.

After a false start in medicine at Edinburgh, Sherrington entered Cambridge and there studied under the physiologist Michael Foster. As an undergraduate in Foster's laboratory Sherrington was caught up in one of the most interesting scientific controversies of the last century. The question being debated hotly was the existence of localized areas of the brain, specific for each function carried out by the body. The setting for the most forthright exchange of views in this matter was the Seventh International Medical Congress, held in London in 1881.

At this congress Professor Goltz of Strasbourg demonstrated a dog from whose brain he had made large tissue removals, and in whose performance he said he found no change. Goltz therefore concluded that there was no real localization of function in the brain whatever.

Goltz's own estimate of the dog's performance was at once challenged by Gerald Yeo, a surgeon who was at that time professor of physiology at King's College, London. Yeo thought the dog did show a deficit, and, in passing, he waxed caustic on the desirability of asepsis in neurosurgery.

Next on the programme came David Ferrier, the neurologist, demonstrating a monkey in which he and Yeo had made a cortical removal seven months previously. As the monkey dragged his limbs along on the side opposite to the removal, the great Charcot remarked, "C'est un malade." But this was not all. A second monkey was shown, from which the auditory cortex, as it is now known, had been removed on both sides, 10 weeks before. Exploding.a percussion cap beside it failed to produce any response, and deafness from the cortical removals seemed proven. As tempers rose over the two views—localization or no localization of function—it was suggested that the animals should be chloroformed forthwith and that a representative committee should report on the state of the brains. Only in England would the committee method have suggested itself. At all events, one hemisphere of the brain of Goltz's famous dog found its way to Cambridge with J.N. Langley of the Committee, and it was on this specimen that Sherrington the undergraduate was put to work. His first publication with Langley appeared in 1884, and in 1885 Sherrington, alone, published a further work concerning it. Sherrington found himself afloat on the sea of neurology, with a full tide running.

For a time Sherrington demonstrated in anatomy at Cambridge under Sir George Humphry who said of him at that time: "He did his work well and the students were much attached to him. His genial friendly qualities made him a general favourite and a most agreeable colleague." Proceeding to St. Thomas' Hospital Medical School, London, where he had his name on the register for some time, Sherrington carried on with his formal medical course, while demonstrating in histology. He qualified as M.R.C.S. in the latter part of 1884 and proceeded to Strasbourg to work with Goltz at first hand.

Returning to Cambridge he completed his M.B. degree with distinction and began his study of pathology. On a combined Cambridge University-Royal Society study of cholera, he, J. Graham Brown and C.S. Roy were sent to Spain to investigate claims that a vaccine against the disease had been perfected. They made many observations and postmortem examinations, but found the vaccine non-existent. In later years it was like a chapter out of *Don Quixote* and his windmills, to hear Sherrington relate the comic opera nature of parts of this adventure.

A year later he travelled to Italy to investigate another outbreak. He wisely used the opportunity to visit art galleries and libraries. (It was probably here that he contracted that expensive disease for which there is no cure, bibliophilia. It has since proven highly infectious, especially among neurologists.)

Sherrington took some of his pathological material to Berlin to examine in the laboratory of Rudolf Virchow. Virchow's life as a pathologist was almost over, so deeply had he become immersed in German politics. Although Sherrington found it more profitable to transfer to Robert Koch's laboratory, he nevertheless admired the manner in which Virchow stood up to Bismarck. Strasbourg had opened Sherrington's eyes to the jackboot of Prussianism, and he never forgot it. During the First World War and throughout the Nazi invasion of Spain beginning in 1936, Sherrington cursed the German dictators.

One apocryphal Oxford story is told in which Sherrington, early in 1914, sent some microtome knives to the Sartorious factory in Göttingen for resharpening. The war intervened and for four years Sherrington ruefully repeated his certainty that the steel blades had been turned into weapons to kill his countrymen. At the end of the war the resharpened blades were returned by post, with a note: "Due to unforeseen circumstances delivery has been delayed."

Instead of a proposed stay of six weeks in Koch's laboratory Sherrington remained until the following year, learning microscopic anatomy and bacteriology, which were later to be of the greatest use to him. While in Berlin he heard lectures by Helmholtz, DuBois-Reymond and Waldeyer. He dismissed the latter as superficial when he pointed out a nerve cell to Sir Charles as "Das Denkorgan." Waldeyer's later popularization of already-known facts as the "Neurone Theory" annoyed Sherrington mightily, and he always came vehemently to the defence of Cajal and Van Gehuchten, as the real authors of the concept.

Returning to England, Sherrington was made a lecturer in physiology at St. Thomas' Hospital Medical School. At the end of the year he was named Professor-Superintendent of the Brown Institution of the University of London as successor to Sir Victor Horsley. (This veterinary laboratory for the care of sick animals and for research into their diseases, was established by the will of Thomas Brown in 1852, but 19 years of discussion ensued before it was constructed.).In this setting Sherrington was to carry out some of his greatest detective work on the secrets of the nervous system. In probing the knee-jerk, he sought answers to the question: How did the spinal cord cause certain muscles to contract, extending the knee, when the patellar tendon was tapped?.He discovered that nerves connecting muscles to the spinal cord were approximately one-third sensory in function, and only two-thirds motor (i.e., causing contraction). Why were there sensitive fibres carrying messages from muscles to the nervous system?.This Sherrington answered with a series of papers on the microscopic pressure and tension receptors concealed within limb muscles. Thereafter, an explanation of posture became possible.

In an unusual incident Sherrington ushered in the use of diphtheria antitoxin in Britain. He had been immunizing a horse when news reached him that his nephew on the south coast had contracted the disease. He bled the horse and rushed serum to the patient in time to save his life. Lister was greatly excited by all this, when the story was told to him the same evening by his young friend.

The University of Liverpool appointed Sherrington to the Holt Chair of Physiology in 1895, and in that capacity he was to become one of the outstanding writers on science in the English-speaking world. With his visitor, Harvey Cushing, he explored the electrical currents on the surface of the brain in orangutangs, gorillas and chimpanzees. His discoveries required the coining of new terms that would be exact and not confusable. The early training at Ipswich Grammar School in language was to guide Sherrington in his choice of such terms as "synapse," "decerebrate rigidity" and "the final common pathway." His Silliman Lectures given at Yale University in 1904 advanced medical knowledge still further as he described "The Integrative Action of the Nervous System."

The Liverpool period was rich in discoveries made and lifelong friendships developed, such as that with the pioneer American neurosurgeon Harvey Cushing. Sherrington's boyish appearance and cycling were probably surprises to Cushing, who was fascinated by the gold spectacles perched precariously on the physiologist's nose, even when he had "lost" them.

The working out of the segmental arrangements within the nervous system, of the reciprocal action of antagonistic muscles, and reflex inhibition, all occurred in this fruitful period. Sherrington astounded some physiologists when he wrote that "Desistence from action may be as truly active as is the taking of action." He welded together neurophysiology and neuroanatomy at every turn, and in no place more successfully than at the "synapse" (from the Greek "clasp"), whose activity, multiplied by hundreds of times, gave rise to the "central excitatory state" or to the "central inhibitory state."

Sherrington often returned to his undergraduate work from Cambridge days, concerning the great centrifugal motor pathway, from the brain's surface to the cells of the spinal cord, known as the "pyramidal tract." So in succession came the experiments on "tonus," "decerebrate rigidity" and "the stretch reflex" which are known today, wherever neurology is practised, as the cornerstones.

In 1913 Sir William Osler, Regius Professor of Medicine at Oxford, convinced the board of electors that they should bring Sherrington to fill the Waynflete Professorship of Physiology there. The bibliophiles in Oxford, the humanists, the philosophers and most of all the students applauded this wise decision, for no single appointment did more to change Cecil Rhodes' gloomy prediction that there would never be an Oxford man at the top of the scientific tree. In the years 1913 to 1935 Sherrington had a succession of pupils who went to the top of the tree in many parts of the world: Penfield and John Fulton from the United States, Cairns, Eccles and Florey from Australia, Denny-Brown from New Zealand and Granit from Finland, to name but a few.

When World War I broke upon the world Sherrington went on a mission for the War Office—to work as an unskilled labourer in a munitions factory, investigating fatigue. No one in the factory knew him, and when he left after three months, the foreman offered him a letter of reference should he ever need it. His report that a 13-hour day, which he (aged 57) and his unskilled colleagues had worked, was too long to be efficient or safe, eventually found a sympathetic acceptance.

The end of the war brought Sherrington a well-earned period of diastole after four years of concentrated systole, and he was able to write his revolutionary book *Mammalian Physiology: A Course of Practical Exercises*. A foreign reviewer complained that the examples in the book were taken from English authorities only, little realizing that the data were those collected by physiology students, many of them American Rhodes scholars, in the laboratory at Oxford over the previous seven years.

The years between the wars were to be Sherrington's happiest and busiest. From 1920 to 1925 he served as president of the Royal Society, and found time to publish his *Assaying of Brabantius and Other Verse*. Some few have heard of it, but fewer still have had a chance to savour its contents. Two short examples follow:

NOW IN THE CLOISTER FEW THE FEET THAT ROAM
Now in the cloister few the feet that roam,
ours that must stay, who little can than wait,
exchange our tidings, good, ill, early, late,
and send our 'god–speed' to them past the foam,
the young folk, splashed with death in the trenched loam.
Ay, oil the hinges of the ancient gate,
keep burnished bright the goblet's silvern state
against the hour shall hail the soldier home.
You stately tower, from high you saw them go,
and have full many doughty scenes and fair
watched and swung bells above, shattering the air
to honour heroes, you too wait as though
of our poor hearth–bound presence scarcely ware,
you heard from far the filial bugles blow. (1916)

One can imagine Sherrington writing from his College, Magdalen, at the river's edge:

OXFORD
The night is fallen and still thou speakst to me,
what though with one voice sole, with accents many,
tongued turret and tongued stream, tracked pasture fenny,
and cloister spirit trod, and centuried tree,
and, bondsmen loosed in Time's tranquillity,
thy bell-dischargèd hours. If wharfage any
thine 'tis where Age shall, nursing late his penny,
smile at long last to hand him Charon's fee.
And now, below, through shadows starr'd, a boat
steals by me laden with singing and young laughter,
and, higher, a wide-flung casement casts afloat
pulses of waltz the which white robes sway after;
vowed Priest of Beauty, these they shrines among,
thou kneelst with old folk, thou that dancest with young. (1914)

Sherrington's literary life ranged from poetry to philosophy. His pupil E.G.T. Liddell relates that a few weeks after the publication of Robert Bridges' *The Testament of Beauty* in 1930, Sherrington, long an admirer of his medical student contemporary, fell to reciting long passages from it while preparing the experimental laboratory for the day's teaching. In the academic term 1937-38, Sherrington gave the Gifford Lectures at Edinburgh, published as *Man on His Nature*. Again because, as literature, this is so narrowly known, there follows an extract from it concerning "the brain and its work":

> A scheme of lines and nodal points, gathered together at one end into a great ravelled knot, the brain, and at the other trailing off to a sort of stalk, the spinal cord. Imagine activity in this shown

> by little points of light. Of these some stationary flash rhythmically, faster or slower. Others are travelling points, streaming in serial trains at various speeds. The rhythmic stationary lights lie at the nodes. The nodes are both goals whither converge, and junctions whence diverge, the lines of travelling lights. The lines and nodes where the lights are, do not remain, taken together, the same even a single moment...
>
> Suppose we choose the hour of deep sleep. Then only in some sparse and out of the way places are nodes flashing and trains of light-points running. Such places indicate local activity still in progress. At one such place we can watch the behaviour of a group of lights perhaps a myriad strong. They are pursuing a mystic and recurrent manoeuvre as if of some incantational dance. They are superintending the beating of the heart and the state of the arteries so that while we sleep the circulation of the blood is what it should be... .At intervals even a gush of sparks wells up and sends a train down the spinal cord only to fail to arouse it. Where however the stalk joins the headpiece, there goes forward in a limited field a remarkable display. A dense constellation of some thousands of nodal points bursts out every few seconds into a short phase of rhythmical flashing. At first a few lights, then more, increasing in rate and number with a deliberate crescendo to a climax, then to decline and die away. After due pause the efflorescence is repeated. With each such rhythmic outburst goes a discharge of trains of travelling lights along the stalk and out of it altogether into a number of nerve-branches. What is this doing?.It manages the taking of our breath the while we sleep.
>
> Should we continue to watch the scheme we should observe after a time an impressive change which suddenly accrues... The brain is waking and with it the mind is returning. It is as if the Milky Way entered upon some cosmic dance. Swiftly the head-mass becomes an enchanted loom where millions of flashing shuttles weave a dissolving pattern, always a meaningful pattern though never an abiding one; a shifting harmony of sub-patterns. Now as the waking body rouses, sub-patterns of this great harmony of activity stretch down into the unlit tracks of the stalk-piece of the scheme. Strings of flashing and travelling sparks engage the lengths of it. This means that the body is up and rises to meet its waking day.

Some thought these lectures his testament of age. Not so those who read them; nor were they surprised to learn of a revised edition being issued in 1951 when Sherrington was 94. The central figure of the early lectures, Jean Fernel (1497-1557), the early physiologist and pathologist, was further studied in Sherrington's delightful *Endeavour of Jean Fernel*, published in 1946.

At the age of 92 Sherrington spoke over the B.B.C. radio in a symposium on "The Physical Basis of Mind." He chuckled as he referred to some penny-in-the-slot theories of thought processes.

Honours failed to change the charming simplicity of this great man. He was awarded the Order of Merit in 1924, and it would have delighted him to know that after his death his place in this illustrious order, limited to a handful of scholars, was to be taken by his pupil Wilder Penfield.

Today the wheel has come full circle and the study that Sherrington made as an undergraduate in 1885 is the basis of today's neurosurgical operation of hemispherectomy to relieve certain cases of cerebral palsy.

The present generation profits by the work of this gifted medical student born over 100 years ago. As Sir Russell Brain's tribute, read at the Royal College of Physicians, expressed it:

> Yet he was the most modest of men who felt, like Newton, that he had done no more than pick up a few pebbles on the shore of the great ocean of truth.

Wilhelm His, Jr. (1863-1934)

His was the son of a famous medical teacher and researcher and was a precocious student at the University of Strasbourg. Before he graduated in medicine at Leipzig he did important work on the metabolism of pyridine in the body. Four years after graduating in 1889 His announced his discovery of the auriculo-ventricular bundle.

John Smyth Macdonald (1867-1941)

Macdonald graduated at Cambridge in 1889 and embarked on the study of medicine that had interested him since reading, as a schoolboy, *The Plague of Thucydides*. He pursued his medical studies at University College, Liverpool, where he served as demonstrator in physiology as a Holt Fellow from 1891 to 1895. His first research was undertaken with Francis Gotch who later became professor of physiology at Oxford. Macdonald achieved his medical qualification in 1897.

His first paper with Gotch was published in 1896 on "Temperature and Excitability," carrying this study through to tissues such as nerves, cardiac muscle and voluntary muscle. His postgraduate work concerned electrolytes affecting nerves and muscles, the injury current, the histology of nerve and muscle, and the heat production of muscle.

Robert Barany (1876-1936)

Barany had a varied and useful life in medical science. He was born in Vienna and graduated there in the year 1900. His M.D. thesis was on rhythmic nystagmus. Barany's clinical training with Emil Kraepelin in Heidelberg was followed by work under Adam Politzer at the University of Vienna otology clinic. He went on to determine the direction of human nystagmus when the outer ear was flushed with cold or with warm water. He recognized that the fundamental work of Santiago Ramón y Cajal had clarified the nerve pathways involved in the organ of balance and its connection with the muscles of the eye. The Barany rotating chair and the "finger-nose" test became routine.

He volunteered for the Austrian Army during World War I in 1914 but by April 1915 he was captured by the Russian Army and placed in a prison camp in Turkistan, where he quickly contracted malaria. At about this time he was awarded the Nobel Prize whereupon he was moved to the university city of Kazan. It took the united efforts of a Russian Grand Duke and the Swedish Red Cross under Prince Carl to bring him to Stockholm to receive his prize. Barany became a Swedish citizen and taught at the University of Uppsala. Another student contributor, C.S. Hallpike, was active in developing a Barany Society. Barany died of a cerebral haemorrhage at the age of 60, his life marked by honours and international recognition. It is sometimes forgotten that in his research he cooled the vestibular area of the cerebral cortex, thus producing vertigo. He was a forerunner in the study of the cerebral cortex long before local cooling of the brain became a recognized clinical research technique.

Thomas Renton Elliott (1877-1961)

Elliott entered Trinity College, Cambridge, in 1896 as a student of anatomy and physiology, among other subjects. However, he suffered appendicitis and typhoid so withdrew for one year. When he graduated with his bachelor's degree in 1901 it was with first-class honours.

Elliott's early student research began with Professor Langley on the ileo-colic sphincter. Thereafter his great work began on the correspondence to be observed between the effects of sympathetic nerve impulses and those of adrenalin. Sir Henry Dale has credited Elliott with being "the pioneer in the field of chemical transmitter function"—despite the "primitive speculation" of early physiologists. The research atmosphere in which Elliott grew up at Cambridge has probably never been bettered. Among those working in the laboratory of physiology were Sir Michael Foster, W.H. Gaskell, J.N. Langley, W.B. Hardy, H.K. Anderson on the autonomic system, Joseph Barcroft on the blood's respiratory function, Walter Morley Fletcher on muscle and Keith Lucas on neuro-muscular conduction.

Elliott delayed his entrance into the University College Hospital Medical School for his clinical training until he was 29. By then his research reputation brought him into contact with such luminaries as Sir Victor Horsley, John Rose Bradford, and Wilfred Trotter, the neurosurgeon turned social philosopher and vitriolic critic of the contemporary medical education. Elliott played a cardinal role in developing an academic unit at University College Hospital Medical School, where the Rockefeller Foundation gave great help with capital grants after the First World War, leading to an exemplary academic unit combining patient care, teaching and research.

Alexander Forbes (1882-1965)

This grandson of Ralph Waldo Emerson was born in Milton, Massachusetts, the eighth child of William Hathaway Forbes, who was president of the Bell Telephone Company.

Forbes received his bachelor of arts degree from Harvard in 1904 and his master of arts degree in 1905. He then entered the Harvard Medical School, graduating in 1910. As a medical student he published four papers, on Mendelian inheritance in guinea pigs, foreign body giant cells, epidermoid carcinoma of the tongue, and on a new method of estimating acidity and alkalinity (with L.J. Henderson). On graduation Forbes immediately joined Professor Walter Cannon in his physiological researches at Harvard and from 1911 to 1912 he worked with Sherrington at Liverpool. At Cambridge he spent a short time with the gifted Keith Lucas, so soon to be killed in a flying accident. Back at Harvard Alexander Forbes' star was rising in the department of physiology. In 1915 he collaborated with one of his medical undergraduates, Alan Gregg, and published their paper in the *American Journal of Physiology* in 1915, "Electrical Studies in Mammalian Reflexes: (1) The Flexion Reflex." Later Gregg became the Director of the Division of Medical Sciences at the Rockefeller

Foundation from 1931 to 1951 and played a key role in helping Wilder Penfield to develop and build the Montreal Neurological Institute.

With the First World War on, Forbes took flying lessons and became a fearless pilot carrying on this exercise into advanced age. He became a U.S. Navy admiral and mapped the coast of Labrador. There was no stopping him. He researched on anaesthesia, fatigue, beta rays, spinal reflexes and the electromyogram. After Forbes' wartime service had concluded he wrote to Sherrington in Liverpool, "Stanley Cobb and I had the good fortune to take an electrocardiogram and an electromyogram of an elephant a few days ago. The circus sent two of them and some other sideshows to amuse the children at the Children's Hospital next door; and I induced the keeper to let one of them stand under my windows while we ran wires out and did the tests. He was well trained and cooperated with us perfectly, contracting his trunk muscle for the electromyogram when told to; altogether the best experimental animal I have worked with."

Forbes was a pioneer in recording electrically from the exposed cerebral cortex of animals. When he could no longer keep track of all the substances alleged to be active in interneuronal transmission he merely described what he called "soup" at the synapse. Whether flying his airplane to scientific meetings, sometimes losing his glasses in the slipstream, or sailing to Bermuda and Naples, Forbes lived to a great age as a most productive researcher and teacher.

Thomas Graham Brown (1882-1927)

Prior to his graduation in medicine at the University of Edinburgh in 1906, Brown worked with the neurologist Edwin Bramwell on "experimental epilepsy in guinea pigs." With this background Graham Brown, as he was known, spent three years as a Carnegie Fellow in Sherrington's laboratory in Liverpool. His undergraduate work with Bramwell was published in 1905 in the *Review of Neurology and Psychiatry*.

Herbert Spencer Gasser (1888-1963)

Gasser was born in Wisconsin and enjoyed good teaching throughout his early schooling. He entered the University of Wisconsin Medical School that had just opened and worked as an undergraduate with Joseph Erlanger in physiology. He transferred to the medical faculty at Johns Hopkins University and spent a great deal of time in the laboratory of Professor W.H. Howell in physiology. Before graduating with the Hopkins M.D., Gasser had co-authored six papers on such subjects as intestinal absorption, stimulation of medullary centres, acceleration of the heart upon exercise, and effects of chemical products of muscular activity on the heartbeat.

Gasser built, with Joseph Erlanger, some of the earliest amplifiers and worked on the action potential of nerve fibres. Gasser spent two years with Nobel Prize winners A.V. Hill and Sir Henry Dale with whom he published several papers. In 1935 he succeeded Simon Flexner as director of the Rockefeller Institute in New York. He shared the Nobel Prize with Erlanger in 1943.

Edgar Douglas Adrian (1889-1977)

Edgar Adrian was born in London and attended the ancient Westminster School. In 1908 a scholarship took him to Trinity College, Cambridge, where he carried on student research with Keith Lucas on the "all-or-none" principle of nerve activity. He took his Cambridge undergraduate degree in 1911 and entered St. Bartholomew's Hospital Medical School in London, graduating there in 1915. He drew on his Cambridge undergraduate experience when he undertook war research on neurological injuries and shell shock. His neurophysiological research covered endorgans, single fibres and pain. He concentrated on the representation in the cerebral cortex of various forms of sensation. He published eight papers on neuromuscular subjects before he graduated in medicine.

Adrian's pioneer contribution was to the recording and interpretation of the electroencephalogram (EEG). He became a statesman of science and was called upon by many bodies for guidance in research policy. His cultural interests were broad and he was a gifted painter. As Master of Trinity College and later as Chancellor of Cambridge University, Adrian carried high public office with distinction. He loved the beautiful gardens along the River Cam and was rowed to his installation as chancellor in an "eight." He never forgot his student years and was always supportive of young people starting out on a research career. He shared the Nobel Prize with Sherrington in 1932...

Patrick Alfred Buxton (1892-1955)

In 1911 Patrick Buxton entered Trinity College, Cambridge, under the tutorship of Walter Morley Fletcher, having prior to that date wasted years on the classics that he hated. By 1914, however, he took a first-class in physiology, zoology and botany. In late 1913 he began medicine but with the outbreak of World War I in 1914 he enlisted as a private in a field ambulance unit. However, the authorities sent him back to medical school, and in 1915 he passed his second M.B. examinations. He haunted the physiology laboratory at Cambridge, learning methods from A.V. Hill and the gifted Keith Lucas. His undergraduate research concerned the nervous system of the primitive moth. The excellence of this won him a fellowship at Trinity College. He completed his medical qualification in 1917 and joined the Royal Army Medical Corps. He was sent to Mesopotamia and to northwest Persia. After some training in the London School of Tropical Medicine, he became entomologist to the Medical Department in Palestine and while there published his book *Animal Life in Deserts*. All of this graduate activity stemmed from the five papers he wrote before he qualified in 1917. As a result of two years in Samoa he produced "The Insect Fauna of Samoa." In 1926 he was made head of the department of entomology in the newly opened London School of Hygiene and Tropical Medicine, which the Rockefeller Foundation had supported. World War II found him dealing in the application of DDT to lice. His greatest publication was the 800-page *Natural History of the Tsetse Flies*, published in 1954.

John Farquhar Fulton (1899-1960)

John Farquhar Fulton was one of the most unusual medical undergraduates that Boston ever saw. Coming from St. Paul, Minnesota, he graduated with his bachelor of science degree at Harvard in 1921 and his medical degree in 1927. In those six intervening.years he spent a great deal of his time at Oxford, first as a Rhodes scholar and later as a fellow of Magdalen College, where he produced a book, *Muscular Contraction and the Reflex Control of Movement*, in which he prophetically discussed a chemical theory of nerve-impulse transmission. Before he graduated in medicine, Fulton wrote more than 30 papers, on subjects ranging from curare, procaine hydrochloride, muscle histology and decerebrate rigidity, to the early phrenological societies and their *Journal*. With Cohn, Minot and Murphy, he wrote a paper on the active principle in liver that was effective in the treatment of pernicious anaemia. This early beginning was but a foretaste of things to come, so that at the time of his death, early in 1960, John Fulton had a bibliography of 500 published items, including some of the most deservedly popular textbooks and scientific monographs in the English language.

Appointed as Sterling Professor of Physiology at Yale University at the age of 31, Fulton and his colleagues set the stage for a complete reappraisal of the function of the human frontal lobes of the brain. From his laboratory at Yale contributions to neurophysiology literally poured forth. Historical volumes such as those on Michael Servetus, the alleged heretic burned at the stake by John Calvin, the early physiologists at Oxford, Richard Lower and John Mayow and an endless array of bibliographies, including one on aviation medicine, stamped Fulton as a major contributor to the literature of medical history. His schedule both at New Haven, Connecticut, and at Washington, D.C., during World War II would have driven most researchers to distraction. He found refreshment and satisfaction in book collecting. With Harvey Cushing and Arnold Klebs he gave Yale University one of the finest collections of the world in medical history. He died of diabetic complications in 1960. He was a great correspondent and kept in touch with his early teachers, especially Sherrington, and with myriad students around the world. At Mill Rock on the height of land above New Haven he and his wife Lucia kept an American "open arms" that rivalled the one kept by Sir William and Lady Osler at Oxford for so many years. Fulton personified the helpful professor in medical schools.

Fulton's epitaph might reflect the introduction to the first edition of his scholarly work *Selected Readings in the History of Physiology* where he says, "For many reasons it is desirable that a medical student be conducted early in his career to the front-line trenches of medical and physiological discovery." John Fulton was such a conductor.

NEUROPHARMACOLOGY

Following are a few student contributors whose early work places them in the general heading of neuropharmacology.

Francis Martin Rouse Walshe (1885-1973)

This neurologist of later years began his career in 1910 when he published his undergraduate paper, "Sulfonal Poisoning: A Case, and Some Remarks on the Symptoms Usually Described." (Garrod and Hopkins published on this earlier.).It appeared in the *University College Hospital* magazine but sounded no trumpet as one of the most brilliant neurologists of his generation appeared on the scene. After taking a first-class honours degree in his bachelor of science work in 1908, he simply revelled in the clinical opportunities that opened up at University

College Hospital in London.

Walshe was probably the severest critic in the field of neurology in several decades, but the brilliance of his writing was awesome. His attacks on John Fulton and the Yale group—who turned out to be correct (concerning cortical representation of function and especially the pyramidal tract in spastic conditions)—were at times vitriolic.

As a Catholic he excoriated "the dreadful miraculist literature with which we disfigure the fair perspectives of our faith." He was a charming friend and a fearsome adversary. When Walshe became editor of the British journal *Brain*, he wrote to Sherrington concerning a volume of his writings: "I look to it to turn my mind sometimes from the grim world that surrounds us all now, and to renew in its pages some of the delight that I found when Bayliss first gave me my copy of *The Integrative Action* some thirty years ago when I was a student. Such as my work has been since, what I got from the book has been the best part." He added, "It would be impossible for me to overemphasize the excitement of mind this book produced in me—and kept alive over many years." One of Walshe's interests, out of many, was in the work of James Parkinson, and Walshe in his beautifully written textbook on neurology reminded his readers that in some cases it was possible, by infiltrating the skin on the back of the hand, with local anaesthetic, to prevent the "shaking palsy" in that hand.

Ulf Svante von Euler (1905-1983)

This student was the son of a German chemist who came to Sweden to work with Svante Arrhenius. Arrhenius won the Nobel Prize in Chemistry in 1903. Von Euler's father, who had the arresting name of Hans Karl August Simon von Euler-Chelpin, won the Nobel Prize for Chemistry in 1930 for his discoveries in plant chemistry and sugar fermentation.

U.S. Von Euler published his first scientific paper at age 17. He began studies at the Karolinska in 1922, graduating in medicine in 1930. For the four years prior to that time he was immersed in pharmacological research in Stockholm with Goran Liljestrand and Robin Fahreaus, the pioneer in the study of red blood cell sedimentation rate. Von Euler discovered many things including the prostaglandins, but in 1970 was awarded the Nobel Prize in Medicine or Physiology for his demonstration that noradrenaline was the neurotransmitter in the sympathetic nervous system. He also measured the catechol amines in pheochromocytomas. (Nerve fibres to those tumours were described by another student, Edith Bülbring.).Von Euler had to wait till 1970 for his Nobel Prize because he had served on the Nobel Committee for Medicine or Physiology and from 1965 was chairman of the Nobel Foundation.

Von Euler, throughout his research lifetime, was interested in the autonomic nervous system. His first paper actually studied vasoconstriction in the blood vessels of patients who had developed a high fever. For the four-year period with Liljestrand he pursued pharmacology of transmitter substances. These he then followed in Henry Dale's laboratory with John Gaddum. On returning to Stockholm he did the basic work on stimulators and relaxers of smooth muscle, leading to his work on prostaglandins. By 1946 Von Euler was able to confirm his earlier hunch of noradrenaline as an important neurotransmitter.

Von Euler was one of the international statesmen of science that Sweden has produced. The thorough undergraduate tutelage and opportunity that he enjoyed made him an outstanding scientist.

Carl Ferdinand Cori (1896-1984) and **Gerty Theresa Cori** (1896-1957)

This dedicated pair shared the Nobel Prize in Physiology or Medicine in 1947. From their university days their research lives were very much entwined. They were of a generation whose lives were severely interrupted by World War I. Carl was born in Prague, but at the age of two moved to Trieste, where his father became director of the Marine Biological Station. Though his father had studied medicine, he then took a Ph.D. degree in zoology and was well fitted for his directorship of that station. In the melting pot of Trieste, as it then was, Carl became fluent in Italian.

Carl's interest in many zoological species inspired him in the summer of 1914 to study the life forms of some of the uninhabited islands off the Dalmatian coast. His collection of insects led to his first publication, and his collection of specimens was given to the Natural History Museum of Vienna. Caught unawares by the outbreak of war while he was out at sea, Carl quickly set about registering as a student of medicine at the German University of Prague. With the war on, he was rapidly propelled through two years of chemistry, physics, biology, anatomy, biochemistry, physiology and pharmacology.

By the third year of his studies he was drafted into the Austrian Army and, because of his ability as a skier, served first with the alpine troops. After a close call he was put in the Sanitary Corps where, after an experience with typhoid himself, he developed a new interest in immunology. Very shortly he was transferred back to the Marine Biological Station in Trieste. His next posting was to the front lines on the Piave River in Italy, where he was enrollled in a course in clinical medicine and pathology given by professors from the University of Budapest. With a horse and buggy he was charged with looking after the Italian-speaking local population. The postwar wave of influenza turned him into a post-mortem expert.

With the Armistice, Carl set off on a freight car roof, which exposed him to low-flying aircraft. By the end of 1918 he was able to resume his clinical studies in Prague where he published a student paper on the effects of adrenalin and vagal stimulation on the excitability of the heart. In 1920 he graduated with his M.D. degree and was married in Vienna to his fellow student of the same age, Gerty Theresa Radnitz.

Gerty was born in Prague in 1896, where her father directed a sugar factory. After an education at home and at a Lyceum for Girls she studied chemistry sufficiently to enable her to register as a medical student with Carl in 1914. In the year of their graduation, 1920, they produced a joint work from the University Medical Clinic, on complement. Their journey from pharmacology to bacteriology was to be expected in a confused wartime situation that they barely survived. The near starvation of people in Vienna was a sad chapter in postwar history. As a clinician Carl was able to receive one free meal a day. Gerty was not so fortunate and developed symptoms of xerophthalmia. With a better diet at home in Prague she recovered. Carl took up work at the Pharmacological Institute despite the violently anti-Semitic atmosphere engendered by the director. It was with relief that he was offered a post at what is today Roswell Park Memorial Institute in Buffalo, New York. The blind officialdom encountered at Buffalo they tolerated for 10 years until 1931 when Carl was made professor of pharmacology at Washington University in St. Louis. There a new world opened to them of which another Nobelist, Professor Severo Ochoa, wrote: "Their lives followed more than just parallel courses; they followed a single, lofty and straight course. This life they shared with their students and collaborators in a spirit of friendship and understanding which, with the integrity and excellence of their scientific leadership, resulted in high accomplishment. Together these scientists survived racial discrimination and most miserable treatment as husband and wife anxious to work together. It says a lot for the human spirit that this pair could survive the indignities of blind authoritarianism mixed with a destructive war when they were undergraduates in Europe." They were the third married couple to share a Nobel Prize in science.

CLINICAL NEUROLOGY

Georgius Zecchius

In 1586 a medical student, Georgius Zecchius at the University of Basel in Switzerland, submitted his graduation dissertation on epilepsy and had it published by the famous printing house of Oporinus who had in 1543 published the work of another medical student contributor, Andreas Vesalius. Zecchius has been brought to modern notice by another graduate of the University of Basel, Dr. Peter Gloor, the scholarly neurophysiologist of the Montreal Neurological Institute.

Thirty years later the medical student Gregor Nymann (1594-1638) wrote his thesis at the University of Wittenberg, "*Disputatio de Apoplexia.*"

In the 18th century a landmark thesis was published by a medical student in Paris, L.F. Bravais. The title of his discourse was "Researches on the Symptoms and Treatment of Hemiplegic Epilepsy." Many years later Charcot coined the term "Bravais-Jacksonian Epilepsy," to denote focal seizures.

Marc Dax (1771-1837)

Dax was born in Tarascon-sur-Ariège and studied medicine at Montpellier, not far distant. In the Year VII of the Republic (1799), he wrote his graduation thesis on A *Record of the Medical Topography of Aigues-Mortes*. It would seem that Dax was a "pensionnaire escolaire" of that ancient walled town on the Mediterranean, near the westerly mouth of the Rhone River. The Middle Ages had seen crusade after crusade set sail from the fortress town, hopefully to return, guided by the great lighthouse surmounting the walls. Today Aigues-Mortes is far inland, its once-active harbour silted up, and its lighthouse no longer a guide to seafarers. The name originally meant, in Provençal, "dead or quiet waters," thus "safe harbour."

Dax's 33-page thesis, printed by Jean Martel of Montpellier, is a thorough account of all the diseases of all the inhabitants of the little walled city for a five-year period. The cause of death is set over against the name of each person dying in that time, and these mortality tables are a model of clarity. As well, Dax attached a set of commentaries, by diseases. He discusses fevers and the convulsions that they caused in children. It is clear that he already had a neurological bias, as he wrote, "Epilepsy seems to be getting more frequent day by day and the convulsions to which children are prone, sometimes leave them with partial paralysis, and sometimes there is added, imbecility."

Important discoveries were being made in that ancient medical school, Montpellier, cradle of the liberal international spirit in medicine. Here, before the Meridional Medical Congress of 1836, Marc Dax read his paper "Lesions of the left Half of the Brain Associated With the Loss of Signs of Thought," or aphasia. He had been studying cases with loss of speech since he was 24 years old, and by the age of 60 he is said to have described 140 patients. Some of these were sent to him for study by Baron Larrey, surgeon to Napoleon's armies. Perhaps because Dax was a legitimist in French politics, he was unpopular in Montpellier at the time of giving his paper. At all events it was not published, but remained in the possession of the dean of the faculty of medicine there. In the controversy concerning aphasia and cerebral localization that developed 25 years later in Paris, the son of Dax, himself a doctor, published the original 1836 manuscript. The work shows that Dax understood very well the import of his post-mortem observations. Though he searched, he was not able to find a single case of destruction of the right hemisphere in a right-handed person suffering from aphasia.

Nathan Strong, Jr. (1781-1837)

This little-known figure published a graduation dissertation at Hartford, Connecticut, in 1810 entitled, "On the Disease Termed Petechial or Spotted Fever." It was as important,in its way, as Elisha North's monograph of 1811 on cerebrospinal meningitis, which is usually quoted as the earliest definitive work.

Asmus Julius Thomas Thomsen (1815-1896)

This physician was born in Brunsholm, Denmark. He studied medicine at the University of Kiel, at Copenhagen, and at Berlin. In 1839 he qualified in medicine and wrote his graduation thesis on dipsomania. He began practice in Kappein, Germany, and all his life suffered from muscle weakness and cramps, which he was sure was an inherited illness. When he was 61 his youngest son, who had the disease, was accused of trying to evade military service by claiming this illness. Thomsen, Sr., therefore set out to clarify this situation and wrote the definitive account of his family's disease, tracing it back to his maternal great-grandmother. His account appeared in 1876. Today the disease is known as myotonia congenita.

Charles Oscar Waters (1816-1892), upon graduating in medicine in 1841 wrote to Professor Robley Dunglison at Jefferson Medical College noting a hereditary chorea with onset in middle life and with "perfect dementia." Five years later Charles R. Gorman (1817-1879) wrote his M.D. thesis at Jefferson Medical College in Philadelphia in 1846, "On a Form of Chorea, Vulgarly Called 'Magrums.'"Unfortunately, that thesis was lost during the demolition of college buildings at Jefferson.

Charles Louis Alphonse Laveran (1845-1922)

Laveran is remembered as the scientist who discovered the malarial parasite and for seemingly endless contributions to tropical medicine during a long and useful life. His father and grandfather had both been doctors and his mother was one of the de la Tour family of army commanders. Alphonse entered the Imperial School of Military Medicine at Strasbourg in 1863 and moved into clinical training in 1865. By the time he graduated in medicine in 1867 he had written an important work on injuries to the nerves and on the regeneration of these nerves.

He began his military service at Val-de-Grace, which had been the home of Napoleon's battle surgeon, Baron Dominique Larrey. Laveran suffered many attacks from people who did not believe in the parasitic nature of malaria. Some were wedded to the bacterial theory. However, Laveran persuaded Pasteur and Emile Roux by personally demonstrating a severe case of malignant malaria in a soldier in Paris. The French Army studiously ignored his great work and sent him to menial administrative tasks. However, the Pasteur Institute in Paris rallied to his defense and support. When, therefore, Laveran won the Nobel Prize for Medicine in 1907 he gave half of it to the Institute to fully equip a research laboratory specifically for tropical medicine.

Professor Pierre Marie (1853-1940) makes reference to his pupil Moutier who wrote a thesis on aphasia at Bicêtre. Another student, A. Amberg, wrote his Berlin thesis for graduation in medicine in 1855, "*Dissertatio de tabe dorsuali*," in which he emphasized the miosis associated with that disease and gives at least a faint intimation of the fixation of the pupil. He also later described *strabismus convergens*.

Edouard Brissaud (1852-1909)

Edouard Brissaud lived a life full to overflowing with clinical observations, on paralysis agitans, medico-legal problems in injuries of the nervous system, history, and folklore. His life was cut short by a brain tumour, which was operated upon in Paris by Sir Victor Horsley—too late. As a medical student he began his neurological writings by discussing, in his graduation dissertation, the paralysis that follows a stroke—otherwise known as hemiplegia. The permanent contractures which ensued, and which so deformed once-flexible limbs occupied most of his attention. It is interesting, in the light of his later medico-legal writings, that his thesis clearly described a type of periodic or remitting hemiplegia found in lesions of the pons, adjacent to the bulbar area. Brissaud was one of the founders of that bible of French neurology, the *Revue Neurologique*.

Otfrid Foerster (1873-1941)

This self-taught neurosurgeon began his medical training at the University of Breslau and graduated there in 1897 with a thesis on agglutination and bactericidal activity of blood serum from convalescent typhus cases. His work was immediately reported in German journals, as was his work on the serodiagnosis of abdominal typhus.

Foerster's life work was in the neurological field and from seeing patients with brain injuries in the First World War he wrote many papers on epilepsy. In 1930 he published in *Brain*, with Wilder Penfield, a landmark paper, "The Structural Basis of Traumatic Epilepsy and Results of

Radical Operation."He is.said to have been the first to carry out electrocorticograms in the operating room to localize cerebral tumours. Professor Zulch has credited him with introducing hyperventilation to provoke epileptic seizures.

Andre Leri (1875-1930)

In 1922 Leri described what is today known as his syndrome, "Une maladie congenitale et hereditaire de l'ossification." However his student thesis was in the neurological world, where he reported on "Eye changes in tabes dorsalis." He then worked with Pierre Marie on ankylosing spondylitis. By 1929 his own bone pain and X-rays confirmed his suspicion that he had cancer. He died a year later at age 55. His syndrome combines small stature, small joint mobility, contractures, and thickening palmar and plantar fascia.

PSYCHOLOGY AND PSYCHIATRY

J.E.D. Esquirol (1772-1840)

Student contributors in the field of psychiatry may have been few but they became the pillars of this important branch of medicine. J.E.D. Esquirol, the favourite pupil of Pinel the reformer, wrote his graduation thesis in 1805 on "The Emotions Considered as Causes, Symptoms and Curative Means in the Field of Mental Illness."The tide was just beginning to turn in the vast sea of torture and abuse to which mental patients had been subjected. The lashing and chaining of patients and the "non-injurious torture" prescribed by Reil among others—such as shooting off cannon and ducking patients in water—was being replaced by Pinel's humane approach. If it took courage on Pinel's part to strike the chains from the incarcerated patients, it probably took more courage on the part of the medical student Esquirol to say that Pinel's controversial treatment was right and had a sound scientific basis.

Esquirol's later life bore out the promise of his early years. He introduced many elements into psychiatry: the use of the statistical method in mental disease; the term "hallucination" as it is understood today; and a saner outlook on responsibility before the law of mentally sick people. Like his teacher, Pinel, he was an innovator in a long-ignored field of medicine. In turn, his own students, such as Baillarger, carried the torch, and campaigned for the rehabilitation of patients discharged from mental hospitals—a labour of love still crying out to be effectively done.

Edward Osler (1798-1863)

This medical student was indentured as a surgeon's apprentice to James Dunn Trevasso of Falmouth, Cornwall, for five years from March 22, 1811. In the documents signed the student had to "faithfully serve his secretes... Tavernes of custome he shall not haunt," etc. As Sir William Osler wrote, "Edward Osler was my father's eldest brother. After serving his apprenticeship he went to the United Hospitals of Guy's and St. Thomas' and took the M.R.C.S."

In the year 1817, at the age of 19, Edward Osler read part of his thesis to the Abernethian Society on the subject "A Dissertation on Nervous Influence. Life. The Will." One year before he wrote in his notes:

"Surgery by Astley Cooper delivered at the Theatre St. Thomas' Hospital in the course commencing October 8, 1816." It deals with Cooper's heroic ligature of the abdominal aorta.

Of his Uncle Edward, Sir William Osler wrote:

> As a boy in the backwoods settlement in Upper Canada, the English post would bring letters from Uncle Edward for whom we cherished an amazing veneration; for on the shelves in father's little study were there not actually books written by him, and poems, and mysterious big articles with drawings about shells, and now and again did we not sing in Church one of his hymns?.The reputation of the family seemed to circle about this uncle, whose letters were always so welcome, so full of news of the old home, and so cheery.

William James (1842-1910)

William James was the eldest son of Henry James, Sr., the leading American disciple of the religious mystic Emanuel Swedenborg, and intimate of Emerson, Carlyle and other British scholars. William grew up with private tutors and with an exposure to progressive schools in England and in France. Central to his later work was his command of European languages and literature. From 1857 to 1858 he was a student at the Collège of Boulogne-sur-Mer followed by a year at the University of Geneva in Switzerland.

His artistic education was furthered by the well-known American portrait painter William H. Hunt at Newport, Rhode Island. At the age of 19 he entered the Lawrence Scientific School at Harvard University, where he studied chemistry under Charles Eliot, later president of Harvard. In Eliot's view, James was not a hard-working student. The study of comparative anatomy was also added to his repertoire and at the age of 21 James entered Harvard Medical School. At the age of 23 he dropped everything and went with the famous zoologist Louis Agassiz to the Amazon basin in South America, expecting to become a naturalist. However, he made a discovery there that was to change his life. He discovered that he was really a philosopher and not cut out for mere observation. He returned to Cambridge, Massachusetts, for more of his medical course, but then went off for one and a half years to Germany. From Berlin he wrote to a friend, "It seems to me that perhaps the time has come for psychology to be a science."

In those years Helmholtz, another student discoverer and Wilhelm Wundt were introducing experimental methods in physiology and psychology. Although William James graduated in medicine at Harvard in 1869, he was ill for approximately three years. However, in 1872 he was appointed an instructor in physiology at Harvard and was able in 1875 to offer a graduate course on "The Relations between Physiology and Psychology" and founded the first psychological laboratory in the United States. He was having such trouble with his eyes that he searched for a volunteer from the medical class who would read to him each day a chapter from Wundt's *Psychologie*. Another student discoverer, Bernard Sachs (1858-1944), volunteered. Sachs was already working on his dissertation, "Comparison of the Fore and Hind Limb in Vertebrates," which won him the Bowdoin Prize and $50. Webb Haymaker reveals that half the money went to purchase a copy of Darwin's *Works*. The remaining half went for a dinner with four of his friends.

This was three years before Wundt founded his institute for the same purpose at Leipzig. By that time William James had signed a contract with his publishers to produce his book on the subject in two years. Due to illnesses of various descriptions, it actually took 12 years.

A full professorship in psychology was given James by Harvard in 1889 and by the year 1907 he resigned from Harvard in order to devote more time to writing. He died at age 68.

William James is quoted in many directions by many scholars. He accused neuroanatomists and physiologists of constructing "a psychology without a soul." Others have described him as a forerunner in fashioning the neurone theory. William Osler recalled that "in one of his Hibbert Lectures last year at Oxford, William James made a remark that clung—'we live forward, we understand backwards...the fleeting moment was as we try to catch it.'" While Osler was saying one thing about Oxford, William James was saying just the opposite. In his Linacre Lecture at Oxford in 1908 Osler said, "Through the centuries the collegiate tail continued to wag the University dog, and to this day in Oxford at least the higher faculties remain to a greater extent unorganized and under the control of the Masters of Arts. The system has worked well for the squire but badly for learning, admirably for the school-master and the parson, but badly for the nation since it permitted the old universities to sleep on for years after science had cried her message from the housetops—Awake! Awake! for the light has come!" At the same time William James wrote, "Let other places of learning go in for the improvements!.The world can afford to keep her one Oxford unreformed. If I were an Oxonian, in spite of my radicalism generally, I might vote against all change there."

Habit is... the enormous fly-wheel of society.
William James

Soon Osler was writing to Professor H.P. Bowditch at Harvard concerning "a delightful three months" in Paris where Bergson paid a remarkable tribute to William James, whom he called "the most distinguished and stimulating of living thinkers in Philosophy."

Emil Kraepelin (1856-1926)

The future leader in the field of psychiatry graduated from medicine at Würzburg. Much criticism has been directed at Kraepelin. Balancing this is the writing of Clarence B. Farrar, of Toronto, the editor of the *American Journal of Psychiatry*, who tells what it was like to study with these giants at Heidelberg. From this delightful, first-hand study, one can see Kraepelin's lifelong drive to contribute. As an undergraduate he won a prize for his essay, "The Influence of Acute Somatic Illness on the Development of Mental Disorder." Very honestly Farrar adds, "No one else competed." At the age of 27, Kraepelin produced a thin *Compendium of Psychiatry* during the Easter holidays; again, as Farrar admits, because Kraepelin needed the money. However, by the end of his career, his *Compendium* had grown to four volumes containing 2,372 pages.

While studying with Wundt, the psychologist, Kraepelin did many experiments on the effects of toxic substances on animal behaviour. He believed in external causes of mental disease, and blamed alcohol first. He had a phobia about this, and was the butt of many pranks by his laboratory colleagues as a result. Metabolic factors, exhaustion and fevers were included in his list. The internal factors or predispositions he saw as sex, age and occupation. The "personal" factors, specific for an individual, were heredity and "faulty upbringing." He had some racial views reminiscent of Morel's degeneration theory. However, Farrar says these never obscured the eye of Kraepelin the great observer. He is dismissed by many as the father of "descriptive psychiatry," as if this were reprehensible. The fact is that he was the father of a revivified psychiatry based on observation. He knew the natural history of mental diseases as few have done since. The classification of the major psychoses as manic-depressive on one hand, and dementia praecox on the other, stems from his own observations and deductions.

At the age of 30 Kraepelin became professor of psychiatry at Dorpat and at age 40 he was made professor at Heidelberg, where he stayed for 14 years, leaving to become head of a research institute in Munich. He died in 1926 at the age of 70 while still working.

Alfred Binet (1857-1911)

Occasionally medical students get off the beaten track, some never to graduate with the M.D. degree. Such was Alfred Binet, who was born in Nice in 1857, the only child of a medical father and grandchild of a grandfather who had been a doctor attending Napoleon. As a child Binet added English and Italian to his native French language. By age 15, in Paris, he was winning prizes at school in French language, composition and discourse as well as in Latin translation. He undertook the study of law and by age 21 was a licentiate. He said, however, "As for the law, that is the career of men who have not chosen a vocation."

As a medical student he became diverted through reading Herbert Spencer, Alexander Bain, Francis Galton of genetic fame, Helmholtz's *Optique Physiologique* and especially John Stuart Mill, who for years was his mentor. The air was full of controversies concerning free will, evolution, the nature of consciousness, and "the principles of association of ideas."

Binet's first paper was published in 1880 in the *Revue philosophique*. As students age 23 are sometimes given to florid and comprehensive theories, Binet sought to explain all of psychology.

He was saved from this environment when, in 1882, Joseph Babinski, his classmate who was on the way to stardom in neurology, took Binet to the Salpêtrière where neurology and to some degree psychiatry were presided over by Jean Martin Charcot. Binet became Charcot's shadow and for seven years observed large numbers of patients in that hospital, particularly those who were hypnotized hysterics, which abounded in Charcot's practice. This caused Binet to focus on disassociation as opposed to his earlier interest, association. With Charcot's colleague, Charles Fere, Binet wrote a book on animal magnetism. He progressed in his writing, which was widely recognized especially after he won a prize of 1000 francs awarded by the Academy of Moral and Political Sciences. Perhaps because it had 511 hand-written pages, the essay was never published. Drawing on his seven years of experience in the clinic, he wrote: "Doctors of psychopathology must start with the normal state before drawing conclusions." The evaluating committee of the Academy wrote in their adjudication, "This is the work of a mind that is very open, curious, searching..., of a man who has frequented laboratories and hospitals... who makes methodical experiments, sometimes on sane subjects, sometimes on those with different degrees of mental illness. The Salpêtrière is his field of study... The paper shows an independent mind and effectiveness as an observer and experimenter."

Binet then plunged into zoology and dissection and a course in botany. He used the term "comparative psychology" to cover the work that he was doing on the behaviour, physiology, histology, and anatomy of insects, culminating in his thesis for the degree of Doctor of Science in 1894. The title of his work was "A Contribution to the Study of the Subintestinal Nervous System of Insects." With the text he supplied beautiful drawings that he had done himself. So much for Alfred Binet the medical student. The rest is history, as his graded tests for mental status have been adopted and elaborated generations later.

Arnold Lucius Gesell (1880-1961)

Arnold Gesell was proud to have been born in a small town that boasted two streets in the state of Wisconsin. At the age of 16 he entered a "teachers' institute." He revelled in the motto of his home state: "Forward." In the Normal School he developed an interest in biology and met a graduate of Clark University. After two years at the University of Wisconsin at Madison Gesell won a fellowship to Clark University, where the Hopkins-trained President G. Stanley Hall was developing studies on children. After taking his Ph.D. in 1906 at Clark University, Gesell served for a year in a settlement house on the East Side in New York. With his wife he then visited training schools for mentally retarded children and taught in California in association with Lewis Terman.

As a result of exposure to these developing areas, Gesell decided to study medicine in order to get a better background for his work with children. He completed his first year of medicine at Madison, Wisconsin, and was then offered an assistant professorship at Yale's new School of Education. He was able to juggle his timetable sufficiently that he could both teach at Yale and graduate in medicine there in 1915. By that time he had to his credit eight publications. He was soon promoted to a full professorship at Yale Graduate School.

During this concentrated struggle to both teach psychology and study medical subjects, Gesell nevertheless as early as 1911 founded the now famous Yale Clinic for Child Development, where medical students could come face to face with problems that would confront them in practice.

With Rockefeller and Carnegie backing, his clinic branched out into cinematography. Gesell said of it, "By itself it bakes no scientific bread, but as a tool for psychological research, its potentialities are inexhaustible." One-way vision screens became popular for child observation and the laboratory launched into the study of twins, macacus rhesus monkeys, chimpanzees, and particularly blind children. Around it the Institute of Human Relations was built, which brought kudos to Yale.

Otto Meyerhof (1884-1951)

Not every Nobel Prize winner in Medicine for his work in biochemistry could say that he began life in psychiatric research. This was the situation for Meyerhof as he graduated with the M.D. at Heidelberg after studying medicine at Freiburg, Berlin and Strasbourg. His M.D. thesis written in 1909 at Heidelberg was published in 1910 as "*Beitraege zur psychologischen Theorie der Geistesstoerungen*." His undergraduate studies were laden with psychology, philosophy and psychiatry.

He had the good fortune to enter the medical clinic of Ludwig Krehl who was a physiologist turned clinician and a pathologist as well. His textbook, *Pathological Physiology*, was translated into English with the help of Albion Walter Hewlett who was a member of the class graduating in 1900 at Johns Hopkins Hospital Medical School in Baltimore along with such worthies as Henry Christian; Clarence B. Farrar, the future psychiatrist; J.B. MacCallum, a short-lived but brilliant student contributor on the heart; Dorothy Reed, after whom an important cell was named; and Florence Sabin, the future anatomist. Because Hewlett had been such a favourite of William Osler, Professor of Medicine at Johns Hopkins, Osler provided for the English translation a very laudatory introduction to Krehl's classic. It was in Krehl's clinic that Meyerhof first met another future Nobelist, Otto Warburg.

Lionel Sharples Penrose (1898-1972)

Coming from 200 years of Quaker ancestry, Penrose chose to serve on Red Cross trains in France in World War I. In January 1919 he was demobilized and entered St. John's College, Cambridge. He took his bachelor of arts degree there in 1921, having studied with Bertrand Russell in mathematical logic, but principally in psychology. In 1921 he enjoyed a year of research with the recognized pioneer in psychology, F.C. Bartlett. Leaving Cambridge he went to Buhler's laboratory in Vienna where his interests were memory and perception. There he met Sigmund Freud, Wagner Jauregg, and Paul Schilder, all student contributors. In Vienna he developed his interest in abnormal psychology and in mental disorders generally.

Returning to Cambridge in 1925, Penrose decided to study medicine and completed his qualification at St. Thomas' Hospital Medical School in London in 1928. He was invited to Canada as Director of Psychiatric Research for the Province of Ontario and in 1945 returned to London as the Galton Professor of Eugenics at University College Hospital, London. This laboratory, endowed by Francis Galton, who died in 1911, was host to many postdoctoral students from the United States of America. In London, it was said that while Penrose was associated with the explosive Professor J.B.S. Haldane, his laboratory was as far removed geographically as possible to minimize the latter's reported "outbursts." Penrose was the first of the Galton professors to have a medical degree. On his retirement, he was given an award by the Joseph P. Kennedy Foundation. His publications numbered 281.

Konrad Lorenz (1903-1989)

Though born in Vienna Lorenz took his premedical training at Columbia University in New York City. Before he graduated in medicine in Vienna in 1928 Lorenz had published a number of studies on "imprinting." He then proceeded to take a Doctor of Philosophy degree in 1933 by which time he was married to a gynaecologist, who found that her house was filled with tame rats, cockatoos and jackdaws.

In 1941 Lorenz began his service in the German Army as a physician, which took him on such duties, especially neurological, into Poland. There he was taken prisoner by the Russians who moved him to

Armenia and then to a camp near Moscow. He was not released until 1948.

In his work with baby ducklings he found that these very young birds recognized him as an individual, in many ways as if he were their mother. During this limited time period he formed the view that the imprinting was genetically determined. He felt that the process was irreversible. He did not meet Tinbergen until 1936, but with that Dutch zoologist he was recognized jointly in the award of the Nobel Prize in 1973.

[1]. His inaugural lecture is remarkable for the broad spectrum of interests it discloses. Besides visual subjects such as dioptrics, it covers skin sensation, and, most importantly, contains the first mention of fingerprints as having individual characteristics.

CHAPTER THIRTEEN

Nutrition

Daniel Whistler (1619-1684)

Whistler was born in the County of Essex and took his bachelor of arts degree at Oxford, being a student of Merton College. On October 18, 1645, at the age of 25, Whistler presented his thesis for the doctor of medicine degree at Leyden. The short form of the title is "*De morbo puerili Anglorum*." Beyond the Latin title Whistler used the term "the Rickets." He speculates upon the origin of the term but says, "However, not to argue further, I would stand godfather, and for the present let the infant name of this infantile disease be 'Pseudo-splanchnosteocaces.'"

What Whistler was trying to do was to bring together all the characteristics and criteria for considering this a single disease. It was only a beginning, but he called attention to the enlarged joint epiphyses, knotty swellings where the bones of the ribs joined their cartilages, and says, "the whole bony system is in truth flexible like wax that is rather liquid, so that the flabby and toneless legs scarcely sustain the weight of the superimposed body." He said that the patients were "too feeble to sit up, much less to stand." He noted the increased head size, the soft ligaments, the late cutting of teeth with many decaying, the narrow chest, difficult respiration, a low fever, slow pulse, thick urine, decreased appetite, dislike of sweets. Some might be bright, even precocious. Some might have scurvy-like skin patches.

Whistler's account came 63 years after a disputation held at Basle in 1582 by Jerome Reusner, who spoke of curved, weak limbs and deformed ribs. Whistler's account clearly preceded the publication by Francis Glisson of the year 1650. This Cambridge man, who served as Regius Professor for 40 years, gave a more complete account of rickets five years after Whistler, and added a fuller description of infantile scurvy.

James Lind (1716-1794)

Indeed, before this subject could be set in a clear and proper light, it was necessary to remove a great deal of rubbish.
James Lind, Introduction to
A Treatise on Scurvy (1853)

James Lind has been called "the father of nautical medicine." He was the son of a merchant and at age 14 finished grammar school in which he was competent in Latin and Greek. Soon after turning 15 James Lind became apprenticed to a well-known Edinburgh physician. After eight years of tutelage Lind joined the Royal Navy as a Surgeon's Mate. No sooner had he done that than war broke out between England and Spain, so that he was certainly kept busy. The writer Tobias Smollett joined the navy in the same year as did Lind. He was later to say of the lowly rank which he and Lind occupied that Captain Oakham "was too much of a gentleman to know a surgeon's mate, even by sight." Sir Sheldon Dudley has added recently, "Surgeons, and *a fortiori* surgeon's mates occupied a very lowly position in the naval hierarchy of those days."

The U.S. naval historian, J.S. Taylor, wrote in 1920 of Lind and his fellow campaigners Trotter and Blane: "They struggled against stupidity, ignorance, prejudice and indifference, in high places and low, the Admiralty and the forecastle; they had the hard task of seeking to break down immemorial custom; dared to challenge 'tradition'; hammered at the walls of a hierarchy as soul-chilling, as rigorous, as iron-bound as any Brahmin caste; preached seemingly frivolous novelties to an insular conservatism that held hardships essential for hardihood." This all sounded very much like the criticism by Florence Nightingale of the British army during and after the Crimean War.

From 1746 to 1747 Lind found himself on the H.M.S *Salisbury* on duty in the English Channel. On May 20, 1747, Lind began his famous controlled experiment on the treatment of scurvy. On June 16 his ship arrived in Plymouth and that ended the experiment.

Seven years before Lind's famous experiment with orange and lemon juice, Commodore Anson set out to circle the world, and en route to plunder any Spanish treasure ships that might be encountered. After four years at sea Anson, who had started off with 2000 men, arrived back in Britain with only 200. Lind was aware of the use of lemon juice by certain explorers and surgeons in the fleet and must have been staggered at the number of myths and anecdotal accounts concerning the alleged cure of scurvy by other means. Everything that a sailor might encounter on a voyage was blamed for scurvy. It was all reminiscent of the fog of nonsense spoken with distinction of various commanders in the past. He probably pondered on this for a long time before he set up his controlled experiment.

Lind tells the story clearly: "On the 20th of May 1747, I selected twelve patients in the scurvy, on board the *Salisbury* at sea. Their cases were as similar as I could have them. They all in general had putrid gums, the spots and lassitude, with weakness of their knees. They lay together in one place, being a proper apartment for the sick in the fore-hold; and had one diet common to all, viz. water-gruel sweetened with sugar in the morning; fresh mutton-broth oftentimes for dinner; at other times light puddings, boiled biscuit with sugar, etc. and for supper, barley and raisins, rice and currants, sago and wine, or the like. Two of these were ordered each a quart of cyder a-day. Two others took twenty-five drops of elixir vitriol three times a-day, upon an empty stomach; using a gargle strongly acidulated with it for their mouths. Two others took two spoonfuls of vinegar three times a day upon an empty stomach; having their gruels and their other food sharpened with vinegar as also the gargle for their mouth. Two of the worst patients, with the tendons in the ham quite rigid, (a symptom none of the rest had) were put under a course of sea water. Of this they drank half a pint every day and sometimes more or less as it operated by way of gentle physic. Two others had each two oranges and one lemon given them every day. These they ate with greediness, at different times upon an empty stomach. They continued but six days under this course, having consumed the quantities that could be spared. The two remaining patients took the bigness of a nutmeg three times a-day, of an electuary recommended by an hospital-surgeon, made of garlic, mustard-seed, horse-radish, balsam of Peru, and a gum myrrh; using for common drink barley-water boiled with tamarinds; by which, with the addition of cream of tartar, they were gently purged three or four times during the course."

Lind concluded, "The consequence was, that the most sudden and visible good effects were perceived from the use of oranges and lemons; one of those who had taken them being at the end of six days fit for duty. The spots were not indeed at that time quite off his body, nor his gums sound; but without any other medicine than a gargle for his mouth he became quite healthy before we came into Plymouth which was on the 16th of June. The other was the best recovered of any in his condition; and being now pretty well, was appointed nurse to the rest of the sick.

"Next to the oranges I thought the cyder had the best effect. It was indeed not very sound. However, those who had taken it were in a fairer way of recovery than the others at the end of the fortnight which was the length of time all these different courses were continued, except the oranges. The putrefaction of their gums, but especially their lassitude and weakness, were somewhat abated, and their appetite increased by it." Lind added that the other treatments were of no avail and there was no sign of recovery in the patients.

Lind recommended in addition to the citrus juices, sauerkraut, onions, possibly in soup, cress, parsley or similar green vegetables grown on board ship, fruit kept in dry bottles, cider or fruit wines such as gooseberry, blackberry, currant, elderberry or orange wine. He set out at the same time to improve the working conditions on board ship and hoped that a fiddler, a singer, "or anyone possessing special talents for entertainment should be utilised to furnish supervised amusement."

One year after this experiment Lind left the Royal Navy to attend the faculty of medicine at Edinburgh, from which he graduated in 1748 with the degree of Doctor of Medicine. By then clinical teaching in the wards of the Royal Infirmary had been established. His thesis, "*De morbis venereis localibus*," has never been translated into English.

Lind's classic, *A Treatise of the Scurvy*, was published in 1753, dedicated to Lord Anson. This great work of 358 pages was prepared while Lind practised medicine in Edinburgh, where he was elected a Fellow of the Royal College of Physicians. He became a charter member of the Royal Society of Edinburgh. In addition to the *Treatise* Lind wrote two other books: *Essay on Preserving the Health of Seamen* and *Essay on Diseases incidental to Europeans in Hot Climates*, the latter going through five editions in his lifetime. In 1758 Lind was appointed as the chief physician to the Royal Naval Hospital at Haslar near Portsmouth. When completed it was certainly the largest hospital in Europe capable of serving 2200 in-patients. In one of his letters he mentioned that it covered 32 acres of ground and had a high wall to prevent desertion. His professional staff consisted of 17 men and 90 "woman nurses." Twenty-four women served in the wash-house, " all these under sober and discreet Matrons." In the first two years, 5,734 patients were admitted, of which 1,146 suffered from scurvy. After 25 years in charge he retired from Haslar Hospital and died in 1794. James Lind was a pioneer in preventive medicine and in the improvement of the lot of sailors in the Royal Navy. To commemorate the 200th anniversary of Lind's publication on scurvy, Dr. Douglas Guthrie, Professor of the History of Medicine at Edinburgh, along with Dr. C.P. Stewart published a reprint of the first edition of Lind's *Treatise on the Scurvy*. Along with that invaluable volume were appended "Passages in Ancient Authors" of 105 pages. This was followed by a chapter, "The Lind Tradition in the Royal Naval Medical Service," by Surgeon Vice-Admiral Sir Sheldon Dudley. He writes of modern times, and reminiscent of Lind's concern for sailors, "It is not the least of Admiral Lord Mountbatten's claims to fame that he was the first great world commander to acknowledge publicly that the Japanese were beaten as much by our greater skill in medicine and hygiene as by our superiority in the art of destroying men."

With no elaborate apparatus, and little but his eyes to guide him, he got nearer to the truth about the nature of scurvy, malaria and typhus than perhaps any single man before.
Professor Douglas Guthrie on the 200th anniversary of Lind's *Treatise*.

Christiaan Eijkman (1858-1930)

Eijkman was born in a small town in Gelderland in Holland, one of seven children. As a subsidized student of the Dutch Army he undertook, in return for his medical training, to serve as a medical officer upon graduation. During his medical studies he served, for two years, as an assistant to the professor of physiology. Under his guidance he wrote his graduation thesis on polarization in nerves. Little did he realize that his introduction to the peripheral nervous system was to be his eventual float to posterity because of what transpired later in the Dutch East Indies.

After acquiring his M.D. degree at Amsterdam on July 13, 1883, Eijkman and his young bride set off for the Dutch East Indies where he was to become Medical Officer of Health.

On the island of Java, Eijkman developed malaria and was forced to return to Holland on sick leave. He undertook studies in bacteriology and worked in the laboratory of Robert Koch in Berlin. There he met two Dutch physicians who had been appointed by the government to proceed to the East Indies in order that they might study the disease called beriberi, which was causing concern in such congregations of troops as could be found in the army, in labour camps and in prisons.

Eijkman's wife having died, he set off again for the Indies where his friends had been isolating a micrococcus which, to them, seemed to be implicated in the disease beriberi. With the return of his friends to the Netherlands, Eijkman was made head of the small laboratory which had been set up by them in Batavia (now Djakarta) and in addition he was given directorship of the Javanese Medical School. He proceeded to look further into the possibility of a bacterial infection causing beriberi. He made no progress in this direction but noted that a flock of chickens maintained at his laboratory were having difficulty flying and walking. It appeared that a paralysis was progressing from the feet upward into the body, and once affected with this problem, the bird could no longer move, eat or drink. In addition to the dark colour of the comb and skin the bird developed a total inability to keep its head up, and the head fell backwards on a retracted neck.

In that tropical setting it was naturally thought that a strange infectious disease must have taken over. On November 27, 1889, a new cook in the hospital to which Eijkman was attached refused to supply leftover cooked white rice any longer for his chickens and he had to be content with a supply of rough chicken feed that contained raw, unpolished rice. Once the paralysed chickens were fed on what the country people ate in the way of unpolished rice, the "epidemic" was over. The paralysis in chickens could be remedied in pigeons and in other birds. The outbreaks of beriberi in the prison system were brought to an end when rough, unpolished rice was part of the diet. This brought to an abrupt end the search for some bacterial cause of beriberi.

Eijkman returned to Holland in 1898 as professor of public health at the University of Utrecht where he continued his work for 30 years. He retired at 70 and to universal applause was awarded the Nobel Prize for Physiology or Medicine, which he shared with the Cambridge biochemist Sir Frederick Gowland Hopkins. Hopkins had played a key role in developing among his Cambridge undergraduate students such vitamin researchers as Sir Edward Mellanby, who launched the studies leading to the discovery of vitamin D, as well as J.B.S. Halldane, the all-round biochemist, and Judah Quastel, one of the fathers of brain chemistry.

One aspect of the research on deficiency diseases and the way in which clinical trials have been carried out is the finite and short periods over which the trials took place. Lind started his famous controlled study on scurvy on May 20, 1747, and completed it on June 16 of that year. Eijkman was able to equate recovery in his chickens to the dictates of an army cook in November 1889. (In more recent times the transforming work on pellagra, by the immigrant who arrived in the United States at age six, Joseph Goldberger [1874-1929], was completed in 1915 in a very short period—given the fact that the disease had been well described by Casál, a Spanish physician, in 1755. Goldberger, like Lind and Eijkman, had to disprove the theory that infection caused scurvy, beriberi and pellagra. With prison volunteers he showed that it was a nutritional disease only. He quickly eradicated the disease, with adequate diet, in three southern orphanages.)

All these crucial trials were short in duration but long on prevention.

CHAPTER FOURTEEN

Pathology and Infection

William Osler (1849-1919)

Thousands of cars course hourly along the highway between Hamilton and Dundas, Ontario. No one in them sees anything remarkable about the little pools and springs beside the road. Yet it was with a study of the microscopic creatures within one such spring that the writing career of William Osler began. His short paper "Christmas and the Microscope," appeared in Hardwicke's *Science-Gossip*, London, 1869, and like so many papers and addresses to follow, it began with a quotation—this one from Horace.

It is hard to believe that a boy scraping the algae off the sides of a barrel with a stick on this December afternoon would some day write the world's greatest textbook of medicine and inspire two of the largest medical foundations ever created. His influence on medical education was world-wide, and his contribution to the literature and history of medicine unequalled in modern times.

Osler was raised in a country manse, one of nine children. Though given to wild escapades as a child he became a close student of nature under the Rev. W.A. Johnson, the godson of the Duke of Wellington, at Trinity College School at Weston, Ontario. The physician to the school, Dr. James Bovell, stimulated Osler's interest in nature and was later to shepherd him into Trinity College Medical School at Toronto, where he was dean. The study of fossils, the grinding of bones and teeth, and the microscopic examination of all manner of water dwellers kept Osler busy. School for him was a mixture of athletics and scientific investigation, though a sound knowledge of the classics was to rub off on him.

Entering Trinity College, Toronto, in theology, Osler eventually transferred to the study of medicine and his naturalist's eye soon fell on the minute cysts of the pork parasite, Trichina spiralis, in the muscles of the cadaver that he was dissecting. From one drachm of arm muscle he isolated 159 cysts, most of which contained live worms, moving sluggishly. These parasites had been discovered and first described in 1835 by James Paget when a first-year medical student in London.

Osler tried to infect animals with these, testing dogs, cats and rabbits, being successful only in the rabbits. He pursued the subject with the help of a veterinary hospital in Toronto, and then put his data aside, to attend to his medical course. (He drew on these undergraduate researches in 1876 when he gave the Somerville Lectures in Montreal.)

In summary, our gleanings of William Harvey's achievements in morbid anatomy are as follows:
"We have it from his own notes that he began recording morbid anatomical observations in his Paduan days, and continued until near his death—that is a period of over fifty years."
"I have found some 63 records of personal autopsy observations and it is probable he performed a far larger number; over a hundred is a conservative estimate.
Kenneth Keele, M.D., FRCP

In the same year (1870) Osler compiled his observations on "Canadian Diatomaceae" and published a first-class paper on them, listing 109 species in 29 genera, found mostly in the Dundas marshlands.

Migrating to McGill medical faculty in 1870 because of the clinical facilities of the Montreal General Hospital, Osler became even further immersed in his undergraduate writing career. In the tradition of the *Lancet*, the *Canadian Medical and Surgical Journal* published, under "Hospital Practice," an account of interesting cases appearing on the hospital wards. The clinical clerks wrote up such reports, Osler, in two years, having six printed. The subjects were: suppurative nephritis, fissure of anus, angina Ludovici, carcinoma mammae, and pleuropneumonia with delirium tremens (Osler doing the autopsy and demonstrating a large renal infarct). Dr. John Reddy read a paper before the Montreal Medico-Chirurgical Society on paralysis with aphasia, in which the post mortem specimen was prepared by Osler, neatly showing the offending blood clot in the arteries of the brain. Meanwhile he carried on with his old Toronto hobby of parasites.

> So often prejudice in favour of established theory suppresses anything resembling heresy, or finds some method for disregarding it. When one looks back, one has to project oneself, not only back into the state of more limited knowledge but also into the mental atmosphere of the time. One has to remember what it was like not to know things which now seem self-evident. ... One believed what one was taught, one accepted theories as if they were facts, and the opinions of eminent people were quoted to clinch an argument as if they were divine revelations. This may have been comfortable for the eminent but it was bad for the progress of science, because real radicals who can think for themselves, despite opposition, are rare, and progress depended on them.
>
> Ross G. Macfarlane (1967)

For his graduation in 1872 Osler prepared a unique thesis. It was a report on 50 post mortems. The faculty were so impressed with what they called its "originality and research," together with the 33 microscopic and other preparations accompanying it, that they awarded Osler a special prize. Only the introduction to his thesis survives, as included here:

> In that Trinity of being—of body mind and soul—which so marvellously make up the Man, each one has its own special ills and diseases. With the first of these—the body—have we here anything to do, leaving the second to be attended to by that class of men whose duty it is, "to minister to minds diseased," i.e. the Psychologists, while those of the third class beyond a Physician's skill seek aid elsewhere. Few indeed are permitted to end their days in a natural manner, by a gradual decline of the vital powers, till that point reached, where nutrition failing to supply the fuel, necessary to keep the lamp of life alight, leaves decay to drag back the fabric to the dust.... The number of avenues through which death may reach us, the natural frailty of our bodies the delicate and intricate machinery which maintains us in a condition of health may well make us exclaim with the Poet
>
> Strange that a harp of thousand strings
> Should keep in tune so long.
>
> To investigate the causes of death, to examine carefully the condition of organs, after such changes have gone on in them as to render existence impossible and to apply such Knowledge to the prevention and treatment of disease, is one of the highest objects of the Physician.

Within a year of graduation, Osler made in London an important discovery on the role of the "platelets" of the blood. Wilburt Davision, on of Osler's medical students at Oxford wrote, "Your comment on Osler's discovery of platelets made me recall a source of great embarrassment to me. Osler had asked me while I was an intern (a medical student pressed into service at the Radcliffe Infirmary at Oxford) to do a platelet count on a patient who had purpura. I looked up one or two articles [this was in 1915] and found that platelet counts were of dubious value and gave that information to Sir William. He quietly took me to the laboratory and showed me how to count platelets and I learned a few months later of his [original] work on platelets."

Osler's name was associated, as was that of Vaquez of Paris, with splenomegalic polycythemia. After discussing this disease in a clinical lecture at the Radcliffe Infirmary at Oxford in 1907, Osler insisted, "But the priority of description rests with Vaquez and if a name is to be associated with the disease it should be that of our distinguished French colleague."

Vaquez published with Quiserne the latter's Paris thesis of 1902 in which the student made the point that there was a continuous increase of red blood cells in the disease they were describing. Osler mentioned this in his description of nine cases of polycythemia in the *American Journal of Medical Science* in 1903.

Rudolf Virchow (1821-1902)

Osler and his generation were to sit at the feet of a revolutionary teacher in the field of pathology, Rudolf Virchow, in Berlin. At age eighteen, Virchow began his medical studies at the Kaiser Wilhelm Academie for Army Surgeons. As a second year student, he began a research project on inflammation in the eye in rabbits sent to him by his father in Pomerania. As his biographer Ackerknecht puts it: "The fact that Virchow did research here on inflammation in a nonvascular tissue determined in a way all his later opinions on parenchymatous inflammation, and therewith on the cellular and not vascular basis of inflammation." His Latin thesis on this work was presented in 1843.

Three years later, he established what has come to be the famous pathological journal, *Virchow's Archive*. He coined the term *omnis cellula e cellula* and rang the death knell of theories of humours, vapours and spontaneous generation. So trenchant did his criticisms of the Prussian government become for it failures in the public health field that he was banished to Wurzberg for seven years, only to be welcomed back to Berlin to a new pathological institute. He served for fifty years in the Reichstag, ever the enemy of Bismarck. He helped his friend Schliemann, who unearthed Troy and Mycenae.

And learn to play the game fair, no self-deception, no shrinking from the truth; mercy and consideration for the other man, but none for yourself, upon whom you have to keep an incessant watch.... If necessary, be cruel; use the knife and the cautery to cure the intumescence and moral necrosis which you feel in the posterior parietal region, in Gall and Spurzheims' centre of self-esteem, where you will find a sore spot after you make a mistake in diagnosis. It is only by getting your cases grouped in this way that you can make any progress in your post-collegiate education; only in this way can you gain wisdom with experience."
Sir William Osler

Osler's influence on medical student researchers was catalytic. During his years at Hopkins he taught many student researchers in whose work he was intimately associated. For instance, William G. MacCallum will be discussed later in this chapter. Closely paralleling MacCallum's work was that of Eugene L. Opie, who graduated with the first class to leave Johns Hopkins Medical School. Between his third and fourth year of medicine Opie became interested in malaria-like parasites in Baltimore birds. He went on, in 1901, to describe "the relation of chronic interstitial pancreatitis to the Islands of Langerhans and to diabetes mellitus." He followed 11 cases to autopsy and concluded, "A relationship has been observed between lesions of the Islands of Langerhans and the occurrence of diabetes mellitus." In the same year Ssobolew ligated the pancreatic duct and found no diabetes. The Islands remained untouched. However, in two diabetic patients he showed that no islets had survived. Two years previously a Paris student, Carnot, showed that toxic or infectious matter could occlude the pancreatic duct.

In 1906 Lydia Maria DeWitt[1] showed in cats that extracts from the Islets of Langerhans, after the pancreatic ducts were obliterated, reduced glucose in the circulating blood. Despite all this and the research of Mering and Minkowski, it was not until 1921 that Frederick Banting and Charles Best were able to produce insulin capable of arresting human diabetes. Plenty of warning had been given at the University of Toronto where William Osler, probably thinking about Opie's work, told the medical profession in 1909, "As our knowledge of the pancreatic function and carbohydrate metabolism becomes more accurate we shall probably be able to place the treatment of diabetes on a sure foundation." His friend Professor A.B. Macallum, Canada's first biochemist, told Banting's graduating class of 1916 that he hoped that some member of that group might unlock the secret of the Islets of Langerhans in the pancreas.

When Osler left Johns Hopkins Medical School in 1905 to become the Regius Professor of Medicine at Oxford, his former students presented to him 12 volumes of their collected reprints to that date. Their dedicatory letter is to be found on one of the left-hand pages bearing special texts in this volume.

Many of the former pupils whose reprints were now gathered together were undergraduate contributors to science. For instance, Thomas R. Brown of the class of 1897 was the first to demonstrate the eosinophilia in trichinosis, "the porkworm disease." A list of the students involved reads like a *Who's Who* of the next century's medicine, many of them in the field of infection.[2]

Two students from Hopkins had the privilege as undergraduates of accompanying Simon Flexner and Professor Lewellys F. Barker on the health commission sent to investigate plague in the Philippine Islands. These were John Marshall Flint and Frederick P. Gay. The plague studies were done by Barker and Flint as they returned home by way of India. An entire volume could be written on the undergraduate research activities of the students at Johns Hopkins University which, from its inception, has strived to offer research facilities and support for medical students.

Of this collection of reprints and what it involved, Osler wrote, "My chief treasure ... A splendid record."

The emphasis at Johns Hopkins on student research was sustained and blossomed. In the class of 1906 alone, four papers were written by students on pathological states in animals that were found accidentally, in the Old Hunterian Laboratory at Baltimore. One of Osler's students, a future dean of medicine at Yale, Milton Winternitz, as a medical student at Johns Hopkins Hospital, in his second year, published his first paper on enzymes in *Hoppe Seyler's Zeitschrift* (1905).

The class of 1904 contained student contributor **Francis Peyton Rous** (1879-1970). During his lifetime he witnessed great changes in medical research. As a young student growing up in Baltimore he had an early interest in living things. After studying premedical subjects at Johns Hopkins University he gravitated to medicine in year 1900. In his long and productive life Rous ran the gamut from cancer research to the preservation of living red blood cells and the early work with J.R. Turner and O.H. Robertson which produced the world's earliest blood banks. After several years preparing himself for a medical research career, Rous was invited to join the staff of the Rockefeller Institute in New York City. That was the beginning of 60-year association with the institution that later became the Rockefeller University. He went to a very productive career in the viral cancer field.

E.E. Tyzzer (1875-1965)

Johns Hopkins Medical School did not have a monopoly on medical student research, as illustrated by the amazing career of Ernest Edward Tyzzer. Born on a farm in Massachusetts, Tyzzer sustained himself financially through a four-year course at Brown University and then a similar length of time in Harvard University by trapping fur-bearing animals such as mink, skunk and weasel. In 1893 he entered Brown University with only $50 from his trapping experience. The following year he financed his studies through working in the college dining room and on scholarships. An inspiring teacher in comparative anatomy persuaded him to stay for his master's degree, working on the central nervous system of the flounder, part of which was carried on at Woods Hole Oceanographic Institution.

In 1898 he entered Harvard Medical School still trapping for a living. In his second year Professor Councilman set him various research projects. In the summer of 1900 he returned to Woods Hole where he studied the relationship of parasites to tumours in fish and there produced his first paper, "Tumours and Sporozoa of Fishes." During the spring recess from Harvard Medical School, and while continuing his trap lines, he found parasites in fox carcasses and brought those to his class to show Professor W.T. Councilman, professor of pathology. In 1901, while he was a senior student, an epidemic of smallpox descended upon Boston, which led to his work on variola and to his classic contribution on the histopathology of varicella. Under Councilman he studied lesions in the cornea of the rabbit. As a side issue he was sent to Gallup's Island in Boston Harbour to collect material from those dying from smallpox. He graduated from Harvard Medical School over the objections of a dermatologist who thought that Tyzzer was deficient in that specialty, despite the fact that Tyzzer had been skinning animals since boyhood and was an expert in the field of rodent infections, the parasites of ruffed grouse as well as equine encephalitis in pheasants. Tyzzer's work had helped to preserve the turkey industry from disaster through his work on "blackhead disease." An echo of the Harvard dermatologist was to be heard years later when McGill's outstanding athlete, George Degnan, was "plucked" by a public health professor. Degnan eventually became one of California's most productive public health practitioners.

TROPICAL DISEASES

Stubbins H. Ffirth (1784-1820)

Born in Salem, New Jersey, Ffirth entered as a medical student at the University of Pennsylvania and became interested in the unusual behaviour of yellow fever, and its infectivity, when compared with measles, smallpox and similar diseases. He wondered why the disease did not necessarily spread to those in contact with a sufferer. His experimental work as a medical undergraduate is detailed in his student thesis of 1804 on "Malignant Fever."

Ffirth placed human black vomit and blood from yellow fever patients into cuts that he made in his legs and his arms in an effort to infect himself. He administered the same vomit to animals and inhaled the fumes from similar material which he heated. He also made some into pills and swallowed them.

A Philadelphia critic termed the experiment as "unnecessary and disgusting." Ffirth replied: "You are pleased to say that the experiment was 'disgusting' as well as 'unnecessary'... but to a person anxious for the investigation of truth, nothing having a tendency thereto, or in any way to elucidate the subject, ought to be considered as such: everything which has this object in view might be encouraged.... It is my opinion.... that the progress of science tends to the extension of human happiness; everything therefore having a relation to this, whether it be disgusting or not, is laudable." He began his work in an attempt to answer the question, "Why was only a small proportion of the community affected by yellow fever?" After this paper he gave up his effort to enlighten the ignorant and took up practice in Charlestown. He died at the age of 36. Although his thesis lay unread for a century, the American researchers Finlay and Reed finally benefited from his early contribution.

Thirty-three years after Ffirth's thesis, **Louis Daniel Beauperthuy** (1803-1871) presented his M.D. thesis in 1837 in Paris entitled "*De la Climatologie*" in which he projected his "*théorie insectile*." The masterly history of this pioneer in both yellow fever and leprosy research has been written by the distinguished British historian of medicine, Dr. Alex Sakula. He tells how the young student in Paris attended courses in botany and entomology and spent his vacations at his West Indies home on the island of Guadeloupe where his father was a physician. There he saw almost endless yellow fever and he began to think of the possibility that mosquitoes and possibly other insects transmitted the disease. Upon graduation he became an explorer of Latin American countries and carried on research in the basin of the Orinoco. In Venezuela he put down his roots in Cumana situated 300 kilometres east of Caracas, the capital. There he qualified for his Venezuelan medical doctorate and began practice. At the age of 63 he transferred to a leprosy hospital in Guyana, where he died of a stroke in 1871.

A decade after his arrival in Venezuela a cholera epidemic struck the area and, because of his experience in the Paris epidemic of 1832, he was made responsible locally. As Sakula writes, "Examining the excreta of the cholera victims he detected the motile vibrios which he described in 1855. This was 28 years before Robert Koch definitively isolated the causative organism of cholera." Among other things Beauperthuy found that when anti-mosquito precautions were taken by using smoke or nets, the infection with yellow fever was reduced. "He came to the conclusion that the mosquito must be the vector by which the infecting agent of yellow fever was transmitted." The culprit in his view was the striped-legged mosquito, now called *Aëdes aegypti*. His paper in a local government publication in 1854 received minimal circulation. Two years later he conveyed his findings to the outstanding medical scientist Flourens in Paris. He reported on Asiatic cholera, yellow fever and malaria. The Academy of Sciences in Paris set up a special committee on which Gabriel Andral sat. (He had been the great teacher along with Laennec of Oliver Wendell Holmes, James Jackson, Jr., and other New England and Pennsylvanian students.)

Twenty-five years after the work of Beauperthuy, Carlos Finlay published his classic work on the role of the mosquito in yellow fever.

Infectious agents became the subject of many student investigations. As a student, the physician ophthalmologist **Jonathan Hutchinson** (1828-1913) began studying the notched teeth in infantile syphilis. In the year of his qualification in medicine he began his observations on inflammation of the eye in infants and young persons who suffered from hereditary syphilis. He continued his interest in the human eye and its problems. In 1910 William Osler wrote concerning Hutchinson: "We all recognize how much science is indebted to general surgeons who have made ophthalmology a study, and to all of us at once will occur the name of that veteran—the greatest general eye specialist of his generation—Jonathan Hutchinson, the last of the polymaths, the man at home in all spheres of medical science."

As detailed in *Young Endeavour*, a Peruvian medical student, **Daniel Carrion** (1859-1885), gave his life in proving that Oroya fever and Verruga Peruana were manifestations of the same infectious tropical disease. In his fourth year of medical school he mapped the regions along the route of the Trans-Andean Railway where, in a single year, 7000 workers had died of the fever and skin eruptions. He was voluntarily inoculated with blood from an acute case and died 38 days later. He is memorialized in the name of the local hospitals and his own medical school.

Charles Gabriel Seligman (1873-1940), as an undergraduate at St. Thomas' Hospital, set out to find the active agent in the tropical disease known as "Madura foot." (Readers will recall that this is one of the many interests Van Dyke Carter had after leaving his friend Henry Gray the anatomist, his classmate at St. George's Hospital, London.) Seligman's microscopic preparations of streptothrix Madurae were part of his publication in his graduation year. Strangely, he had also, as an undergraduate, studied the colour of the hair and the eyes in the families of his fellow students and nurses, in several generations, which introduced him to the study of anthropology. After graduation he joined a Cambridge expedition to the Torres Straits. Eventually he moved from the pathology of tropical disease to endocrinology and to anthropology in New Guinea and Egypt. He was really a field worker not a theorist and his medical training certainly shone through. As scientist and good citizen he served on committees to relocate refugees in the medical profession.

A pioneer in the search for causal agents in infectious diseases was **Dr. George Richards Minot** (1885-1950), son of Dr. James Jackson Minot of Boston. He was a gifted observer of natural history in his youth and published his first paper on butterflies at the age of 17 (as did Frederick Gowland Hopkins in Britain in his youth).

As an undergraduate at Harvard Medical School Minot became interested in haematology under Dr. J. Homer Wright and studied anaerobic bacteria and blood platelets with Frank Mallory.

Minot received the Nobel Prize in 1934 for his work on liver therapy

The scope of an able man is increased through association with the right youngsters who become almost a part of him, and he of them, in turn. It is one of the finest things human beings do as social animals.
No need to remark on that blessed self-hypnotism, wherewith the investigator convinces himself that what he tries to do is worth while. Without it he could scarcely get on.... The greater the theme the more it helps him.
Peyton Rous

In this book disease is studied as a perversion of physiological function. The title `Clinical Pathology', expresses well the attempt which is made in it to fill the gap between empirical and scientific medicine. Every few years the laboratories seem to run ahead of the clinics and it takes time before the facts of the one are fully appreciated by the other."
William Osler's introduction to the English translation, by A.W. Hewlett, of his teacher Krehl's textbook at Tubigen

in pernicious and other forms of anaemia. In turn, one of Minot's students, **Robert Frederick Loeb** (1895-1973) became a contributor to medical science while a student at Harvard Medical School, which he entered at age 20. (He was the son of the biologist Jacques Loeb.) His first year of medicine at Harvard went rather badly, and his marks in anatomy were so poor that he thought of changing course and taking geology. However, he graduated at the top of his class in 1919, having been given a prosectorship in anatomy. As a second-year student he was chosen by Otto Folin, the biochemist, to assist in the teaching of first-year medical students. Loeb wrote his first paper with G.R. Minot on methods of curbing the frightful spread of influenza in the epidemic of 1918 among Harvard students. Of Loeb's subsequent career it has been said that he rejected trivia for the more substantial problems. At Columbia University he became well- known for his work on proteins, blood elements and the kidneys. He was equally well-known for his work also on Addison's disease, and studies on the diagnosis of acute rheumatic fever.

What it comes to in practice is this. The phagocytes won't eat the microbes unless the microbes are nicely buttered for them. Well, the patient manufactures the butter for himself all right; but my discovery is that the manufacture of that butter, which I call opsonin, goes on in the system by ups and downs - Nature being always rhythmical, you know - and that what the inoculation does is to stimulate the ups or downs, as the case may be. Drugs can only repress symptoms; they cannot eradicate disease. The true remedy for all diseases is Nature's remedy. Nature and Science are at one, Sir Patrick, believe me; though you were taught differently. Nature has provided, in the white corpuscles as you call them, in the phagocytes as we call them - a natural means of devouring and destroying all disease germs. There is at bottom only one genuinely scientific treatment for all disease, and that is to stimulate the phagocytes. Stimulate the phagocytes. Drugs are a delusion. Find the germ of the disease; prepare from it a suitable anti-toxin; inject it three times a day quarter of an hour before meals; and what is the result? The phagocytes are stimulated; they devour the disease; and the patient recovers - unless, of course, he's too far gone. That, I take it, is the essence of Ridgeon's discovery.

George Bernard Shaw, *The Doctor's Dilemma*, after a visit to Almroth Wright at St. Mary's Hospital, London, 1905

BLOOD ELEMENTS

John Hughes Bennett (1812-1875)

At the age of 17 Bennett was apprenticed to a surgeon named Sedgwick in Maidstone, England. Four years later he entered the University of Edinburgh Medical School and while an undergraduate there published two papers that were forerunners of well over 100 career papers published on medical subjects. He received his M.D. degree at Edinburgh in 1837. The importance of Bennett's eventual career was that he gave "the first definite description of leukaemia" in the *Edinburgh Medical and Surgical Journal* of 1835. His paper was "Case of Hypertrophy of the Spleen and Liver, in which Death Took Place from Suppuration of the Blood." He is said to have discovered the parasite of aspergillosis, and in addition published a book on the medicinal values of cod-liver oil.

John Eason did undergraduate work on "The Pathology of Paroxysmal Haemoglobinuria." His M.D. thesis at Edinburgh in April 1905 was awarded a gold medal and part of this is reproduced with the above title in the *Journal of Pathology and Bacteriology* for 1906. In it he cites the Paris thesis of 1903 on the same subject by Camus. It is clear that Eason's experiment began in 1903 and that his results were first communicated to the Galenian Society in Edinburgh in January 1904. Camus' work published in 1903 in his thesis in Paris showed that the liver cannot hinder the occurrence of haemoglobinuria.

Another Scottish contributor was **Carl Hamilton Browning** (1881-1972). While still a medical student at the University of Glasgow, Browning was put to work by Professor Robert Muir on a specific problem—the development of the granular leucocytes. Though he graduated in 1903 his paper was not published until 1905 in the *Journal of Pathology and Bacteriology*. Browning then studied in Paul Ehrlich's laboratory at Frankfort on a Carnegie scholarship. There he worked on "the necessity for discovering defined substances that would destroy disease-producing organisms without damaging their host." This was a recurrent theme of Browning's work during World War I when he showed that acriflavene and proflavine were active against gram-positive and gram-negative aerobic or anaerobic bacteria. These drugs were tried out in war wounds and it was held that the main tissues were unaffected. The Biographical Memoirs of the Fellows of the Royal Society for 1973 concerning Browning state, "that these substances were adopted so late by the British Army was largely due to the opposition of Alexander Fleming in England.... Fleming was at that time under the influence of Almroth Wright and the opsonic index, and later conceded the value of these acridines."

Another future professor of microbiology to have some German training was Cyril Leslie Oakley (1907-1975). At the age of 19 he was publishing on "*Copepoda*" (fish lice). With proficiency in Latin, Greek, Hebrew, French, German and Chinese, Oakley entered University College, London, with a Kitchener Memorial scholarship. He took his bachelor of science degree with a first-class in zoology and at the same time managed to qualify in medicine in the year 1930. He studied in Aschoff's laboratory in Freiburg and then spent 19 years with the Wellcome Research Laboratories at Beckinham in England. Thereafter he was made professor of microbiology at the University of Leeds and became editor of both the *Journal of Pathology* and the *Journal of Medical Microbiology*. He was a pioneer in the study of clostridia. As a hobby he took up the study of ecclesiastical architecture.

In these days of aggressive self-assertion, when the stress of competition is so keen and the desire to make the most of oneself so universal, it may seem a little old-fashioned to preach the necessity of this virtue [humility] but I insist for its own sake and for the sake of what it brings . . . for its own sake, since with it comes not only reverence for truth, but also a proper estimation of the difficulties encountered in our search for it.... Start out with the conviction that absolute truth is hard to reach in matters relating to our fellow creatures, healthy or diseased, that slips in observation are inevitable even with the best-trained faculties, that errors in judgment must occur in the practice of an art which consists largely in balancing probabilities;—start, I say, with this attitude of mind, and mistakes will be acknowledged and regretted; but instead of a slow press of self-deception, with ever-increasing inability to recognize truth, you will draw from your errors the very lessons which may enable you to avoid their repetition.
Sir William Osler,
The Grace of Humility

ANTIBIOSIS

Ernest Duchesne

On December 17, 1897, a French medical student subsidized by the army presented his thesis for graduation at the University of Lyon on the relationship between microorganisms, and especially the antagonism between moulds and microbes, as he phrased it. In 54 pages, Ernest Duchesne reviewed the literature in considerable detail and related the protection that penicillium glaucum conferred on the test animals who had been simultaneously inoculated with B. coli or B. typhosus. He found that moulds were "capable of attenuating to a remarkable degree the virulence of the bacterial cultures," which he had injected intraperitoneally into the animals. On graduation he was required to return to the French Army, but humbly said that he hoped that others would follow on with this work because he had been able to make only a modest contribution. (In this he echoed another student discoverer, Langerhans.) He added that these discoveries and others might be directly useful and applicable to prophylactic hygiene and therapy. It was just over 40 years later that Howard Florey and Boris Chain, working in the Sir William Dunn School of Pathology at Oxford, carried out a similar experiment that set the stage for the whole new chapter in the antibiotic control of infections that has changed human history. Florey later said that his face would be forever red for having accepted the Nobel Prize, along with Chain and Fleming, for the development of penicillin, in view of the early work by the student Ernest Duchesne.

TYPHUS vs. TYPHOID

William Wood Gerhard (1809-1872)

Osler was always keen to give credit to his old pupil of Philadelphia days, Gerhard, for identifying the difference between typhoid fever and typhus. Gerhard, Stillé, and Pennock did this 10 years before Sir William Jenner of University College, London, proclaimed it, and have since been given the credit. Gerhard described the typhus fever that occurred at Philadelphia in 1836, and showed the distinction between that disease and typhoid fever.

Gerhard was a pupil in Paris of the great P.C.A. Louis, along with Henry Bowditch, Stillé and the earlier group, notably Oliver Wendell Holmes and James Jackson, Jr., of Boston. As a medical student in Paris, Gerhard had been a member of the Society for Medical Observation. His groundwork in Paris laid the foundation for his first accurate clinical study of tuberculous meningitis. His student work encompassed the endermic application of medicines and his description at the age of 23 of the serious cholera epidemic in Paris while he was a student of Louis. Also in 1832 he wrote his important paper on smallpox.

OTHER APPROACHES TO MEDICINE

Alexander John Haddow (1912-1978), at the age of seven was making detailed pencil drawings of yellow fever mosquitoes. He entered the University of Glasgow in honours zoology in which he graduated with a first-class. However, Professor Edward Hindle, F.R.S., interested him in yellow fever work with the result that in 1938 Haddow qualified in medicine. Before that time he had published five papers on agents of human myiasis and the infestation of tissues and bodies by fly maggots. He also worked on marine species and his wide base of preparation enabled him to undertake an expedition to the Inner Hebrides.

Another unusual training was that of Charles M. Carpenter, born in 1895. Not only did he take his Doctor of Veterinary Medicine degree, but also a Ph.D. before entering medicine. It was not long before he undertook work on brucellosis and, in 1930, a study on the effects of fever and fever therapy. This he carried out with Stafford L. Warren, Ruth Boak and Alice D. Leahy.

Next, a discussion of four student researchers who lived most unusual lives. The first of these was **Paul Gordon Fildes** (1882-1971). Paul was the son of the distinguished artist Sir Luke Fildes who painted the well-known portrait "The Doctor" sitting by the bedside of a very ill patient. This was exhibited at the Royal Academy in 1891.

At preparatory school Paul was taught by an ex-medical student and gradually became interested in physiology, especially gastric physiology. He wrote a paper on "The Passage of Food to the Stomach" while still at Winchester. He proceeded to Trinity College, Cambridge, where he studied under Walter Morley Fletcher (later the secretary to the Medical Research Council of Great Britain). Fildes had exotic friends, such as Wilbur Wright, the early aviator. In 1904 Fildes entered the London Hospital on the recommendation of Sir Frederick Treves (of Elephant Man fame). At the London, Fildes worked with Professor Leonard Hill among other things on explosive decompression, which they authored together. Then in 1907 as a fourth-year medical student Fildes worked with Professor William Bulloch, the noted historian of bacteriology, for two years before taking his medical qualification. Bulloch put Fildes to work reviewing 120 families of "bleeders" going back over eight generations, some back as far as 400 years. In his paper, Fildes cited 940 references, of which he was able to consult all but three. This paper appeared in the *London Hospital Gazette* in 1909, the year in which he achieved his Cambridge medical degree.

Fildes became Bulloch's assistant at £25 sterling per year, having replaced F.W. Twort, who left to become superintendent of the Brown Institution, a post originally held by Sir Victor Horsley and later Sir Charles Sherrington.

During his war service Fildes worked on anaerobes and on typhoid, paratyphoid, and cerebrospinal fever. He became one of the founders of the *British Journal of Experimental Pathology* and later worked on tetanus. Thanks to Howard Florey, Fildes was able to develop virus research supported by the British campaign for cancer. Before he died he was moving in the direction of molecular biology and bacterial genetics.

Graham Selby Wilson (1895-1987)

This charming academic lived 92 useful and benign years. In 1912 he entered Kings College, London, but by 1914 was caught up in World War I. He was sent to Charing Cross Hospital Medical School and in the war emergency was graduated in 1916. While a student at Charing Cross he undertook, at the suggestion of Professor W.W.C. Topley, his first research project on the serological diagnosis of typhoid fever. Wilson won the Governor's Gold Medal at Charing Cross as well as the University of London Gold Medal in his final school year. He then spent four years in the Royal Army Medical Corps, the last year as a bacteriologist in India. He worked then with Topley at Manchester and finally at the London School of Hygiene and Tropical Medicine.

In the Second World War he joined the emergency hospital service and headed its laboratory division by 1941. He "retired" in 1963 having been made a Fellow in the Royal Society and a Knight.

Wilson's work embraced many fields, such as salmonella, brucella, tuberculosis, milk-borne diseases, and the control of diphtheria. Topley and Wilson's *Principles of Bacteriology and Immunity* developed from their conjoint work in Manchester, 1923-1927, where they had given a diploma course as a beginning. The last edition appeared 61 years later.

Wilson was born to ride a bicycle. He could be found at the early morning communion services at Westminster Abbey, having cycled six miles from Highgate. From the Abbey he would cycle to the Athenaeum on Pall Mall for a sparse meal and chiefly for conversation. If he were inspecting laboratories at a distance, he took his bicycle on the train with him. He eventually had a serious cycling accident resulting in multiple fractures, but that did not prevent him from completing in his ninety-first year his large biographical study of history from the 16th century to the 1870s. He was a gentle man, trusted by all, and especially a friend of students.

John P. McGovern

As an army medical student entering Duke University in 1942, McGovern fell under the spell of that great pediatrician Dean Wilburt Davison, one of Osler's former students at Oxford. The pediatric world was aware of the fact that nearly a thousand American infants were dying of whooping cough each month, many of them without protective inoculation against Pertussis — then directed only to those aged six months or more. This upset McGovern, and with the industry and dedication that were to characterize his later career as an outstanding allergist, he set out to change things.

With wartime shortages abounding he bred his own test mice, borrowed equipment and supplies, and induced the Eli Lily Company to provide him with the test vaccines needed. With a unique intraperitoneal mouse protection test to monitor the immune response of very young infants he showed, through his controlled study, that immunization of three month old children was safe, effective and practical.

For this well-conceived research, McGovern, the overworked student in the truncated three-year wartime medical course was given, on graduation, the first Borden Award for Undergraduate Medical Research.

Baruch Samuel Blumberg (1925-)

This 1976 Nobel Prize winner was born in New York City in 1925. In 1943, straight out of high school, he joined the U.S. Navy, in which service he remained for three years. He became a deck officer on landing crafts during the war and while in the navy completed his college work. He was granted a bachelor of science degree by Union College, Schenectady, in fields of bacteriology, pathology and physics. Instead of pursuing an advanced degree in physics at Columbia as he intended, he broke that off and entered Columbia Medical School. Between third and fourth year medicine he went to Surinam to conduct research on filariasis, malaria and intestinal parasites. He qualified for his M.D. degree in 1951. Thereafter he interned at Bellevue Hospital in New York until 1953. One of his mentors was Professor Dickinson Richards. After two years at Columbia-Presbyterian Hospital in New York he worked with Professor Karl Meyer on hyaluronic acid. He then spent two years in the department of biochemistry at Oxford, after which he journeyed to Nigeria. He says that he learned a great deal from the two students who were under his tutelage in Nigeria.

Strangely, Blumberg interrupted his work at the Fox-Chase Cancer Laboratory in Philadelphia to become Master of Balliol College, Oxford, reputedly the first scientist in 700 years to hold that post. However, he was the fourth American scholar to head an Oxford college. He has more than 400 publications to his credit. He says that in Surinam he had time to ponder the question, "Why do some people get sick and others do not?" His question is reminiscent of the statement, repeatedly made by a Nobelist, Wagner Jauregg: "It is necessary for physicians to study the healed cases of supposedly incurable disease." Gulliver Blumberg had one of the most unusual careers of his generation of medical undergraduates.

VIRUSES

Jules Jean Baptiste Bordet (1870-1961)

Having attended secondary school at the Atheneé Royal de Bruxelles, this young man entered the Free University of Brussels at age 16. He already boasted a chemical laboratory in his attic. Instead of the usual seven years required, he qualified in medicine after six years. He had already done research on the defence which capsules provide for bacteria even in immunized animals. This was published in his year of graduation, in the *Annales* of the Pasteur Institute. On moving to Paris Bordet was made an assistant to the famous Metchnikoff and remained in that laboratory until the year 1901. Part of his work was in the Transvaal where, to combat rinderpest, he injected cattle with small amounts of serum from convalescent animals, and thereafter exposed them to the natural infection with only a mild attack of the disease.

From Paris he returned to Brussels and founded the Institut Pasteur de Brabant.

With his brother-in-law Octave Gengou he studied the role of specific antibodies, and used complement fixation for differentiating between normal serum and serum that contained specific antibodies. Their methods greatly simplified the detection of cholera, anthrax, and typhoid fever. Bordet was made a Fellow of the Royal Society of London and won the Nobel Prize in 1919.

A brilliant and hard-working medical student, Bordet began his research career while an undergraduate. As William Bullock, of University of London, wrote, Bordet was, at the time of receiving the Nobel Prize in 1919, "by common consent... the greatest living exponent and worker on immunology."

Albert Claude (1899-1983)

This outstanding contributor to the knowledge of viruses was born in Belgium and at the age of 12 went to work in a steel factory near the French border. When World War I erupted, Albert joined the Belgian underground and worked with British Intelligence. He was later cited for valour by Winston Churchill. As a veteran he was permitted to enter the medical school at the University of Liège and graduated in 1928 with the M.D. degree. His thesis concerned the fate of a mouse tumour following its grafting into a rat. For a time he worked in an institute whose director believed that bacteria helped in the development of cancer. Claude showed correctly that the fluid injected into the test animals by the director actually was contaminated with bacteria. On making this clear, Claude was asked to leave. He then went to the Kaiser Wilhelm Institute in Berlin with Dr. Albert Fischer, to work with him on tissue culture. He was keen to characterize the agent found in the sarcoma that Peyton Rous sought in chickens.

Claude was determined to emigrate, and sent a hand-written proposal in "basic English" to Simon Flexner, the director of the Rockefeller Institute in New York. In September 1929 Flexner accepted Claude who stayed for 20 years. There he produced his sub-cellular fractionation technique based on high-speed centrifugation. In 1974 Claude shared the Nobel Prize in Medicine with Christian de Duve and George Palade.

William Barry Wood, Jr. (1910-1971)

Wood was born in Milton, Massachusetts, and attended the local academy as well as the Thatcher School in California. His years from 1928 to 1932 at Harvard College were heavily slanted to football, baseball, hockey and tennis. After a chance encounter with President James Conant, Wood had an opportunity to work with Professor L.J. Henderson. He did honours thesis work with Henderson on changes in white blood cells before, during and after strenuous exercise, having to procure blood samples from his fellow athletes. From the resting count of 5,000 white blood cells he might find as many as 24,000 after sustained effort. This was published as "A Study of Leukocytosis in Exercise," with H.T. Edwards.

Many years later Wood wrote about his choice of Johns Hopkins Medical School, where his father-in-law had studied medicine. He learned of the increased time set aside for research by medical students there. However, he was still not sure and, as he wrote: "So I went to talk to some of the Boston Brahmin physicians. And they told me I was crazy! They said that Johns Hopkins was a second-rate place, that there was no medical school that could measure up to Harvard.... But despite that advice I decided to go to Hopkins, and I never regretted it."

Once installed at Hopkins, Wood spent time with Mansfield Clark in biochemistry and metabolism and spent one summer at the University of Wisconsin in microbiology. The next summer he spent as a student clerk at Boston City Hospital with Soma Weiss, William Castle and Chester Keefer.

In 1936 Wood received his M.D. from Hopkins having already published two papers, one on the reducing action of glucose and the other on the relation of the oxidation reduction potential to the growth of anaerobic microorganisms. This was his springboard to work with Hans Zinsser and with the virologist John Enders. Eventually he became vice president of Hopkins, where he was closely associated with the microbiology club, and with its members Paul Beeson, René Dubos, and Walsh McDermott.

Thomas Weller (1915-)

Weller was born in 1915 and pursued a master of science degree at the University of Michigan which he received in 1937. His research was on parasitic organisms. Unlike Wood, he entered Harvard Medical School, keeping up his work in the laboratory of two well-known parasitologists.

In 1939 he began work with John Enders on viruses in tissue culture. He achieved his M.D. degree in 1940 and took clinical training at the Children's Hospital in Boston. Thereafter he served in the Army Medical Corps and in Puerto Rico pursued his interest in bacteriology, virology and parasitology. On his return to the United States he joined the research division of the Children's Hospital in Boston. From his medical student's research and publication with Enders and Feller on roller tube culture of a virus, to the Nobel Prize in Medicine in 1954, his career was one long series of successes. The Nobel Committee wished to award the Prize in Medicine or Physiology to John Enders in 1954, but he informed them that he could not accept it unless Weller and Robbins shared it with him. The Committee met his request.

We hear too much of `breakthroughs' in these days, for in my opinion, such language tends to obscure the fact that all of us depend on the work of our predecessors. This to my mind is nowhere more clearly demonstrated than in the steps that lead to the elucidation of the complicated changes of pathological processes."
Howard Florey, 1962 President's address to Royal Society, London.

In many parts of the field students continue to make important findings. For instance, R.W. Goltz, born in St. Paul, Minnesota, in 1923, during his studies in the University of Minnesota developed an interest in dermatology that led to his work on papillomata of mucous membranes. He was the first professor of dermatology at the University of Colorado. Similarly, Joseph E. Murray, born in 1919 in Massachusetts, and after taking his B.A. at the College of the Holy Cross in Worcester entered Harvard University. While a student in the medical school there he engaged in a research effort, sponsored by Arthur Hertig, with an investigation of the newly introduced Papanicolaou smear of cervical epithelium cells. Upon graduation Murray introduced the procedure clinically at the Peter Bent Brigham Hospital. In 1958 Allan Sherwin at the Montreal Neurological Institute began his outstanding research on allergic encephalitis. In 1993 Yun-Kang Chow, working at the Massachusetts General Hospital, produced a new strategy involving three drugs at one time, to combat the HIV that causes AIDS. The viral field will certainly attract many more student contributors in the future.

[1] She showed in her 1906 paper, in the *Journal of Experimental Medicine*, of 46 pages and excellent illustrations, that digestive activity of the pancreas was unrelated to the survival of the Islands of Langerhans, which she considered to be "vascular glands with a sinusoidal circulation." She found in the cat that when the pancreatic duct was closed by ligation, section or obstruction, the islets remained unaltered. She concluded that the Islands "have a secretion which is probably poured into the blood vessels; this secretion has no digestive action on starch fibrin or fat, but has a marked glycolytic."

[2] Others among his students contributed undergraduate studies as well: W.J. Talbot; Mabel Austin, on endocarditis; Dorothy Reed, after whom a special type of cell has been named; Florence Sabin, the anatomist; Adelaide Dutcher, on tuberculosis; F.C. Goldsborough, on diseases of the cerebral arteries; Louise Tayler-Jones, on kidney worms in swine; and Benjamin Schenk, on sporotrichosis.

CHAPTER FIFTEEN

Physics and Vision

Jean Fernel (1497-1557)

Jean Fernel was born in 1497 in Montdidier in the diocese of Amiens. His father was both a substantial innkeeper and a furrier. When Jean was 12 his family moved to Clermont in Beauvoisis, a distance of 20 miles from Paris. After a thorough schooling there, he proceeded, with his father's help, to the University of Paris, entering the progressive Collège de Ste. Barbe, the history of which dated from 1460, when it was established by the Collège de Navarre.

Fernel took his master's degree in arts at age 22. He was invited to join the faculty of the college and teach dialectics but declined. The recent advent of printing had brought the great books within reach of many for the first time and Fernel chose, rather, to learn more of the humanities. The further he went with his self-education the more violently he reacted to his recently completed training. He classed some of his tutors as "barbaric," and resolved to go back over all his work systematically and alone. For five years he did nothing but devour humane letters and treatises on mathematics. He drove himself so hard that he was taken ill with a quartan fever, and required a long convalescence.

At 27 he embarked upon the four-year course in medicine at the University of Paris. He had serious financial difficulties since his father could no longer support him, there being others in the family in need of education. As a result, Fernel gave lectures in philosophy at the Collège de Ste. Barbe in order to support himself. As a third-year medical student he published his first book, *Monalosphaerium*, in which he described an astrolabe that he had invented for calculating the hour of the day, and for measuring elapsed time. This work contains a considerable amount of what today would be termed astrology, but which in 1527 was thought to represent the necessary setting for such discussions. Fernel composed an album of illustrations to accompany the main volume.

In the final year of the medical course, Fernel produced his second book entitled *Cosmotheoria*. It is chiefly remembered by mathematicians for the measurement of a degree of meridian that Fernel made from his own observations and his triangulation covering the territory lying between Paris and Amiens. One hundred and forty years later Jean Picard was to establish a value almost identical through observations made in the same part of the countryside.

In the same year (1528) Fernel's third book appeared, *De*

Proportionibus, in which he discourses on the theory and use of fractions.

In 1530 he received his licence to practice. His biographer records: "Fernel's practice became very large. It left him scant time even for his mid-day meal. His patients were of diverse rank, attendants of the court, dignitaries, officials and visitors to Paris, and many of the poor. He never neglected the poor."

Fernel wrote many medical books, among them an *Anatomy*, of which Sherrington says, "The absence of 'pictures' from Fernel's 'Anatomy' may be connected with Fernel's expressed opinion, reported by Plancy, that young physicians misspend hours in looking at pictures in anatomy books when, what should be done was to go do actual dissections with a concise manual in the hand." Fernel made his *Anatomy* a concise manual. It was a preface to his account of the working of the body. "Anatomy is to physiology," he says, "as geography is to history, it describes the theatre of events."

His textbook, *Physiology*—the term that he coined—was most popular, and even posthumously 31 editions of it were issued over a 100-year period. Embarking on something akin to a modern system of medicine, he produced his *Pathology* and *Therapeutics*. His special pathology even today would be considered as modern. In the 18th century, Boerhaave recommended Fernel's pathology as the best available. Thirty-six editions of it were to appear over the next century.

At his death, Fernel left a manuscript on syphilis, which unfortunately was not printed until 1579. He complained that the French called it the Neapolitan disease and the Neapolitans called it the French disease. Because printing was becoming widespread, many of the victims of the disease wrote poems on their symptoms and miseries, dedicating them to cardinals and rulers—which led among other things to the erroneous view that it was a disease of poets. Fernel put an end to this sort of pseudo-scientific speculation in his work, *De Luis Venereae Curatione*.

Fernel's life in medicine is one of the most absorbing in the history of science, and has been chronicled by Sir Charles Sherrington, O.M., published in 1946. The restless spirit and the drive to probe into causes, which so possessed Fernel as a student, persisted throughout his life. His simply stated views have a modern ring to them.

Fernel was not a fractious medical reformer nor a political gadfly. He was an excellent and busy practising physician who was indefatigable in his teaching of students. A description of Fernel's day, by his biographer Plancy, reads:

> Four o'clock found him risen and in his study, to read or write until daybreak. Then he went out, to visit patients or to the School to lecture. Then back to his study until the midday meal, which he sometimes did not sit down to take. The meal over, he was off again, to visit the sick. At the day's end he supped with his family and after that withdrew again to his study to read or write. He went to bed at one hour before midnight.

In Fernel's words:

> Many tell us that the art of healing, discovered by the labours of our forefathers, and brought to completion by dint of Reason, has now attained its goal. They would have us, who command it,

> tread in the same footsteps as did the Past. It were a crime, they tell us, to swerve a hair's breadth from the well established way. But what if our elders, and those who preceded them, had followed simply the same path as did those before them? . . . . Nay, on the contrary, it seems good for philosophers to move to fresh ways and systems; good for them to allow neither the voice of the detractor, nor the ways of ancient culture, nor the fullness of authority to deter those who would declare their own views. In that way each age produces its own crop of new authors and new arts....

Concerning medicine as a calling, Fernel wrote:

> Is there a greater blessing vouchsafed to mankind than Medicine is? Life is our dearest possession, by which we breathe and enjoy the company of our fellow-beings. Can any calling be worthier than that which preserves and maintains life itself? Is wealth or fortune, in whatever measure, in the last resort more estimable than is good health? Is any misfortune or disaster more grievous than ill-health? He who succours the sufferer and the sick exercises a knowledge which deserves the admiration and affectionate regard of all men.

Sir Charles Sherrington said of Fernel: "He was one of the relatively few who as they enter advanced years grow more modern."

Galileo Galilei (1564-1642)

Galileo was born February 15, 1564, at Pisa, the eldest of seven children. Many of his ancestors had been physicians. His father was a musician, mathematician and linguist. His early education was at Pisa and at the age of 12 he was sent to school at Vallombrosa near Florence for study in the humanities. This provided a good basis in Greek and Latin and in the natural sciences and philosophy. Galileo became a novitiate of the order that maintained the school at Vallombrosa but his father withdrew him and sought to raise him for the cloth trade of Florence. However, the precocious boy was already well-known as a maker of toy machines and models of great ingenuity. He had also learned to play the organ and the lute. He had developed certain skill in drawing and painting and in later life seems to have been a helpful critic to rising painters. He wrote poetry, essays on Dante and Tasso as well as a play.

The father next looked to a scientific career for his son and because he thought medicine offered some financial stability, he enrolled him in the medical school of the University of Pisa on September 5, 1581, at age 17. The father tried unsuccessfully to get one of the 40 free places for needy students at the University in Galileo's first year and again in the third year. Galileo's first contact at the medical school was with the great physician-botanist Andrea Cesalpino, who taught as professor of medicine at Pisa from 1567-1592.

Galileo was a discerning student who sought proof of everything. In this he reflected his father's temperament for the father had already stated in some works of literary criticism, "It appears to me that they who, in proof of any assertation, rely simply on the weight of authority, without adducing any argument in support of it, act very absurdly. I, on the contrary, wish to be allowed freely to question and freely to answer, without any sort of adulation, as well becomes those who are sincerely in search of truth."

His fellow students called Galileo "The Wrangler." He applied his own yardstick to Aristotle, Plato and St. Thomas Aquinas—not a popular pastime with those in authority. As one biographer said, "A philosopher needed only to know Aristotle by heart; to understand him was a secondary consideration; to contradict him was blasphemy."

Galileo made his earliest scientific discovery as a first-year medical student in 1581. In the cathedral of Pisa he saw the lamplighter pull back a large hanging lamp in order to light it. Once lit it was allowed to swing freely in the air. Galileo noticed that though the pendular excursions diminished gradually, the duration of each excursion remained the same. He proved this by reference to his pulse, his only timepiece. He experimented at the home of Muzio Tedaldi, a relative with whom he lived in Pisa. There he devised his Pulsilogia, or Protoclock. This had an immediately favourable reception from the physicians of Pisa.

Drawings of three models of Galileo's Pulsilogia are shown in the illustrations for this chapter, and were taken from the work of Sanctorius, the founder of the physiology of metabolism and professor of medicine at Padua, who in 1607 incorporated them in his book, *Methodi Vitandorum Errorum in Arte Medica*. Fahie's description follows:

> Figure 1 consists merely of a weight at the end of a string, which is held at the top of a graduated scale. The string being gathered up into the hand until the vibrations of the weight coincide with the beatings of the patient's pulse, the length is ascertained from the scale, which if great indicates a languid, and if small a more lively action. In figure 2, the improvement is introduced of connecting the scale and string; the length of the latter is regulated by turning a peg, and a bead on the string shows the measure. Figure 3 is still more compact, the string being adjusted by winding or unwinding upon an axle at the back of the dial plate.

In the year 1582-83 Galileo listened to lectures at Pisa by a Florentine friend of his father's, Osrilio Ricci, a mathematician and tutor to the Court of Tuscany. Soon Euclid replaced Hippocrates and Galen in Galileo's interests. Galileo's father set out to prevent any further shift towards mathematics by his son. He petitioned the Grand Duke Fernando I a second time for help for his son from the foundation for poor scholars but to no avail. This may have been due by then to the unpopularity of "the wrangler" with officialdom. By the summer of 1585 Galileo was withdrawn from the University of Pisa without his degree and he returned home to Florence. There he plunged into mathematics and physics and examined in great detail the works of Archimedes.

In 1586 he constructed his hydrostatic balance with which to analyze alloys. This is reminiscent of Archimedes' detection of fraud by the goldsmith who was making Hiero's crown long since. Galileo then turned to his work on the centre of gravity in solid bodies. His paper brought him immediate and favourable notice in Italy. Despite this the next two years were to see five unsuccessful applications made by him for vacant chairs of physics. As a result Galileo made ready to set out with another

Florentine for the East, when he was accepted at the University of Pisa as a professor with the annual salary of £13.

Once installed at Pisa, Galileo began to re-examine the scientific teachings of Aristotle. Leonardo da Vinci had, unknown to Galileo, done exactly this. Aristotle's teaching, which was nearly 2000 years prior to Galileo, was that if a heavier and a lighter piece of the same material were dropped from a height simultaneously, the heavier piece would strike the ground first. Galileo went up to the top of the leaning Tower of Pisa one morning, while students and professors crowded around. He rolled a 10-pound shot and a one-pound shot over the overhanging edge simultaneously. They struck the ground together, disproving Aristotle's view.

There was, in this demonstration, no timing problem. However, when Galileo sought to prove experimentally that in falling the final velocities are proportional to the times, and the spaces fallen through are proportional to the squares of the times, he had to find an accurate way of measuring time, so he went back to his student invention, the pulsilogia.

Before Galileo's analysis of Aristotle's theories had proceeded much further the narrow minds of Pisa proceeded to castigate Galileo. Galileo went on to ever greater triumphs at Padua, and Pisa forgot their brilliant young scholar. As late as 1613 Father Cartelli, Galileo's first pupil, wrote to him from Pisa, "Of our controversies (on the earth's motion) not a word is allowed to be said, a thing which astonishes me. Your marvellous discoveries are scarcely known here even by name."

Galileo's later works were many and varied: on the telescope, the microscope, the thermometer, geometrical and military compasses, fortifications, mechanics and especially astronomy. They form the basis of his fame as a great contributor to science. His observations on natural phenomena and their forthright interpretations brought him into conflict with all manner of entrenched temporal power. Some who had their tenuous theories rocked to the foundations by Galileo's discoveries, accused him of blasphemy. Others, perceiving the great worth of his inventions and generalizations, stole them. Much of his time was spent in self-defense and in proving plagiarism by his academic colleagues.

The University Senate in Padua, under great pressure in 1599, gave Galileo a niggardly increase in his stipend, from 300 to 320 ducats annually, observing that, "the professors should eke out their income by their private lessons." In addition they told Galileo that, "The Senate does not choose to make his case a precedent for every learned and needy foreigner who might think fit to press his claims, and that the usage of Bologna with regard to her professors was not to be set up as an example, as Bologna had a larger amount of money at the disposal of her University than the Venetian capital Senate had."

Galileo was twice called before the Inquisition for his Copernican views on the earth's status in the universe and was imprisoned at the age of 68. All his works were proscribed. Borelli considered himself a pupil or disciple of Galileo, although he had never seen him. He came from Messina to visit him shortly before he died. Galileo died on January 8, 1642, surrounded by his son Vincenzio and his wife, by Toricelli, his long and faithful disciple, and the youthful Viviani, who was to be his first biographer. Even in death Galileo was persecuted and his friends were forbidden to bury him in consecrated ground. In 1683 Viviani dared to erect the first memorial to Galileo, and when Viviani died in 1703 he left all his estate for the building of a further memorial. Thirty years more were to elapse before it was thought safe to proceed with this.

Jacobus Hovius

In 1702 Hovius wrote his graduation thesis at Utrecht, "*Tractatus de circulari humorum Motu in Oculis*" in which he described the circulus venosus Hovii. In 1715 he added his *Epistola* in which he defended his priority against Ruysch who described the same circuit in 1706.

Franciscus Bourdon

In 1760 this Montpellier medical student published his *Dissertatio de Amblyopia*. This is a very rare publication today. In it the author analyzed the causes and characteristics of each anomaly and the possibilities of correction, using optical means. Bourdon in his little classic went back to Boerhaave for some of his authorities.

Allvar Gullstrand (1862-1930)

Gullstrand was born in Landskrona, Sweden, where his father was a physician. His early schooling demonstrated his great ability in mathematics and in 1880 he entered the University of Uppsala in technical and medical sciences for five years. He spent a year in Vienna, but returned to Uppsala in 1888 to gain his medical licence. In 1890 he took his M.D. in Stockholm.

His thesis, defended in May 1890, was entitled "*Bidrag till astigmatismens teori*." Thereafter he became a lecturer at the Karolinska in Stockholm and eventually moved up through clinical posts. He carried on his research as professor of ophthalmology at Uppsala beginning in 1894. However, in 1913 a special chair in physiological and physical optics was created so he might have more time to devote to research.

One of his researches was published in 1900 on the intracapsular mechanism of accommodation. He developed better methods of identifying precisely which individuals, in cases brought before him, might exhibit paralysis. A new view was taken of the post-surgical needs of cataract patients. Gullstrand greatly improved the ophthalmoscope, the precursor of the slit-lamp.

After being awarded the Nobel Prize in 1911 he joined the Foundation's Committee on Physics.

Hamilton Hartridge (1886-1976)

Born prematurely, Hartridge lived 89 years. In 1905 he entered King's College, Cambridge, where he studied chemistry, physics and physiology. In the years 1908-1909 he made his most famous invention, the reversion spectroscope, thanks to the time he was able to spend in the laboratory of Joseph Barcroft. He achieved his M.D. in 1914. During the First World War, from 1915 to 1919, he was the problem-solver at the National Airship Construction Station. He returned to Cambridge to teach physiology and produced 70 papers in 30 years. His research in the sensory field covered the physiology of vision from bats to humans.

William Rushton (1901-1980)

Though Rushton entered Emmanuel College, Cambridge, in 1921, he did not achieve his medical qualification until 1937. The reason was that during those years he published 18 papers. He was awarded his bachelor's degree at Cambridge in 1925 and then began research with Edgar Adrian, who shared the Nobel Prize with Sherrington in 1932.

Rushton's first paper was published in 1927, on the threshold for nervous excitation. He went on to take his Ph.D. in 1928. His next project was to measure visual pigments in living eyes. He was also a pupil of Hamilton Hartridge, of whom he wrote: "He generated an atmosphere of excitement where the answers seemed to be waiting just 'round the corner to be picked up by a well-designed experiment."

When Rushton shifted his research interests exclusively to vision, he published another 147 papers.

Haldan Keffer Hartline (1903-1983)

Hartline was born in Pennsylvania and in 1923 carried on his research at the Woods Hole Marine Biological Station where he met Jacques Loeb. Loeb offered to publish his undergraduate work on "Influences of Light of Very Low Intensity on Phototropic Reactions of Animals." Then Hartline became a medical student at Johns Hopkins in Baltimore, where he carried on intensive research using his string galvanometer to record retinal action potentials in frogs, rabbits and cats. The active lead was on the cornea. He published two papers on this research in 1925. In that year he extended his investigations to human subjects and to decerebrate preparations.

Hartline graduated with his medical degree in 1927. While Johns Hopkins gave him his medical degree, it was felt that a considerable amount of his time was spent at Woods Hole and at Cold Spring Harbour. His laboratory was once described as "slightly disorganized but extremely fertile chaos." Actually, he revelled in this situation.

After an Eldridge Johnson Foundation travelling fellowship, Hartline joined the University of Pennsylvania as a fellow in medical physics from 1931 to 1949. Thereafter he researched at Johns Hopkins and at the Rockefeller University in New York.

In 1967 he shared the Nobel Prize in Physiology or Medicine with Sherrington's pupil Ragnar Granit of Sweden. Also sharing the prize was Professor George Wald of Harvard. The curiosity that he exhibited at so young an age carried on through a very productive career of research on the visual system, much of it done as an undergraduate.

Franz Anton Mesmer (1733-1815)

After six years at the University of Vienna, Mesmer graduated in medicine and produced an amazing doctoral dissertation in 1766. It was entitled, *Dissertatio physico-medica de planetarum influxu*.

It was probably plagiarized from Richard Mead's (1673-1754) "Treatise Concerning the Influence of the Sun and Moon upon Human Bodies and the Diseases Thereby Produced."

In his doctoral thesis Mesmer quotes 23 cases, of which 22 belong to Mead. Mead's description included cases reported by others. There is an old story of a female patient who was being observed by several physicians during an eclipse of the moon. As they left her in order to view the eclipse she fainted, and remained in that state until the eclipse was over. There's also a story retailed of epileptic sailors who had their seizures set off by the moon. The term "lunatics" was long used in the United Kingdom.

Nine years after Mesmer's thesis talked of "animal gravitation" he began to speak of "animal magnetism" with hypnotic overtones and séances, which brought him into Vienna and Paris drawing-rooms, but finally, into obscurity.

Mesmer, as has been shown by Dr. J.S. Jenkins, was an accomplished musician and a very close friend and supporter of the young Mozart. One of Mesmer's patients was the blind pianist to whom Mozart in Salzburg dedicated his piano concerto in B flat major. In 1778 Mesmer deserted the wealthy widow who had become his wife in Vienna and fled to Paris, and with the help of Queen Marie Antoinette he became wealthy for a time. Mozart's *Cosi fan tutte* made great fun of Mesmer and his magnets.

Thomas Young (1773-1829)

In every age there is a rare individual who stands out as a universal genius, gifted in many directions, and able to penetrate with clarity and apparent simplicity the very depths of little-understood secrets of nature. Thomas Young was such a giant and his Cambridge student title, "Phenomenon Young," fits him well. In 1793 he began his studies in the Great Windmill Street school of John Hunter in London—the last year of Hunter's unparalleled life. By September of 1793 Young had moved over to St. Bartholomew's Hospital Medical School and was dissecting the freshly removed eye of an ox when he observed that the ciliary muscles (later to be described microscopically by another student, Joseph Lister) were still active and, on being stimulated to contract, changed the shape of the lens. This acute observation brought to an end the spurious though official view, taught for centuries, that focusing of vision on near and distant objects was achieved by a shortening and lengthening of the eyeball itself. The publication of this discovery earned him his Fellowship in the Royal Society of London at the age of 21.

After a year in London Young decided to enter the Medical School in Edinburgh and began his studies under Joseph Black the chemist—that quiet, simple man who lived only to discover and train discoverers. On his journey to the north Young visited Erasmus Darwin and stopped in Leicestershire to learn the newest methods of stall-feeding cattle, of cross-breeding sheep for wool or for meat, and of irrigating the land.

As a small boy Young had been introduced to oriental studies, Hebrew, colour-mixing, book-binding and copper-plate making. Later his summers were spent with his grandfather in measuring the height of hills with a quadrant, in lens grinding, lathe turning, in making his own microscope and in meteorological observations. Before going up to London from his native Somersetshire he studied French, Persian, Chaldee, Syriac and Samaritan, together with botany, chemistry, optics and mathematics. The accomplished Young was thereafter sought by the Duke of Richmond, Master-General of Ordnance, as his private secretary, a post that would have foreshortened his career, as such posts always seem to do.

Young's medical studies in Edinburgh were spiced with considerable literary activity. He had already turned his hand to translating Shakespeare into Greek, and now he assisted the professor of classics in editing an *Anthology of Greek Poets*.

For Wren, to study the anatomy of the eye was to study Nature's architecture. He dissected the eye, and 'exactly measur'd and delineated the Spheres of the Humours in the Eye, whose Proportions one to another were only guess'd at before.... He contrived an artificial Eye truly and dioptrically made—(as large as a Tennis-Ball) representing the picture as Nature makes it: the Cornea and Crystalline were glass, the other Humours Water. He took an exact Survey of a Horse's Eye, measuring what the Spheres of the Crystalline and Cornea were, and what the Proportions of the Distances of the Centres of every Sphere were upon the Axis.' As late as 1682 we find Wren, when President of the Royal Society, commenting on communications concerning the anatomy of the eye and of refractive errors.

William C. Gibson,
Creative Minds in Medicine

Before long Young decided that a doctoral degree in medicine from a German university had much to recommend it and he therefore enrolled at Göttingen for his clinical work. He has recorded an example of one of his student days there, which included: history of Europe, materia medica, acute diseases, dancing lessons, music lessons on the clavichord, drawing, physics and medicine. This busy round did not keep him from original work, however, and his thesis, on the human voice, was a study of sounds of all sorts. The culmination of his experimental work was his presentation of a universal alphabet, comprising 47 letters. The combinations of these letters would, he held, reproduce any sound which the human voice could utter. The importance of this invention lies not in the fact that it predates George Bernard Shaw's alphabet, but rather in the train of thought that it started in Young's ever-fertile mind. He reasoned that the combining of sounds might have a counterpart in the field of light, and this analogy he pursued for much of his remaining life. The laws governing the interference of light, and his theory of colour vision (now referred to as the Young-Helmholtz theory) were to be his greatest contributions to science, and rank with Newton's discoveries.

The presentation of Young's thesis in the public auditorium in Göttingen, together with his oral examinations, led to his degree as "Doctor of Physic, Surgery and Man-midwifery." The oral examination he described as follows:

> I made no preparatory study, as is usual here, and also at Edinburgh not uncommon, under the name of grinding. The examination lasted between four and five hours; the four examiners were seated round a table, well furnished with cakes, sweetmeats and wine, which helped to pass the time agreeably; the questions were well calculated to sound the depth of a student's knowledge. . . We were all previously obliged to give a summary account of the manner in which our lives had been spent.

Young often returned to the question of language and its potential for communicating ideas. His apprenticeship as a schoolboy was rich in foreign languages and his work on sound formation and conduction, while a medical student, complemented this early interest. Young did not miss a chance to remark: "It is also one of the spurious arts of becoming popular, to affect innovations in language," and he said of Emmanuel Kant, "His language is unpardonably obscure." Perhaps Young foresaw the verbal nightmare into which the language of some sciences would degenerate in less salubrious times.

Whatever Young thought of these products of the human tongue divorced from the brain, he grasped firmly his theory of a universal alphabet tuned to the human ear and representing all possible human voice sounds, usable by all lands. It was no accident that the basalt slab known as the Rosetta Stone, brought to the British Museum after the collapse of Napoleon's forces in Egypt, engaged Young's attention in 1814. It was known that the hieroglyphic inscription was written in 195 B.C., contained a decree by Ptolemy Epiphanes, and had a weathered Greek translation beside it that he was able to handle with ease when it was restored.

Possibly because the hieroglyphs on the stone brought to mind Young's own 47-character alphabet, he made the great initial discovery that Egyptian hieroglyphs were phonetic symbols, and that they were a type of "shorthand for sound." He applied this to deciphering the Rosetta Stone, and independently discovered the special designations used for proper names and for the name of a goddess. Champollion, usually given credit for these discoveries, actually did his work seven years later.

Prior to this work, however, Young had lived his most productive years. He intended to qualify to practice medicine but the Royal College of Physicians required him to stay two consecutive years in one place. His uncle, Dr. Brockleby, died leaving him his house in London and £10,000. Young decided to keep his terms at Emmanuel College, Cambridge, returning to London at the end of 1799 to practise in Welbeck Street. It is unlikely that Young spent his time at Cambridge, as it is alleged young men do at Oxford, in "learning to talk nonsense with distinction," for he was soon writing in the Transactions of the Royal Society on his wave theory of light. In his first year of medical practice he wrote the first account of astigmatism.

Young became interested in capillary attraction and from this subject developed his methods of measuring the size of ultimate particles, which as Lord Rayleigh said nearly 100 years later, establishes Young as the first to measure the size of atoms. He wrote on the theory of the tides, on bridges and construction, providing "Young's modulus," now used daily by engineers in computing the strength and elasticity of materials. He measured the size of the blood corpuscles and of pus cells, and wrote on the dynamics of the blood circulation and the pulse. In the field of life insurance he worked out "A Formula for Expressing Decrement of Human Life." He standardized the imperial gallon, and contributed to the techniques of gas lighting and of ship-building. He was secretary of the Board of Longitude, Conductor of the Nautical Almanac, Foreign Secretary of the Royal Society for 27 years and Volta's successor in the French Academy of Sciences.

At the age of 31 Young married Eliza Maxwell of Lanarkshire, "a woman of sound common sense." As Sir Thomas Lawrence's portrait, painted three years before Young's death, suggests, he was a handsome man. He was a universal genius, at home in many fields of study. This capable man also had a great sense of humour, as revealed in his letters to friends at home and abroad. It would doubtless tickle his fancy to know that a sober medical historian of the early part of the 20th century concluded that, "Young was fond of dancing and good society, but was not regarded as a successful practitioner because he studied symptoms too closely."

Franz Cornelius Donders (1818-1889)

Few men have contributed to as many fields in science as did Franz Cornelius Donders. He was a forerunner of Charles Darwin in evolutionary theory; his works paralleled those of Helmholtz in physics; and his classic description of the anomalies of accommodation and refraction of the human eye stamped him as one of the great clinical investigators in the field of ophthalmology.

He was born in Tilburg, North Brabant, in the Netherlands on May 27, 1818. He was the only boy in the family and followed eight girls. His father was an unbusiness-like man whose interests lay in music, chemistry and literature, and who died of so-called "congestion of the brain" soon after the birth of his son. As a result there was little money available for Franz's education.

It is recorded that Franz, as a precocious child, would be sat upon a table in the local pub and given half-pennies for doing mental arithmetic before the marvelling locals. Even as a child he was paymaster to a large concern nearby. His mother wrote of this: "Imagine the little boy with dark eyes peeping out of the black locks, sitting behind the desk to give the coins to the big workmen!" Another of his duties was the regulation of the city clock. By the age of 11, "Master Franz," as he was called, was employed as a salaried tutor at the school he attended.

Proceeding to the seminaries at Tilburg and Boxmeer, he learned to converse in French, Latin, Greek and English. He also took up the violin. At one stage he was contemplating entering the ministry, but gave this up for medicine, from which calling he never looked back, despite financial difficulties and the unsettled political situation brought about by Belgium's struggle to break away from Holland.

At age 17, Donders entered upon his medical course at the University of Utrecht, being attached as a pupil at the military hospital. In later years he wrote of this period:

> Indescribable was the impression made upon me here by the chemical lectures and experiments of Nicolas de Fremery. When for the first time I mastered the notion that all that exists, in its infinite variety, is composed of a relatively small number of elements, which in certain proportions unite and reunite, it seemed to me as if, with the creation of the elements, the whole of nature had been given, and my imagination worked this out in its own way. Later I became especially interested in physiology.

Because Donders finished his course before he was old enough to graduate at Utrecht, he transferred to the University of Leyden where he presented his graduation thesis: "*Dissertatio inauguralis sistens observationes anatomico-pathologicas de centro nervoso.*" This thesis, based on original work, Donders presented in 1840, at the age of 22. It was well received by his elders and Donders became a man marked for his intelligence. When he commenced his military service, it was not long before the Director General of the Dutch Medical Services singled him out for special duties. By dint of his unceasing labour in the hospital wards and post-mortem rooms at Flushing and at The Hague, he achieved the chair in anatomy, physiology and histology in the reorganized Military Medical School, at the age of 24. It is sobering to think of the teaching duties that he assumed: 18 lectures per week for 46 weeks each year. Only one who had been a tutor since the age of eleven could handle such a load.

At the age of 26 he began considering the possibility that there was a law of the conservation of energy in all of nature. (Another future ophthalmologist, Helmholtz, at age 26, was to enunciate his famous theory on this subject.) Early in 1845, Donders read his paper to the Society of Sciences in Utrecht, on "A Glance at the Change of Matter of Epitellurian Life as the Source of Proper Heat of Plants and Animals." His undergraduate musings in the field of chemistry recurred as he wrote:

> All working in Nature, all life on earth, rests on the change of the elements from which it is formed, but side by side with this

> change of matter stands a change of forces. Both are inseparably bound up together. No one molecule of matter can be destroyed, but neither can a minimum of Energy... Determinate quantities of movement, heat, light, electricity, magnetism, and nervous force respond to each other, and can pass from one into the other.... There is therefore a sum of energy, just as much as there is a sum of matter; both are proportionate to each other, both remain always the same.

On becoming professor extraordinary at the University of Utrecht in 1847, Donders gave an inaugural address on "The Harmony of Animal Life, a Manifestation of Laws." He shows clearly in this discourse how truly he was a forerunner of Charles Darwin, whom he later came to know and whom he visited at Down. Briefly, Donders stated the laws to be those of habit, exercise and inheritance. He wrote:

> Already some light dawns in science on the causes of the phenomena we referred to, the laws of habit and of exercise; and thus, ascending from cause to cause, without ever losing ourselves in dreams about the purpose, we approach, slowly it is true, but with firm step, the ideal point of view, according to which all the phenomena of nature will be seen proceeding from the attribute of the elements and elementary forces. And if once by an All-wise Omnipotence these elements and forces have been created for a predetermined purpose, and if the conditions of the whole future have been enshrined in their attributes, then, also, not a single drop of blood flows without purpose through our veins, but it is a purpose which lies outside the science of nature.

Donders wrote to Darwin in 1871 about the state of the subject in the year 1847:

> I tried to show how the infinite harmonical relations, on the one hand between animals and surrounding nature, on the other hand between the different parts and organs of every organism, are to be deduced from the laws of adaptation by habitude and by exercise, and from the laws of transmission... but still was not aware of the influence of natural selection, your great and immortal discovery, the mighty factor, which alone allowed [one] to give a full and special demonstration of the theory of descent.

Donders' work in physiological optics developed, and he undertook enough clinical practice in this field to eke out a living for his growing family. He was given a temporary hospital in which to work, and did not tell the University of Utrecht until years later that this had determined him to remain there at the moment that the entire medical faculty at Bonn had invited him to fill Helmholtz's chair. He developed his practice and research to such a degree that in 1864 he was able to encompass the whole of one of the principal fields of ophthalmology in his classical work, "On the Anomalies of Accommodation and Refraction of the Eye, with a Preliminary Essay on Physiological Dioptrics." Donders went on to investigate pitch in vowel sounds, "Reaction Time," "Muscular Work and Development of Heat in Relation to the Necessary Elements of Food," "The Influence of the Vagus Nerve on the Cardiac Movements," and "The Chemical Phenomena of Respiration."

Snellen, his pupil, succeeded him in the hospital and Donders was given the chair of physiology in the university. There, he wrote on colour sense and colour blindness, and personally examined without remuneration many of the railway personnel of Holland in the interests of his campaign for safety on railroads and at sea. He took on many public duties and became rector of his university.

On his retirement in May 1888, the Royal Society of London sent as its representatives to the Jubilee Celebration, Joseph Lister, Jonathan Hutchinson and Hughlings Jackson, a tribute to any man. A very large subscription was taken up in his honour, and at his request was used to found a series of travelling fellowships for work in physiology and ophthalmology. He died within a year of this testimonial.

Adolf Kussmaul (1822-1902)

The noisy, gasping respiration of a diabetic patient in coma is known to medical students still as "Kussmaul's air hunger," having been described in 1874 by an erudite German physician. Kussmaul came from a medical family in Karlsruhe and graduated in medicine at Heidelberg at the age of 23. While an undergraduate he became interested in the problem of the colour of the pupil in the human eye, especially the variations noted in patients with glaucoma. He noted that the darkness of the pupil merely reflected the lack of light within the globe. By every means Kussmaul tried to illuminate the interior of the eye, as by immersing it in water, whereupon the vessels of the retina became visible. The ophthalmoscope that he designed failed to meet the requirements, but the determination displayed, and the clarification of the problem achieved, mark Kussmaul as a true forerunner of Helmholtz in ophthalmology. Kussmaul's student work won for him the Karl Fredrick Gold Medal, which was awarded at the rededication ceremonies of the University of Heidelberg.

After graduation in 1845 Kussmaul served as an army doctor and general practitioner for several years until he was struck down with a disease resembling poliomyelitis, which affected his legs. He returned to academic life at Wurzburg where the youthful Virchow was revolutionizing pathology. Thereafter Kussmaul served in the chair of medicine at Heidelberg, Erlangen, Freiburg and Strasbourg. He was the first to describe progressive bulbar palsy, periarteritis nodosa, and the visual inspection of the oesophagus and stomach by a lighted tube.

Kussmaul wrote his *Recollections of Youth by an Old Physician* in 1899, and from it one may get an unforgettable impression of the changes that occurred over the period of Kussmaul's long and useful life. Osler wrote of Kussmaul:

> How true sometimes is the paradox of the Gospel that to save his life a man must lose it! . . . In that best of all medical autobiographies . . . Kussmaul tells the story of his student days and of the happy beginning of a busy life as district physician in the Black Forest—plenty of work, good health, and a happy home with wife and children. Then the overwhelming disaster—sudden paraple-

gia, a long struggle in adverse circumstances, and a final Victory wrought out of the very elements of defeat.

Hermann Von Helmholtz (1821-1894)

Hermann Ludwig Ferdinand von Helmholtz was born at Potsdam, Germany, on August 21, 1821. His father was a teacher of philosophy and philology in the Gymnasium and was a man respected for his ability and integrity. His mother was the daughter of an artillery officer from Hanover, named Penn, a descendent of William Penn, the founder of Pennsylvania.

Growing up as a sickly child and spending much time in bed, Helmholtz learned to read early and widely. With the wooden blocks which his parents provided for him he began to develop rudimentary geometric skills. Though he had early difficulty with languages, he was able by the age of eight to read Homer, and by the age of 12 was reading Arabic fables.

His health improving, he attended the Gymnasium in Potsdam, where he astonished his teachers with his knowledge of geometry. Among his fellow students was Du Bois Reymond, later to distinguish himself in the field of electrophysiology. Helmholtz soon became an avid nature observer and savoured the full range of his father's excellent library. While his classmates in the Gymnasium studied classics he, by subterfuge, drew many diagrams of the pathway of light through the lenses of telescopes. Using some old botanists' magnifying glasses, he set up a great variety of optical systems for his own diversion.

Helmholtz's father wished him to study medicine because there were three other children to consider in the family and some economic independence was thought essential. Helmholtz himself wanted to do physics, but once admitted to the Royal Medical-Chirurgical Friedrich-Wilhelm Institute in Berlin, took up his studies with great enthusiasm. The rector of the Gymnasium in Potsdam provided him with the following certificate of entrance to university:

> His exceptionally calm and reserved disposition is combined with great intellectual enthusiasm. In it we recognize an excellent combination of clear and prudent understanding and deep good nature. His manners bear witness to a carefully preserved, exceptionally pure, and genuine childlike innocence. These peculiarities, along with the richness and power of his mental development give an agreeable and captivating impression, and justify the hope that such a ground-soil of intellectual life will only bring forth the best of fruits.

In return for the army subsidy that he was receiving at the University of Berlin, the agreement was that Helmholtz, along with the other subsidized graduates, would return to the army for service. At the University of Berlin, Helmholtz came under the all-pervading influence of one of the greatest physiologists of all time, Johannes Müller. Helmholtz served him as a student demonstrator, as did such future giants as Du Bois Reymond, Brucke and Rudolf Virchow. Under the influence of Johannes Müller and Gustav Magnus, the professor of physics, a great impetus to investigation was imparted to these young men. The medical course was broadly conceived and basic enough to serve as a foundation for three brilliant careers in quite separate parts of the scientific field.

The stimulating atmosphere that Helmholtz found is best described in his own words: "My own original inclination was towards physics; external circumstances obliged me to commence the study of medicine. It had, however, been the custom of a former time to combine the study of medicine with that of the natural sciences and, whatever in this was compulsory, I must consider fortunate; not merely that I entered medicine at a time in which anyone who was even moderately at home in physical considerations found virgin field for cultivation, but I consider the study of medicine to have been that training which preached more impressively and more convincingly than any other could have done, the everlasting principles of all scientific work; principles which are so simple and yet are ever forgotten; so clear and yet always so hidden by a deceptive veil."

Helmholtz's mathematics were entirely self-taught. He never studied under any great mathematician and yet he became very much at home in this subject, thanks to his excellent grounding.

Ever since the discovery by Ehrenberg, in 1833, of nerve cells, Helmholtz had been anxious to explore these building blocks of the nervous system. In his final year of medicine, he suffered an attack of typhus fever and, in true army fashion, he was hospitalized without expense, and able to save up a small sum of money. With this he bought the microscope that he used to make the discovery embodied in his thesis. What Helmholtz discovered—the fact that the nerve cells were actually connected with the peripheral nerves—seems elementary today. However, it is to Helmholtz that is owed the proof, given with his primitive compound microscope, that the "corpuscles" in the ganglia of leeches and crabs were actually the origin of the nerve fibres. He immediately proceeded with the generalization that the axis cylinder proceeds from the axon hillock or pole of the nerve cell and is continued out into the periphery as the nerve fibre.

Just before he completed his undergraduate work, he read a paper on venous tumours before the Institute for the Education of Army Surgeons. Thereafter Helmholtz published several papers annually until his death in 1894, a total of 217 papers and books.

In 1842 Holmholtz graduated from medical school and served his year as an assistant physician in La Charité Hospital in Berlin. In 1843 he became assistant surgeon to the Red Hussars Regiment. The great Alexander von Humboldt had Helmholtz relieved of some of his military duties at Potsdam so that he could become assistant to the anatomical museum, lecturer on anatomy to the Academy of Arts, and Extraordinary Professor of Physiology to the Albert University.

From this time began his work on the heat of contraction of muscles. He also accurately measured the heat lost from the body through expiration and evaporation from the skin. He devised the "myograph" or the muscle writer, to measure what Thomas Young had always called for, the exact time relations of muscle activity.

It was while library assistant in the Frederick Wilhelm Institute that Helmholtz read the chief mathematical works of the 18th century. At the age of 26 he wrote his essay on "The Conservation of Energy," which he read before the Physical Society of Berlin. Most of the members of the society were openly hostile to the ideas expressed in his paper. However, George Ernst Reimer, the publisher, was so impressed with the author that he put the essay in print and even paid for it himself. Helmholtz's superior officers in the German Army were so impressed that they relieved him of most of his military duties and gave him still more time for research. It is typical of Helmholtz that he never ceased to praise the Heilbronn general practitioner, Robert Mayer who had independently and, at an earlier date, demonstrated the first law of thermodynamics—that all types of energy are transformable but indestructible. Mayer's demonstration applied only to the physiological sphere. Helmholtz applied it as a generalization to all spheres of experience.

At the age of 29, Helmholtz was appointed to the chair of physiology at Königsberg; at 35 to the chair in Bonn; at 38 to Heidelberg; and at 50 he was called to the chair of physics in Berlin, where he served until his death in 1894.

In 1850, a mere 10 years after Johannes Müller opined that the speed of transmission of the nerve impulse could never be measured, Helmholtz succeeded in measuring it. In 1851, Helmholtz invented the ophthalmoscope, for which contribution alone humanity should remember him. Bearing upon the two discoveries above mentioned, Helmholtz said, "A teacher in a University is subject to excellent discipline, in that he is obliged each year, not only to give at least an outline of the whole of his science, but also to convince and satisfy the clear heads among his hearers, some of whom will be the great men of the next generation. This necessity was most beneficial to myself. In preparing my lectures, I was led to devise a method of measuring the velocity of the nerve impulse and also the conception of the ophthalmoscope." Charles Babbage in England, the mathematician who built cogwheel calculators almost as complex as the present electronic computers, showed the British ophthalmologist Wharton Jones how to use a small silvered mirror to reflect light into the eye, the eye being observed through a small central peephole. The application of a lens system to Babbage's suggested instrument might well have established the priority of the British scientist, but nothing ever came of it. In December 1850, Helmholtz gave his first report of his instrument before the Berlin Physical Society. The response was immediate and tumultuous.

In the succeeding years Helmholtz did pioneering work in the fields of acoustics, dynamics, convection, and electrical energy, and he even regarded chemical atoms as basically electrical entities. In Helmholtz's laboratory, his pupil Hertz discovered the waves that eventually led to wireless communication. Helmholtz published his *Handbook of Physiological Optics*, which was produced from the years 1856-1867 and has become a classic. He revived Thomas Young's theory of colour vision and thought of it as a very specialized application of Johannes Müller's law of specific nerve energies.

Helmholtz was interested in all natural phenomena and wrote on such diverse subjects as cloud formations and the effect of wind on the length of waves in the sea. He was also interested in the study of glaciers. He even wrote a paper on hayfever and, in his own case, its apparent control by the application of a dilute solution of quinine sulphate to the nasal mucous membrane.

He loved to play Bach on the grand piano given to him by the Steinway Company of New York in recognition of his services to music. Above all, Helmholtz liked to be regarded as a teacher. As a writer in the *Edinburgh Medical Journal* for 1859 said, "He treats every subject with which he is engaged with a most masterly and philosophical spirit and investigates all things independently for himself, never resting content with the tradition of the early physiologists." This independent mind-set runs through the lives of many in this volume.

Thirty-five years after graduating from the Army Medical Institute in Berlin, he returned to give what was one of his finest lectures, "Thought in Medicine." Here he summed up his philosophy of medical discovery and medical change. Speaking in the same hall in which he had reported his early student papers he said: "Medicine was once the intellectual home in which I grew up; and even the emigrant best understands and is best understood by his native land."

The most succinct obituary notice on Helmholtz appeared soon after his death in London's famous *Punch*:

> What matters titles, Helmholtz is a name,
> That challenges alone the award of fame.
> When Emperors, Kings, Pretenders, shadows all,
> Leave not a dust trace on our whirling ball
> Thy work, O grave-eyed Searcher, shall endure,
> Unmarred by faction, from low passion pure.

Henry Woodward

Woodward was a medical student at the Trinity College, Toronto when, in 1873, he produced light in a bulb by heating a carbon filament, employing its resistance to electricity to bring about illumination. This took place six years before Edison announced the discovery of his light bulb. In fact Woodward was more advanced than Edison, in that he used nitrogen within the bulb, as is done today.

Woodward's accomplice in this endeavour was Matthew Evans, a Toronto hotel keeper, whose role was to provide development funds. The *Canadian Electrical News* noted: "Woodward and Evans were neighbours who frequently got together to experiment with Woodward's large battery and induction coil. At dusk on a late winter day in 1873 they noticed the light from the spark at the contact post. Woodward stated: `If one could only confine that in a globe of some sort, what an invention we would have. It would revolutionize the world.'"

The Canadian patent that they received noted that the bulb was "filled with rarefied gas that will not unite chemically with the carbon when hot." The Toronto pair recorded the situation: "There were four or five of us sitting around a large table. Woodward closed the switch and gradually we saw the carbon become first red and gradually lighter and lighter in colour until it beamed forth in beautiful light." While the Toronto pair struggled for financing, Edison boldly sought $50,000 for experimental work in his Menlo Park, New Jersey, laboratory where he had invented the phonograph. The Canadians, as history was to repeat, lacked the capital to proceed and Woodward sold out, disheartened. Woodward went to England and gave up further work in the electrical field.

Niels Ryburg Finsen (1860-1904)

Finsen was born in the Faeroe Islands off the coast of Scotland and, as a child, suffered from fatigue and anaemia. He early formed the idea that sunlight, when it was visible at all, was beneficial to him.

He went to Copenhagen to study medicine in 1882 where it became evident that he was suffering from Pick's disease of the connective tissues of the liver, spleen and heart. Nevertheless, he graduated in medicine in 1891. Though Finsen as a child suffered from jaundice and measles, not to mention pneumonia and kidney disease, he was forced to leave a Danish preparatory school because he exhibited "small ability and total lack of energy." He therefore pursued his education in Iceland, the home of his parents. At medical school he continued to consider the idea that bright sunlight was helping his condition, and that there must be some scientific reason for this.

After receiving his medical degree at the University of Copenhagen in 1890 and after a short period as a demonstrator in anatomy, he went back to the question of beneficial effects of light. By 1896 he had established a Light Institute in Copenhagen.

Finsen conducted research on the prevention of scarring of the skin in smallpox cases where the patients were exposed to red light. His first group of eight patients came through the trial period with no scar formation, despite smallpox. He then applied light therapy to lupus vulgaris. He sought to replace skin lesions with normal tissue through concentrated ultraviolet rays.

In 1903 Finsen was awarded the Nobel Prize but increasing illness prevented him from attending the ceremonies in Stockholm. He died at the age of 44, though as Professor Joel D. Howell has said, "He was dedicated to his work, so much so that he chose to share freely the fruits of his insight, rather than go into private practice, a decision that earned him the praise and admiration not only of his countrymen, but of people throughout the world."

Frederick Robert Miller (1881-1967)

Miller entered the University of Toronto in 1899, taking his bachelor of science degree in 1903. He achieved first-class honours with such gifted teachers as Ramsay Wright, A.B. MacCallum (Canada's first professor of biochemistry), and R.R. Bensley. In the summer of 1904 Miller was given space at the Marine Biological Laboratory at Woods Hole in Massachusetts, where he conducted research on galvanotropism in living aquatic organisms. Those were the days of Jacques Loeb, Ajax Carlson and R.S. Lillie.

On returning to the University of Toronto Miller decided to take a medical training, which was made possible financially by a demonstratorship in the laboratories of Professor MacCallum and Professor V.E. Henderson. In 1907 Miller's work on galvanotropism was published in the *Journal of Physiology* just as he was graduating with the M.D. degree at Toronto. He moved on to Vienna, Munich, Paris (observing the clinics of Dejerine and Babinski), and most importantly to Liverpool, where he spent the year 1911-1912 with Sir Charles Sherrington. He joined Sherrington at Oxford in 1914 when that pioneer neurophysiologist was made Waynflete Professor of Physiology.

After World War I, Miller became professor of physiology at the University of Western Ontario, in London, Ontario, where a new medical school was in the process of development. He was joined by Dr. Frederick Banting who, after doing orthopaedic surgery in the war years and later at the Toronto General Hospital, was starting a specialty practice in London. He had a long wait for patients and so spent a great deal of time with Miller, and lectured for him on such matters as carbohydrate metabolism to the medical students.

Banting's first research paper on the cerebellum listed him as co-author with Professor Miller. They were able to show that cooling or cocainizing the cerebellar cortex would abolish in animals a neurological state known as "decerebrate rigidity."

On a fateful night in 1920, while preparing for the next day's lecture on the pancreas in relation to blood sugar, Banting came upon a paper by Dr. Moses Barron, a pathologist at the University of Minnesota. In that paper Barron related the shrivelled appearance of the pancreas after a stone had lodged in its exit duct to the duodenum. Barron, who had been trained in pathology by Dean F.F. Wesbrook at Minnesota, introduced his paper with a thorough review of the literature on the role of the islands of Langherhans of the pancreas in diabetes. After a sleepless night Banting approached Professor Miller with the idea of reproducing this situation in laboratory animals. He hoped that by extracting the active principle of islets of Langerhans, they could ameliorate the condition of diabetic patients. After lecturing, Banting discussed with Professor Miller the possibility of carrying out such experiments in his department. Miller had to beg off because there were as yet no adequate laboratories, and his own office office was filled with cats. However, he did suggest that Banting proceed to the University of Toronto, where the professor of physiology was a world-authority on carbohydrate metabolism. So it happened that a one-time medical student researcher came to the rescue of a would-be researcher who was on his way to the Nobel Prize. This Banting received in 1923, for his work on insulin for the relief of diabetes.

Harold R. Novotny and **David L. Alvis**

Harold R. Novotny, while a medical undergraduate at the University of Indiana, published, in 1961, his research, with Dr. David L. Alvis, on "A Method of Photographing Fluorescence in Circulating Blood in the Human Retina." This meticulous work with patients, and with superb instrumentation, was a sensation, for it showed in the most minute detail exactly what was transpiring in the retina in many ocular diseases. The "cotton wool haemorrhages" were sobering to behold.

Perhaps one noteworthy aspect of this report was that it had been rejected by the senior cardio-vascular American journal in the field, and was soon published with much satisfaction by the newcomer, *Circulation*, in 1961.

Not to be forgotten is the work of Stafford Warren, who as a medical student working with Professor G. H. Whipple at the University of California, "did some fundamental work on the systemic intoxication related to exposure to sizeable doses of the X-ray." This was the beginning of Warren's career in the field of atomic research. He later became dean of medicine of the University of California at Los Angeles.

CHAPTER SIXTEEN

Respiration

Jean Pecquet (1622-1674)

The work of Jean Pecquet of Dieppe and Paris, student of medicine at Montpellier was discussed in the chapter on lymphatics. On the respiratory front Pecquet is again encountered, where Sprat in his *History of the Royal Society of London* describes the work of this amazing medical student. Sprat states that "the elasticity of the aire was fully proposed by J. Pecquetus."

John Mayow (1641-1679)

This Cornish student entered Wadham College, Oxford, in 1658, and in 1660 was elected a Fellow of All Souls College. He would have been a contemporary of Christopher Wren, though younger by some years. It is not clear where Mayow acquired his medical knowledge or training, but as Osler says dryly, "He practised at Bath in summer." In 1668 he published an account of his experiments on respiration, and at the same time his tract on rickets. Mayow demonstrated that what is now called oxygen was vital to the life of animals. The fascinating language of his communication is reproduced in the reader's margin of this page. Mayow was elected as a Fellow of the Royal Society of London in 1678. He died a year later at the age of only 38.

Daniel Bernoulli (1700-1782)

This student graduated in medicine at Basel in 1721 with a dissertation on "De Respiratione." In the introduction he said that he proposed to do a mathematical analysis of the problems of physiology. Actually, two years later he became a Professor of Physiology at the St. Petersburg Academy of Science in Russia. His research projects included muscular movement, blood vessels of the eye, optical phenomena, expulsion of moisture and the circulation of the blood. Having written his "system of physiology" he returned to mathematics. He was succeeded by Leonard Euler (1707-1783).

The first medical dissertation to be defended in Russia was by Foma Ivanovich Barsuk–Mosseyer (1768-1811). This took place in front of a large audience at Moscow University in 1794. The subject of the dissertation was "On Respiration."

ON RESPIRATION

The lungs are placed in a recess so sacred and hidden that nature would seem to have specially withdrawn this part both from the eyes and from the intellect; for, beyond the wish, it has not as yet been granted to any one to fit a window to the breast and redeem from darkness the profounder secrets of nature. For of all the parts of the body, the lungs alone, as if shrinking from observation, cease from their movement and collapse at once on the first entrance of light and self—revelation. Hence such an ignorance of Respiration and a sort of holy wonder. Still, let me draw near to the inmost vitals, and concerning so obscure a matter, make at least a guess.

In discussing Respiration I shall follow the method pointed out by nature and begin therefore with inspiration. . . .

With respect, then, to the entrance of the air into the lungs, I think it is to be maintained that it is caused in the following manner by the pressure of the atmosphere. For as the air, on account of the weight of the superincumbent atmosphere, not only rushes into all empty places, but also presses forcibly upon whatever is next to it (as Boyle's experiments have put beyond doubt), it follows that the air, passed through the nostrils and the trachea, up to the bronchia or gates of the lungs, presses against the lungs from within and seeks an entrance into them. Hence it is that when the inner sides of the thorax (which by compressing the lungs from

continued next page

without were resisting the pressure of this air) are drawn outwards by muscles whose function it is to dilate the chest, and the space in the thorax is enlarged, the air which is nearest the bronchial inlets, now that every obstacle is removed, rushes under the full pressure of the atmosphere into the cavities of the lungs, and by inflating them occupies and fills the space of the expanded chest.

The structure of the lungs is adapted for their inflation as thus described, for their substance is composed, as the eminent Dr. Malpighi has noted, of very fine membranes, which form an almost infinite number of spherical vesicles whose mutual connection is such that there is easy access from the trachea to those nearest to it, and from these again to others. Consequently when these vesicles are inflated by an inrush of air, the whole substance of the lungs must necessarily expand....

John Mayow, 1668

John Oswald

This South Carolina medical student chose as the subject for his inaugural dissertation in 1802 "An Experimental Inquiry into the Phenomena of Suspended Animal Life from Drowning, Hanging and the Action of Noxious Airs, Together with the Most Certain and Expeditious Mode of Recovering Animals in that State." This appeared in Philadelphia and contained 72 pages of text. The thesis described 44 elaborate experiments in which he was assisted by two physicians and two fellow students.

Johannes Müller (1801-1858)

The great Johannes Müller, the inspiration for much of Germany's physiological science in the 19th century, produced a graduation thesis at Leipzig at the age of 21 entitled "De Respiratione Foetus, Commentatio Physiologica." At the age of 25 he enunciated the principle of "specific nerve energies," which put him on centre stage in the world of medical research. Thereafter his research on vision, the vocal cords, voice and hearing were of great importance. His name is remembered in connection with the Müllerian duct described in his publication at Bonn University. He was at odds with John Mayow, previously discussed, on the question of the respiration of the foetus. With his microscopic work he set the stage for the future of German embryology and histology.

Theodore Schwann (1810-1882)

Schwann began his student work at Bonn University and because he was unsure of his future, started with philosophy, mathematics and sciences. His mentor Johannes Müller was there working on the spinal cord of frogs.

However, Schwann studied medicine for two years at Wurzburg and then went to Berlin to rejoin Müller. In turn, his own thesis was on respiration, "De necessitate aëris atmosphaerici ad evolutionem pulli in ovo incubito," which was published in Berlin. Thereafter he helped Müller on his H*andbuch* which could be said to have changed physiology. Those were the days when "spontaneous generation" was in the air, so to speak, but Schwann announced that infusoria were definitely not developed in that manner. With Schleiden he launched "the cell theory."

John Snow (1813-1858)

On December 16, 1837, while still a student of medicine, Snow reported to the Westminster Medical Society, which was later to merge with the Medical Society of London, the results of his experiments on the effects on animal life of combustion of candles containing arsenious acid.

Snow qualified in medicine in 1838 and within a year had performed and reported his experiments that suggested that carbon dioxide gas was toxic when inhaled, and that any decrease in atmospheric oxygen was dangerous to life. He continued that if both aspects were combined, the effect would prove rapidly fatal.

Snow is remembered as a student of anaesthesia. He had to his credit 4000 cases in which he had used chloroform without a single death. History has cast him as the great lifesaver in the cholera epidemic of 1854 in London where he brought a local epidemic to an end by removing the handle from the Broad Street pump which was serving up water from a polluted source. An excellent pub, the John Snow, on the same site today in London has its walls covered with photographs depicting that history.

Alphonse Gal

This inquisitive medical student began in 1868 to spend his summers serving on a sponge fishing boat off the coast of Turkey. By 1872 he was ready to present his thesis for graduation in medicine at Montpellier, that oldest of medical schools in the world still teaching. The title of his dissertation was "Des dangers du travail dans l'air comprimé et des moyens de les prévenir." He records 240 observations which he made on the physiological changes in divers who had been in an atmosphere of compressed air.

His description of "the bends," as these symptoms are now called, began sometimes with "the fleas" under the skin, then muscle and joint pains lasting from hours to two days. He tried rubbing into the skin "soothing balm." He recounts one case of spinal paralysis, with a cure. Another case of paraplegia was less successful in a 20–year–old man "given to drink." He was highly critical of "the bad habit of the Greeks" who hoisted up divers from 37 meters below the surface with very rapid decompression. Gal was faced with a problem in that the only Italian doctor available was 100 miles away. On one occasion the doctor gave a cathartic to a patient who died on the ninth day, paraplegic and uncatheterized.

The sponge ships on which Gal made his observations went as far across the Mediterranean as Bengazi. His autopsies showed diffuse softening of the spinal cord in its lower section in some paraplegics. He raised in his thesis questions for further research, such as inflammation and capillary haemorrhages. For those who were interested in decompression sickness in World War II, this was a veritable textbook.

Gal made excellent clinical observations. Among others he noted that the deltoid muscle heavily used by divers was likely to be most affected with muscle pains on surfacing. He set out to prevent these cases by prescribing shallower depths and, above all, slower decompression, with a gentler ascent to the surface. He noted finally that his preventive measures did decrease the occurrence of paraplegia in his men.

Claude Gordon Douglas (1882-1963)

This student was born in Leicester into a family boasting many generations of physicians. After schooling at Brighton and at Wellington College he entered New College, Oxford, to study for a degree in the Honours School of Natural Sciences (Animal Physiology). In 1904 he secured a first-class at the bachelor's degree level and proceeded to a research degree under the celebrated John Scott Haldane, F.R.S., a world authority on human respiration. Haldane was famous for the respiration experiments he did on his son, John Burdon Sanderson Haldane, the future biochemist.

In 1905 Douglas entered upon his clinical courses at Guy's Hospital Medical School in London and achieved his B.M., B.Ch. in December 1907. He had, while there, carried on research with A. E. Boycott. However, his principal undergraduate research had been with Haldane at Oxford where he developed the method of estimating the total haemoglobin in the body, and thus the total blood volume, by the dilution principle, using carbon monoxide as a marker. He used his method to calculate the volume of red blood corpuscles, and of plasma in rabbits, in anaemia, subsequent to haemorrhage, and after blood transfusion.

He accompanied J. S. Haldane, first to the top of the Peak of Teneriffe, and later to the 14,000–foot top of Pike's Peak in Colorado (which Pike never reached). Then Douglas sought a compressible container for gases used in respiratory research, and recalled the rubberized bags which he had seen at a "magic lantern" show, as a child, in which the oxygen and the "fuel gases" needed for the limelight were stored. The "Douglas Bag" was born, which medical students carried on their backs as they trotted about Oxford. Douglas applied the bag in his studies on the energy expended and the gaseous metabolism of steelworkers, housewives, miners, barrowmen, swimmers and even cricketers.

In 1914 Douglas was quick to volunteer for the armed forces and after a short period at the Netley Hospital was then catapulted into the frightful carnage of the Ypres salient, where in 1915 the German forces used chlorine gas. Douglas was awarded the Military Cross in 1916, and the Cross of St. Michael and St. George in 1919, having been four times mentioned in dispatches. He was by then regarded as "the chief living authority on gas sickness."

Douglas the teacher brought on several generations of research–minded students, among them Dr. Fred Kergin, a Rhodes Scholar in 1930 from British Columbia, later professor of surgery at Toronto; Dr. Carleton B. Chapman, a foremost American medical educator; and Roger Bannister, the four–minute–miler, who joined in a paper on the arterial CO2 after heavy exercise. Douglas in his later years carried on research on silicosis, coal dust, on miners' nutrition (with R. A. Peters and R. McCarrison). He was made a Fellow of St. John's College, Oxford, while still a medical undergraduate, and remained a Fellow for 66 years. For a time he was Dean of the College and quickly put down noisy revels in the quadrangle after dark by fining the first student he encountered. Any miscreant damaging college property was assessed the highest possible cost of its replacement. Douglas lived for the notable college gardens.

Dickinson Woodruff Richards (1895—1973)

Thanks to André Cournand's survey of Richards' contributions, historians can trace the research interests of this first-class American scientist beginning with his graduation from Yale University in 1917.

Richards went to Columbia University in New York for his medical training and as a medical student, in 1922, took his master of arts degree in physiology while working with the perceptive Lawrence J. Henderson. He graduated with the M.D. degree in 1923.

Richards' educational background is interesting. At the Hotchkiss Preparatory School Richards is memorialized as the student who in 1913 made an average in his subjects of 93.4 per cent. Thanks to his Greek teacher there for two years Richards entered Yale University with a prize for Greek, having made the highest grade ever recorded in his entrance examination. At Yale he studied mathematics, the natural sciences and especially the humanities. He led his class in each year.

His student work with Henderson on pulmonary and circulatory physiology he returned to after graduation, internship and a year at the National Institute for Medical Research in London. Throughout his life he worked with distinguished colleagues such as A. L. Barrach and Cournand, and shared the Nobel Prize in Medicine or Physiology in 1956 with Cournand and Werner Forssman. Richards was an outspoken man on the need for improved health care for the aged and for addicted patients.

CHAPTER SEVENTEEN

Surgery

Thomas Greenhill (1681-1740)

At the age of 24 Greenhill published what has been called "a very creditable work for so young a man and its information is still useful." This work was "The Art of Embalming... With an Account of the Particular Opinions, Experiences and Inventions of Modern Physicians." In this work he included "a better method of Embalming and a pharmacopeia." It was in three parts "adorn'd with... sculptures." In it he has a letter to Sir Hans Sloane, 14 plates, one of them a map of Egypt, and a commendation of Sir Thomas Browne's "dormative" hymn. He was one of 39 children born to one mother, thanks to one husband. All were born alive and baptized, a fact which is recognized in the arms of the family, modified in 1698. Greenhill practised surgery in London.

Jacques René Tenon (1724-1816)

In 1755 Tenon read a paper in which he propounded his view that it was necessary to destroy the crystalline capsule if the cataract operation was to be successful. This formed the basis for his thesis in 1757, "*De Cataracta*."

Tenon was born in 1724, the son of a surgeon. The anatomist Winslow soon spotted his ability and pressed him into anatomical research. With other professors he made his mark in botany and did research in natural history. At the age of 20 he became an army surgeon and fought in Flanders. He became chief of surgery at the Salpêtrière, served as a professor of pathology, and sat in the first legislative assembly. He was given the Legion of Honour. His most important work was "*Mémoire sur les hôpitaux de Paris*," which appeared in Paris in 1788. It was so graphic that it raised a tremendous storm, particularly at the Hotel Dieu. This explosion caused reforms in hospitals of Paris that were long overdue in the 18th century. Before he concluded his work he founded a special hospital for children.

John Jones (1729-1791)

Jones was America's first professor of surgery and has been called by some "the father of American surgery." He was born in Jamaica, Long Island, in 1729. His father and grandfather were medical practitioners.

In 1747, after a private education in New York, Jones became apprenticed in Philadelphia to his cousin Dr. Thomas Cadwalader, who had trained in London under William Cheselden and then received his M.D. at the University of Rheims. In 1750, following his preceptor's example, Jones studied with Cheselden in England along with Percival Pott and William Hunter. He then enrollled at Rheims and was soon awarded his medical degree. His thesis title was "Observations on Wounds." Jones went to Paris and made rounds with the surgeons at Hotel Dieu, where he saw exactly what Tenon was to write about in 1788. Jones' impression was this: "It is impossible for a man of any humanity to walk through the long wards of this crowded hospital without a mixture of horror and commiseration at the sad spectacle of misery."

Before returning to the colonies, Jones studied in Leyden and in Edinburgh briefly. In 1755 he was involved in defeating the French forces near Lake George where he treated the captured French commander, Baron Dieskau.

On returning to New York to practice he was associated with John Bard, his son Samuel and three other colleagues in petitioning the governors of King's College hoping to start a medical school. It opened in 1767 and Jones became the professor of surgery.

Jones, Samuel Bard, and Peter Middleton founded the New York Hospital and designed well-ventilated eight-bed wards. Later Jones moved to Philadelphia where in the Pennsylvania Hospital he had, in his large practice, his friends Benjamin Franklin and George Washington.

Christopher Weber

Weber was born in Prussia, the son of a merchant. For his medical education he attended universities in Halle, then Helmstadt, and finally Göttingen where he received his M.D. degree.

His thesis presented in March 1758 was entitled "Some Observations Made Upon Diseased Bodies of Infants." It was one of the earliest published studies of pyloric hypertrophy of the stomach. He noted that newborns suckled well, but vomited stomach contents. One died on the sixth day and the post mortem showed a "pylorus that was hard to the touch like cartilage, and contracted." He found that the duodenum contained no food whatever but that bile was found in it up to, but not beyond, the pylorus.

Johann Friedrich Dieffenbach (1792-1847)

With the ease of transfer between universities in Europe in his time, Dieffenbach studied at the University of Bonn, then in Paris, then Montpellier, and finally at Wurzburg where he graduated in 1822. His thesis was "N*onnulla de regeneratione et transplantatione*." After his training at the Charité in Berlin from 1829 to 1840, he succeeded the famous von Graefe as professor of surgery.

There are few fields in which Dieffenbach did not excel. He successfully treated, in 1829, a strabismus by modifying the affected tendons of the eye muscles. He went on to skin grafting, a natural development from his thesis, and to orthopaedic surgery. Transplantation, the transfusion of blood and operative surgery were the fields in which he made great advances. He was keener upon native invention than upon statements in books.

William-Benjamin Amant Duchenne (1806-1875)

Better-known to the world simply as "*Duchenne de Boulogne*," this student took his baccalaureate at Douai in 1829. He developed a great interest in natural science, but his father, a fisherman, wanted him to succeed in his trade. However, he was able to study medicine at the University of Paris with such teachers as Laennec, Dupuytren, Magendie, Velpeau and Cruveilhier. He graduated in April 1831 with a thesis on burns.

Following his student habit Duchenne wrote daily notes about what he had seen on the wards, as well as what he had been able to read in books and journals. Strangely, he had no university post and no hospital appointment. He was nevertheless a great student of the neuro-muscular diseases and, it is said, "brought order out of confusion." His friends Trousseau and Charcot helped him to publish his work. He introduced muscle biopsy as a diagnostic procedure. He clarified poliomyelitis as a single disease. Appropriately, he is memorialized by a monument at the Salpêtrière in Paris.

Just Marie Marcellin Lucas-Championnière (1843-1913)

This champion of Joseph Lister's work on antisepsis, journeyed to Scotland in 1869 to see Lister at work. He published in his student thesis a study of the first principles of defense against gangrene. Those were "extreme and minute care in the dressing of wounds." As one of his biographers has said, "But his isolated voice was not heard." On his return from Glasgow he wrote his excellent summary, *Journal de Médicine et de chirurgie pratique*. He is highly praised in the *Life of Pasteur* by R. Vallery Radot in which Sir William Osler provided the introduction. He introduced antisepsis into France, and made a great reputation for himself in the surgery of hernia. He assisted his teacher Paul Broca in trephining the bones of the skull. In this connection he produced a book *Trepanation néolithique* in Paris in 1912.

Claude Bernard (1813-1878)

In 1846 Bernard observed, independently, but one year after Weber brothers, slowing of the heart on stimulation of the vagus nerve. The slowing was determined by listening to the heart sounds. This fact was not published by Claude Bernard but by one of his students, Lefevre, in his thesis in 1848.

Professor J.M.D. Olmsted, in his excellent biography of Claude Bernard, tells the story of how he was invited by the Emperor to discuss his science at one of Empress Eugénie's six-day retreats at Compiegne. The Emperor ordered the Minister of Public Instruction to give Claude Bernard what he most needed. He asked for a laboratory but was given instead a first assistant, Paul Bert, as his "préparateur." When Bernard received new laboratories at the Museum of Natural History he gave his chair at the Sorbonne to Paul Bert. Even as an undergraduate he had shown the manual dexterity that enabled him to produce a superior pancreatic fistula, to trace out the chorda tympani and the fine vasomotor nerves. The commissioner of police, who came close to arresting him for experimenting on his stolen dog, later became one of his greatest supporters.

Paul Bert (1833-1886)

Bert was born in Auxerre in 1833 and entered the College of Saint Barbe founded in 1460 and, as Sherrington says, "of old and good repute." The father of physiology, Jean Fernel, had been a student there.

Paul Bert began to study engineering but changed to law and actually passed his licensing examinations. However, he met Gratiolet, Director of Practical Anatomy at the Museum, who turned him in the direction of medicine. Paul Bert graduated in medicine in Paris in 1863. His thesis, "*De la greffe animale*," launched him as a pioneer in skin grafting. The specialty of plastic surgery during the war of 1870 with Germany had certainly been fostered by Bert's original work. He submitted it for the prize offered in experimental physiology by the Académie des Sciences in 1865, which he won.

Bert was an outspoken republican and in 1871 was elected as a Deputy. Ten years later he was made minister of public instruction in Gambetta's ministry, and fell with him after a short time in power.

In some ways Paul Bert could be considered the father of aviation medicine. His classic "*La Pression Barometrique*" raised this subject to the level of international scientific interest. Not only did he build decompression chambers, to study the phenomenon of anoxia, but he sponsored the famous "Zenith" balloon expedition.

Bert doubted the value of vaccination against smallpox. Nevertheless, he had himself vaccinated and two weeks later at the Charité Hospital he inoculated himself with smallpox virus from a man dying of the disease. No ill effects ensued, so he became a vociferous advocate of vaccination. Early in 1886 he was sent out to Tonkin as Resident General to deal with French colonial problems which civilians had with the military. He had almost completed his task when he was struck down with dysentery and died in November 1886 at age 53 at Hanoi.

Paul Bert regretted that in his 1863 thesis, his work could not cover the many fields upon which he had entered. His student Georges Martin wrote his thesis at the University of Paris in 1873 on the subject *De la duré de la vitalité des tissus et des conditions d'adhérence des restitutions et transplantations cutanées (greffes animales)*.

Paul Bert conducted an exhausting number of experiments during his life. In 1863 he surgically united a rat and a cat on six occasions and was convinced that vascular communication had been established between the animals. For instance, atropine instilled per rectum in the cat caused dilation of the rat's pupils. He went into problems of nerve grafts and those of periosteal tissue. In all his work he noted the abundance of uncritical views abroad in the world, and hoped not to add to them. He lacked nothing in perseverance. He was a pioneer in tissue transplants and in organ transplants. On the question of nose transplants or repairs he cited the fact that the French parliament had declared the nose as part of the body. He said that any transplant depended for its success upon the age of the donor, nature of the replacement, the recipient, comparative zoology, the establishment of new connections, nutrition, secretions and innervation. His student thesis contained 60 references to other authors. His experiments in the course of preparing his thesis covered more than 100 animal investigations. He went into the results of duels fought at Heidelberg, and discussed the replacement of teeth.

David Newman (1853-1924)

In 1883 the *Glasgow Medical Journal* published an article by David Newman entitled "Malposition of the Kidney." As a medical student he wished to determine the function of separate kidneys and devised his cystoscope for this purpose. This was the first to use an incandescent electrical lamp along with the cystoscope. The lamp was passed into the bladder separately as were urethral catheters or other instruments used. His publication contained excellent illustrations.

W. Scott Lang

In his Edinburgh M.D. thesis in 1886 this student wrote on his own research, on "Internal Diseases of the Knee Joint." It was published in the *Edinburgh Medical Journal* in the same year. Lang had a tear or a rupture in the semilunar cartilage in his knee-joint and was operated upon by Thomas Annandale, who had been John Goodsir's demonstrator and Lister's successor as professor of surgery in Edinburgh. Lang and two of his classmates may have been soccer players, for all suffered from the same problem. By experimenting on a cadaver, Lang found that twisting could cause the lesion from which he suffered, but pulling could not. He stated that given a good description of an accident, that is, the position of the upper versus the lower leg, the diagnosis could be made. If the patient had a torn internal cartilage, the foot toed in. If, on the other hand, the external cartilage had ruptured, the foot toed out.

Christopher Wren once successfully carried out a splenectomy on a dog. In describing his technique he implored successors to "have a care of the guts." Little did he imagine that a medical student in Paris in 1898 would report in the *Hospital Gazette* on 274 cases of splenectomy with 170 survivals. The student J. Van Verts was indisputably thorough.

Joseph Erlanger (1874-1965)

Erlanger, who shared the Nobel Prize in Medicine in 1944 with Herbert Spenser Gasser, lived a productive 91 years.

He was born of immigrant parents who barely had an elementary education. Joseph was the sixth of seven children born in San Francisco, California. He attended an elementary South Cosmopolitan school where both German and French were offered. He chose German, which was to be of great service when he went to Johns Hopkins University in research and when he did postgraduate work in Germany. In high school he chose the Latin option over the Greek.

He and his neighbour, Albion Walter Hewlett, decided to try to enter the University of California, Berkeley, after only two years of high school instead of three. They succeeded.

In 1891 they entered the College of Chemistry, which they thought would take them towards medicine. They were sergeants in military training. Erlanger's home was just around the corner from Cooper Medical School, but a senior student at Harvard Medical School, Herbert Moffitt, told them of the opening recently of the Johns Hopkins Medical School in Baltimore. That is where Erlanger was determined to go. At the last minute Hewlett chose to stay in San Francisco and attend the Cooper School. A year later Hewlett applied to the Johns Hopkins Medical School and was accepted, but he had to repeat the first year and was therefore in the class graduating in 1900.

Erlanger used highly recommended German textbooks at Hopkins, but in physiology used Michael Foster's three-volume work. He already had a research background beginning with his undergraduate work at the University of California at Berkeley. In his final year there he had studied vertebrate embryology that was a research course in which he worked on the ova of the newt Amblystoma punctatum. He received a top grade in his thesis project there. In his second year at Hopkins Erlanger published "A Study of the Metabolism in Dogs with Shortened Small Intestines." This he did with his friend A.W. Hewlett, and it appeared in the *American Journal of Physiology* in 1901. This paper had 50 references to the literature, five tables and four figures. Most references were in German. The dogs that he studied had been used in Professor Halsted's search on the length of gut that might safely be removed in surgical situations in humans, by analogy. Erlanger, with Hewlett, found only a slight disturbance in the digestive processes apart from interference in the absorption of fats. That work indicated that between 70 and 83 per cent of the gut could be safely removed. After one year's internship at Johns Hopkins he received an assistantship in Professor Howell's department of physiology, where he worked on the projection of nerve action potentials of a frog's beating heart on a visual screen. Between first and second year he spent six weeks in Germany in Professor Hofmeister's biochemical laboratory in Strasbourg. On returning to Hopkins Erlanger studied the circulatory aspect of orthostatic albuminuria in a fellow student. In his third year at Hopkins he was lecturing to medical students on digestion and metabolism. Soon after Wilhelm His, Jr., had described the A-V bundle in the heart, Erlanger invented a clamp that, when applied to that bundle, could cause complete heart block. In this work he was joined by another medical student researcher, Arthur Hirschfelder. On graduation he was off to the University of Wisconsin and eventually to the revived medical school at George Washington University in St. Louis, Missouri. Then, like Gasser, he took up the cathode ray tube in his work on nerve fibre stimulation. Together they were awarded the Nobel Prize in 1944, "for their discoveries regarding the highly differentiated functions of single nerve fibres."

It might have been thought that the atrocities and indiscriminate destruction of life in Spain were those which are prone to characterize the internecine strife of a people in the throes of civil war, but most of the bombs let loose by aircraft were dropped by Nazi and Italian airmen who used Spain as their practice ground for future exploits already envisaged. It is a sad commentary on the world 'Kultur' and on modern civilization that in Spain the use of the Red Cross on hospitals had to be abandoned, since it was found that this emblem no longer gave sanctuary, but invited, nay, provoked air attacks by those brought up in the countries of a Hitler or a Mussolini.

Surgeon Rear Admiral, G. Gordon-Taylor's foreword to Douglas Jolly's *Field Surgery in Total War*. (1941)

Wilder Penfield (1891-1976)

Penfield was born in Spokane, Washington, where his father was a physician. After his preparatory schooling at Galahad, Wisconsin, Penfield entered Princeton University, from which he went to Oxford on a Rhodes scholarship. In the summer vacation of 1915 he worked as a "dresser" at a Military Hospital in France. He had planned to return to France the next summer and was on the S.S. *Sussex* that was torpedoed between Dover and the French coast. The explosion was so great that he was thrown in the air and, on landing on the deck, broke his leg. When Sir William Osler, the Regius Professor of medicine at Oxford, learned that one of "his boys" was injured, he had him brought to "The Open Arms," his home at 13 Norham Gardens overlooking the Parks in Oxford. There Penfield convalesced while at the same time becoming a bibliophile in that book-laden house.

With a letter from William Osler, Penfield returned to the United States and became a medical student at Johns Hopkins in Baltimore. There he produced an 11-page research paper entitled "The Treatment of Severe and Progressive Haemorrhage by Intravenous Injections." This appeared, with five figures, in the *American Journal of Physiology* in 1919.

As he developed as a neurosurgeon at Columbia University in New York, he was given six months study leave to work with Professor Rio-Hortega in Madrid on the development of scars from penetrating wounds of the brain as well as the basic make-up of brain tumours. He later worked for several months with Professor Otfrid Foerster in Breslau on the relief of epilepsy in damaged brains.

With the help of Alan Gregg, Director of the Medical Sciences Division of the Rockefeller Foundation, Penfield built the world's most modern Neurological Institute in Montreal, which opened in 1934. Under his guidance this became a mecca for neurological education and research.

During World War II Penfield became chairman of the National Research Council of Canada Committee on Neurosurgery, and expeditiously wrote an army manual for use in the field. With returning casualties and with the end of the war Penfield did for Canada what Harvey Cushing tried to do in the United States in 1918—that was to keep brain-injured veterans together for study. He achieved this in the military annex that was built at the Montreal Neurological Institute.

Penfield's literary career was extensive and he has written *The Torch*, about Hippocrates, having spent some months on the Island of Cos with his wife. His volume, *The Difficult Art of Giving—The Epic of Alan Gregg* was a masterpiece. A standard work of reference today remains his three-volume *Cytology and Cellular Pathology of the Nervous System*. His knowledge of German and Spanish, added to his long-standing ability in French, served him well. He gave opportunities without number to young medical students to come to Montreal and carry out researches in neurology. Upon Sherrington's death Penfield received his teacher's mantle and joined the small band recognized in England with the Order of Merit. His legacy continues in the institute that he initiated in Montreal. It has become a veritable United Nations of neurology for training and research.

Lester Reynold Dragstedt (1893-1975)

Dragstedt was born in Anaconda, Montana, of Swedish parents. As a boy he had great ability to memorize poetry, long parts of the Bible and great speeches.

Professor A.J. Carlson, the University of Chicago physiologist, told the father, "Send the boy to Chicago. They will find out in three months if he has any brains and, if he does not, you can bring him back to Anaconda and put him to work in the copper smelter." Although Dragstedt, Jr., thought of studying physics, he took up physiology with Carlson, achieving his bachelor of science degree at the University of Chicago. For his master's degree he did graduate student work in physiology and pathology. In 1920 he achieved his Doctor of Philosophy in physiology in the same laboratory. Before graduation in medicine in 1921, Dragstedt produced several papers on toxaemia in intestinal obstruction, the gastric juice and ulcers. He studied also closed intestinal loops and even did research on parathyroid tetany.

En route Dragstedt served as assistant professor of physiology in the University of Iowa until, in the First World War, he did military service. His Iowa research on intestinal obstruction was a milestone. He was able to keep dogs alive after complete duodenectomy. It is said that his operation gave Allen Whipple at the Presbyterian in New York the idea for Whipple's eventual radical operation for cancer of the pancreas.

The war service already mentioned was strenuous. Dragstedt was first sent to Washington, D.C., to work on typhoid, then to Yale to work with Milton Winternitz on toxic substances, then to New Jersey to do post mortems from morning till night for eight months. He was still a medical student when all this was happening, and he had the honour of addressing the Chicago Surgical Society on his student work on intestinal obstruction as well as parathyroid surgical problems. After serving at Northwestern Medical School he joined the revived University of Chicago where Rockefeller funds produced a new type of medical school. There he joined Professor Phemister, who held the view that it would be easier for a scientist to be a surgeon than for a surgeon to learn to be a scientist. After a surgical tour of Europe he returned to Chicago to try to determine if duodenectomy might cause pernicious anaemia. In the new Billings Hospital in Chicago he began his notable studies on gastric fistula, vagotomy and the pancreas. In 1947 Dragstedt succeeded Phemister as professor of surgery at the University of Chicago and in retirement at the University of Florida worked on secretions in the stomach and the physiology of the liver and pancreas, producing eight papers. He received many prizes and medals during his lifetime, including recognition by Sweden. There was no return to Anaconda to work in the copper smelter.

Ernest L. Wynder (b. 1922)

This medical student at the George Washington University School of Medicine in St. Louis undertook a study with the professor of surgery, Evarts Graham (1883-1957), on tobacco smoking as a possible etiological factor in bronchogenic carcinoma, in 684 proven cases. This was reported in the *Journal of the American Medical Association* in 1950 and caused a sensation. This was particularly true for Evarts Graham, who was known to be a heavy smoker. He was not enamoured of Wynder's theory. The authors had made a preliminary report to the National Cancer Conference in 1949. Graham gave up smoking.

Not far away in American terms was the University of Minnesota in Minneapolis where in 1912 Dr. Moses Barron had done his internship in the University Hospital under Dr. Frank Wesbrook. (Wesbrook was about to return to Canada to become the first president of the University of British Columbia.) Barron was impressed with the number of cases of cancer of the lung that he as a young intern was seeing. After returning from World War I he wrote an article in the medical press concerning what he thought to be an increasing number of cases in heavy smokers. He was also the man who fired Frederick Banting's imagination, leading to a method of extracting insulin from the pancreas.

Wynder's undergraduate study was well planned. Of the 684 proven cases, 634 were personally interviewed and another 33 responded by mail. The remaining 17 cases were described by intimate acquaintances of the patients concerned.

Wynder was thorough in his methods. He questioned the patients concerning their past 20 years of history and did the same with the controls. Both physicians and hospitals were of great assistance in digging out the facts. Moreover, he wanted to know everything about the occupations and the possible lung hazards of his cases over the years. All tissue was examined histologically. His controls were non-smoking patients in the hospital clinics and hospital in-patients.

He found that 96 per cent of those who suffered from cancer of the lung had been smoking 20 years. Eighty per cent had been smoking more than 30 years; 19.1 per cent of the males were chain smokers. Only two per cent were females. As to non-smokers, there were only two per cent suffering from cancer of the lung. Today, few cases go undetected, thanks to the work of Sir Richard Doll, formerly the Regius Professor of Medicine at Oxford and his associates in the Royal College of Physicians of London. Doll built at Oxford, post-war, one of the world's most celebrated medical schools. The Queen recently made him a Companion of Honour, one of a handful of scholars.

Michael E. DeBakey

Michael DeBakey gives an excellent description of his medical student contribution in the form of a roller pump:

> When I was a senior medical student, I worked part-time as an assistant in the experimental laboratory of a young internist on the full-time faculty at Tulane University [New Orleans]. He was interested in the physiology of the circulation, and gave me the assignment to develop a pump which could simulate the pumping action of the heart, which could provide him with a means for changing the character and pattern of the pulse wave. I began by doing library research on pumps, which I found have been used by man for thousands of years, mostly in early days for moving water and for irrigation. After rubber was developed, there were several efforts to use the "milking tube" principle, but these devices were generally bulky and impractical and had the added objectionable feature of "creeping" of the tube to the pump mechanism.
>
> I finally developed a rotary pump of relatively simple design, and with a fixed rubber flange on the tube, the "creeping" factor was completely obviated. Although there was a slight pulsation in the outflow, it was almost a continuous flow pump.
>
> When I became an intern at Charity Hospital in New Orleans, I began using the rotary pump for direct blood transfusion. Venipunctures were performed, and the respective needle adapters fitted into the needles of the donor and the recipient, and the transfusion began by turning the crank in the clockwise direction. Each complete revolution gave 2 cc. of blood, so that it took approximately 250 revolutions to transfuse a unit of blood. I had the opportunity to use it in hundreds of cases with complete success.

At the same time a new blood transfusion needle was developed by DeBakey and reported in the 1934 volume of the *American Journal of Surgery*. This was a considerable improvement on the ingenious grooved brass plate that Christopher Wren had designed at Oxford at age 24;

once the vein was trapped by the overlying groove, a needle or a quill was introduced through a small hole in the superior surface of the brass plate, to allow penetration of the firmly held vein. Robert Boyle described the procedure: "Our dextrous Experimenter ... conveyed a small dose of the Solution or Tincture into the opened vessel, whereby setting into the mass of blood... The Dog... not only recovered but began to grow fat so manifestly that 'twas admired: but I could not long observe how it fared him: for this Experiment having made him famous, he was soon after stolen away from me."

While DeBakey was improving intravenous techniques, Francis Moore was entering Harvard Medical School. As a student, on the way to becoming professor of surgery there, he wrote a college musical that was performed with Alastaire Cooke as director. This contribution and many more are recounted in Moore's recently published autobiography.

CHAPTER EIGHTEEN

Cultural Activities

Contributors are presented in the following groups: writers, poets, musicians and sculptors, clinical presentations by undergraduates, the rise and fall of student societies and journals, publishing and translation.

WRITERS

Elias Friedrich Heister (1715-1740)

This short-lived medical student was the son of the distinguished Lorenz Heister (1683-1758), the founder of scientific surgery in Germany and author of a two-volume work on surgery published at Nuremberg in 1718. Among other things he originated the term "tracheotomy." His son, at the age of 21, wrote an amazing *Apologia* for Sir Thomas Browne. Sir William Osler said of it, "I have not met with an eighteenth-century writer who knows so well and quotes so often the *Religio Medici*." He also noted that this medical student gave "a very good account of Vaninus (1585-1619), burnt for atheism at Toulouse in 1619." Osler added, "Among the natural theologians he places his father, to whom he pays a touching tribute."

Not every man fits every hour.
Goethe

Elisha Bartlett (1804-1855)

Osler christened Bartlett "A Rhode Island Philosopher," when he addressed the Rhode Island Medical Society at Providence in 1899.

Bartlett began his extensive writing career at the age of 17, when he contributed a paper to the *Worcester Spy* in Massachusetts. Born of Quaker parents, and incidentally born with transposition of the viscera without sequelae, Bartlett became an avid early reader of the *Arabian Nights*, *Robinson Crusoe* and other available literature. After preliminary schooling in Rhode Island, he then attended the Friends' School in New York. After four years of apprenticeship to physicians in Rhode Island, he took his M.D. degree at Brown University in 1826. That was one year before the "untimely end of the Medical Department" there. William Osler, in speaking to the Rhode Island profession in 1899, called on them to help raise $1 million dollars for the preclinical department. However, until the end of World War II it was not possible to mount a full medical school.

Soon after taking his M.D. degree Bartlett went to Paris, Italy and London to study. He noted in his letters home that the great French clinician Laennec, another student contributor, had died on August 13, 1826. Bartlett selected his lecturers very well, attending those of Cuvier at the Jardin des Plantes. He also attended Dupuytren's clinical lectures, where work on the wards began at 6:30 a.m. by candlelight, and served long days in hospitals. At the age of 22 Bartlett was listening to lectures by the great P.C.A. Louis, to whom Bartlett dedicated his book on *Fevers* and his "Essay on the Philosophy of Medical Sciences." He also wrote in the *American Medical Students' Gazette*, which lapsed, however, after three numbers were issued. In his address Osler described the stage in American medical education in which "there was in this country a group of peripatetic teachers who, like the Sophists of Greece, went from town to town staying a year or two in each, or they divided their time between a winter session in a large city school and a summer session in a small country one." He noted that Bartlett had taught in a succession of nine schools in this manner, but went on to call one of Bartlett's essays "as a masterpiece worthy of Walter Savage Landor—exceeded by few word-pictures in the English language."

Arthur Conan Doyle (1859-1930)

At the age of 17 Conan Doyle entered the medical school of the University of Edinburgh, where he became well-known for his activities in rugby and boxing. He paid for his education by writing his first short story, "Sassassa Valley." During his time at Edinburgh he was an assistant to a local practitioner and served for several months as a ship's surgeon on an Arctic whaler. Late in 1881 he qualified in medicine in Edinburgh and chose as his thesis subject, "On Vasomotor Influence in Tabes Dorsalis."

Thereafter Conan Doyle tried his hand at medical practice, but so unsuccessfully that he set out for West Africa as a ship's surgeon. Then for a time he tried practice in Portsmouth but was soon off to Berlin, where he did postgraduate work in Koch's laboratory. Next he studied in Paris and Vienna and briefly contemplated a possible future as an eye specialist.

Sherlock Holmes and Dr. Watson burst upon the world in 1887 and continued for 40 years. Conan Doyle attempted to end this long series and killed off Holmes only to find such protest that he had him reappear in *The Hound of the Baskervilles*. In addition he organized what was really the forerunner of the British Home Guard, of World War II fame.

Henry Havelock Ellis (1859-1939)

Ellis was born in Croydon near London, the only son of sea captain Edward Pepper Ellis. At the age of seven he accompanied his father on a voyage around the world. He was a precocious student, especially in reading. At the age of 16 he went to Australia where he taught four years as a teacher at Sparks Creek. In relative isolation there, he read some of the works of James Hinton (1822-1875). Hinton's volume, *The Mystery of Pain: A Book for the Sorrowful* was first published in 1866. This London surgeon had already written in 1859 *Man and his Dwelling Place* on science and religion, to be followed by *Life with Nature* in 1862. Late in the year 1880 Ellis entered St. Thomas' Hospital. While he failed the University of London entrance examination, he was allowed to enter as a medical student on the basis of the matriculation that he had earned through

Sir Lauder Brunton to Colonel Fielding Garrison at the Surgeon General's Library, Washington, D.C., concerning Thomas Laycock (1812-1876): "The man was very interesting personally. He had a most profound confidence in himself and I have heard him say 'Twenty-five years ago, gentlemen, I wrote a book which was then half a century above its age, but the age is now gradually beginning to appreciate it.' The odd thing was that in saying this he understated the truth... Laycock was really the original of Sherlock Holmes. Conan Doyle got the idea from Joe Bell, but Joe Bell got his ideas from Laycock, who was Bell's teacher as well as mine. He used sometimes to make very brilliant diagnoses, and at others, great mistakes. I have known him to diagnose waxy degeneration of the capillaries of the small intestine, and post-mortem examination proved the correctness of the diagnosis. He has also been known, simply on walking through a ward to look at a man and say 'This patient has cancer of the pancreas.' Again he was correct. One day he was telling the students a great deal about a child and he said to them 'Gentlemen, I know all this from my observation of the mother.' 'Please, Sir,' said the woman, 'I am only his stepmother.' Another time he was saying, 'This I can tell, gentlemen, from the condition of the patient's teeth.' 'Please, Sir, shall I hand them round?' said the patient, taking the teeth out."

the University of Sydney in Australia. As a medical student Ellis hated the preclinical courses and in his off-hours set out to explore London's museums. He began to feel that he should be writing, and his earliest publication was a review of a book on Rubens, the painter, published in 1880, in *The Pen*. Nothing diverted Ellis from his writing on science, fiction, art, theology, poetry, politics and "the woman question." One of his early articles provided the subject for his book *Little Essays of Love and Virtue*, published 40 years later. Another early contribution was *James Hinton as Religious Thinker* in 1881.

The *Westminster Review* next saw an article by Ellis on "The Novels of Thomas Hardy." So impressed was the editor, Dr. John Chapman, that he offered Ellis a job as theology editor of the journal, with the result that Ellis wrote 53 book reviews on religion in the next 18 months. This brought Ellis into contact with many of the aspiring young members of the Social Democratic Federation, such as William Morris, Sidney Webb and George Bernard Shaw.

During this exciting time Ellis was still struggling through his medical education. Nevertheless, he undertook the editing of cheap reprints of classics in the Camelot Series and then he published unexpurgated versions of Ibsen, Zola, Flaubert and Montpassant. Soon Ellis was taking on the science editorship of the Mermaid Series. The titles included Karl Pearson's *The Grammar of Science*, Lloyds Morgan's *An Introduction to Comparative Psychology* and for good measure Ellis translated Lombroso's *The Man of Genius*. It took seven years for Ellis to complete his medical education, which he did in March 1887 when he acquired the Licenciate in medicine, surgery and midwifery from the Society of Apothecaries. As soon as that was over, he published *The Criminal* in 1890 and *Man and Woman* in 1894.

The power of writing one fine line transcends all the Able-editor ability in the ably-edited Universe.
Edward FitzGerald

His activities as a medical student came to occupy him for the rest of his life, in which he published over 50 volumes of essays and monographs, including a long series on *Studies on the Psychology of Sex*.

W. Somerset Maugham (1874-1965)

Generally acknowledged as a great writer, Maugham grew up as a shy stammerer who rebelled against the narrowness of his Anglican foster parents. He was glad, therefore, to enter St. Thomas' Hospital Medical School in London in 1892. During his work in the slums of that area, as an extern from his hospital, he delivered 50 babies. As a result of his experiences he drafted his first novel, *Liza of Lambeth*. It was published in 1897, the same year in which he qualified as a practitioner. One of his biographers, Joanne Trautman, has commented upon "his admiration for Maupassant," and notes that his first novel "starkly evokes the health conditions of slum women, for whom yearly pregnancies, miscarriages, babies and dead children are the common lot."

In 1907 Maugham wrote his first play, *Lady Frederick*, which was very successful. Thereafter he wrote another 24 plays. In fact, he had four of them running in London theatres at one time. His classic *Of Human Bondage*, published in 1915, led to a large public in the United States of America discovering Maugham. When he died his beautiful home at Cap Ferrat on the Mediterranean was sold to provide a foundation to assist young writers.

POETS

Mark Akenside (1721-1770)

Akenside is best remembered for his poem "The Pleasures of Imagination," which he began to write in 1738 at the age of 17. It was published soon after he had acquired his M.D. degree, the first edition being in January 1744.

Erasmus Darwin (1731-1802)

While still a medical undergraduate, Erasmus Darwin (the uncle of the evolutionist Charles Darwin) published his first poem, "The Death of Prince Frederick," in 1751. This Cambridge graduate proposed his own theory of evolution in Zoönomia (1794) and was well-known for his work *Loves of the Plants*, which appeared in 1789. Darwin was a country practitioner with advanced scientific ideas. He even wrote on transfusions in Volume 64 of *Philosophical Transactions of the Royal Society* with a paper entitled "Experiments on Animal Fluids in the Exhausted Receiver." His nature poetry was well received.

John Keats (1795-1821)

John Keats was the eldest of five children. His father was an ostler at the Swan and Hoop Inn in Finsbury, London. When Keats was eight years old he lost his father, who died after a fall from a horse. When he was 15 his mother died of tuberculosis. His brother Tom died in 1818 of the same disease, so the dice were loaded against John Keats.

Since the age of 14 Keats was smitten by books which, as he said, he "devoured." Among his favourites were Spenser's *Faerie Queene* and the works of Milton, Byron and Wordsworth. At a young age he wrote his own poem, "In Imitation of Spenser."

From 1811 to 1815 Keats was apprenticed to a surgeon at Edmonton and left to enter Guy's Hospital in London in order to finish his medical course. This he did on July 26, 1816, when he received his qualification known as the Licenciate of the Society of Apothecaries. By then he was 21 years old.

His writing career really began at age 18 with the writing of verses that were later published in Leigh Hunt's *Examiner*. In those years he met Shelley, Reynolds, Lamb and Severin. His first volume of poems was published in 1817 and represented about 18 months of work. With his friend Cowden Clarke, whose schoolmaster father had befriended the orphaned Keats, he spent an evening admiring a folio copy of Chapman's Elizabethan translation of *The Iliad*. Sir George Newman said, "Keats went back to his rooms in Dean Street and wrote the most famous poem any medical student has ever produced and sent it forthwith to Clarke for breakfast the next morning: `Much have I travelled in the realms of gold, / And many goodly states and kingdoms seen,' ending with the famous words, `Silent upon a peak in Darien.'"

Keats' fellow student Stephens wrote that "Keats attended lectures and went through the usual routine, but he had no desire to excel in that pursuit. . . . Poetry was to his mind the zenith of all his aspirations." While living in St. Thomas's Street above the shop of a tallow chandler, Keats wrote part of the "Endymion"—"a thing of beauty is a joy forever."

Boston, January 21, 1889

My dear Sir,—I have rarely been more pleased than by your allusions to an old paper of mine. There was a time certainly in which I would have said that the best page of my record was that in which I had fought my battle for the poor poisoned women. I am reminded of that Essay from time to time, but it was published in a periodical which died after one year's life and therefore escaped the wider notice it would have found if printed in the American Journal of the Medical Sciences. A lecturer at one of the great London Hospitals referred to it the other day and coupled it with some fine phrases about myself which made me blush, either with modesty or vanity, I forget which.

I think I will not answer the question you put me. I think oftenest of the 'Chambered Nautilus', which is a favourite poem of mine, though I wrote it myself. The Essay only comes up at long intervals, the poem repeats itself in my memory and is very often spoken of by my correspondents in terms of more than ordinary praise. I had a savage pleasure, I confess, in handling these two Professors—learned men both of them, skilful experts, but babies as it seemed to me in their capacity of reasoning and arguing. But in writing the poem I was filled with a better feeling, the highest state of mental exaltation and the most crystalline clairvoyance, as it seemed to me, that had ever been granted to me. I mean that lucid vision of one's thought and all forms of expression which will be at once precise and musical which is the poet's special gift, however large or small in amount or value. There is some selfish pleasure to be had out of the poem, perhaps a nobler satisfaction from the life-saving labour.

Letter from O. W. Holmes to William Osler

Upon graduation Keats wrote about the nightingale "not born for death." However, he knew that his eventual fate was decided and he went to Italy to die, first to Naples and then to the Spanish Steps in Rome. Despite the overriding problem of tuberculosis he produced some very fine poetry, such as "Hyperion" and "Odes." Rosetti spoke of Keats as "the one true heir of Shakespeare."

Keats the medical student looked at day-to-day occurrences from a slightly different perspective than did his classmates. In his student notebook that has been preserved, he wrote: "The other day, during a lecture there came a sunbeam into the room, and with it a whole troop of creatures floating in the ray and I was off with them to Oberon and fairyland."

Keats was also a realist. Here he describes a hospital ward:

> The weariness, the fever, and the fret,
> Here where men sit and hear each other groan;
> Where palsy shakes a few, sad, last grey hairs,
> Where youth grows pale and spectre-thin and dies;
> Where but to think is to be full of sorrow
> And leaden-eyed despair.

He described "The Lungs through which all of the Blood must necessarily pass that it may come in contact with the air and undergo decarbonation in which process useless and hurtful Matter is expelled from the Body....Above 10 ounces of Carbon are given off daily."

John Keats' anatomical and physiological N*ote* B*ook* has been reproduced in 67 pages with illustrations. In it he discusses dislocation of the jaw and its remedy. He wrote, "Cover the Thumbs with an handkerchief and depress the lower part of the jaw, elevating the chin with the fingers." So much for what he was writing down in the body of the page, but the entire left margin was decorated by delightful small sketches of individual blossoms. Keats' summation was this:

> I mean to follow Solomon's directions, 'Get learning—get understanding.' I find that I can have no enjoyment in the world but continual drinking of knowledge. I find there is no worthy pursuit but the idea of doing some good in the world. Some do it with their society; some with their wit; some with their benevolence; some with a sort of power of conferring pleasure and good humour on all they meet—in a thousand ways, all dutiful to the command of great Nature. There is but one way for me. The road lies through application, study, and thought.

Robert Seymour Bridges (1844-1930)

Bridges' life has been well summarized by Theodore James, the South African physician: "There has not been an English poet more interested in prosody, nor a physician more taken to medicine for its human contact, nor a philosopher who lived closer to the tenets of his belief than Robert Bridges."

John Potter, the Oxford neurosurgeon, has written of the student timetable Bridges set for himself. Potter writes: "Few doctors can have started as medical students with the program devised for himself by

Robert Bridges who subsequently became Poet Laureate. His intention was to study and practice medicine for a limited period of about 15 years only and then to retire at the age of 40 and use for the purpose of his art the knowledge of men that he had so acquired." Because of a chest malady Bridges actually finished practising medicine at the age of 37, but he continued writing great poetry until the age of 85, when he produced his masterpiece, "The Testament of Beauty." Coincidentally with its publication Bridges was awarded by King George V the Order of Merit, which is limited to a small group of distinguished scholars.

He had an excellent classical education at Eton before going up to Corpus Christi College at Oxford. Bridges was no mere dabbler in medicine. He served his time at St. Bartholomew's Hospital as a casualty physician. In one year in that post, according to Osler, Bridges saw 30,940 patients and gave 200,000 doses containing iron.

Poetry and music were bound up together in Bridges' interest. For instance, he became very active in the reform movement concerning psalms and canticles. Living at Yattendon in Berkshire, he had much to do with the Yattendon Hymnal. In 1911 he wrote to a friend, "I think that the intelligent hymn-singer is getting much too squeamish. . . . I do not find an occasional disagreement between accent of words and of music offends me in a hymn. A fine tune is an unalterable artistic form which pleases in itself and for itself. The notion of its giving way to the words is impossible." One wonders what he would think of the work of another Oxford graduate, Henry Francis Lyte, who is said to have composed the hymn "Abide with Me" in one hour, whereupon the village music teacher composed, in 20 minutes, the beautiful tune, which is still revered. Among other things Bridges established and presided over the Society for Pure English. He also rescued from obscurity such poets as Gerald Manley Hopkins. Bridges was widely appreciated and had many friends, one of whom presented him with a clavichord for his eightieth birthday. However, Bridges' crowning achievement, at age 85, was his work, *The Testament of Beauty*. When it appeared in 1929 it took his readers by storm. Sir Charles Sherrington, O.M., used to recite this in his physiology laboratory at Oxford as he was carrying out experiments with his students on the transmission of the nervous impulse. Sir John Eccles has remarked upon the ability of Sherrington's assistants to fill in the gaps in reciting the poem as Sherrington would take a breath. Sherrington loved to tell the story of Bridges sitting an early examination in which it was required to translate a passage from the Greek and a passage from the Latin. Bridges confounded his examiners by translating the Greek into Latin and the Latin into Greek.

It would be wrong to think that Bridges merely favoured his poetry, with occasional references to medical conditions. Far from it. One of his poems, published in 1903, ran to more than 32 verses, reflecting with realism the very facts and conditions of the practice of medicine. The summary by Theodore James already quoted is certainly borne out by the facts of Bridges' productive life. Even in far-off Vancouver his name is perpetuated on a little brass plaque on a chair in the Sherrington Room of the Woodward Biomedical Library at the University of B.C.

Charles Robert Richet (1850-1935)

Richet was the son of the professor of surgery in Paris, and while studying medicine at the University of Paris published his first volume of verse in 1875; a year later he graduated in medicine. Not only did he publish his poetry, but also novels, fables and comedies. He wrote an essay, "*Du somnambulisme provoqué*." His M.D. thesis in 1877 was entitled "*Recherches experimentales et cliniques sur la sensibilité*." One of his first studies in hospital was a young man who had swallowed lye by accident and thereafter had a surgical opening to the outside through the stomach wall. Immediately after graduation Richet produced a French translation of William Harvey's *De Motu Cordis*.

While working on respiration in dogs, Richet showed that the dog, lacking sweat glands, was forced to regulate body temperature through panting. He went on to discuss passive immunity and showed that blood from a recovered animal, when injected into an animal suffering from infection, could bring relief.

He was one of the first medical bibliographers and compiled a large dictionary of physiology. He modestly set out to review the entire world literature in that field.

Richet's poetry was substantial and he gloried in the prize awarded by the Académie Française for his 1922 poem concerning Louis Pasteur.

Ronald Ross (1857-1932)

The life of this self-taught musician, poet and painter has been memorialized by Professor Leonard C. Wilson in *Nobel Laureates in Medicine or Physiology—A Biographical Dictionary*. Most medical students associate Ronald Ross with his demonstration of the transmission of malaria by *anopheles* mosquitos. Too few, however, know of his poetry. In reviewing that aspect of his contribution, Sir D'Arcy Thompson has written: "In the long history of medicine and poetry, we can call to mind many a physician who has been also a poet. No great physician has ever likewise been that rare and wonderful thing, a great poet, for the toilsome life of the one is not to be combined with the fine freedom and the careless rapture of the other. But there is a certain excellence which, though it fall far short of supreme satisfaction, is still a very fine and splendid thing and to such excellence I think Sir Ronald Ross has certainly attained."

Ross was born in Nepal, the first child of a British Army officer. At the age of eight he began his formal education in England. In 1875 he entered St. Bartholomew's Hospital in London to study medicine. While he had great teachers, such as Sir James Paget, another student discoverer, Ross immersed himself in more poetry and music than medicine.

Some of Ross's poetry was published in India. His poems "Edgar, or the New Pygmalion," and "The Judgment of Tithonus" were published at Madras in 1883. Other plays, in verse, included *The Deformed Transformed*, which was published in Bangalore in 1890. "Fables" was printed in Liverpool in 1907 and other poems such as "Philosophies" appeared in London in 1910. His great poem "In Exile," published in Liverpool in 1906, was hailed by John Masefield as "by far the most splendid poem of modern times." His interest in poetry sustained him throughout his varied life. Ross was awarded the Nobel Prize for Medicine in 1902.

George Frederick Still (1868-1941)

The term "Still's disease" has been known since the classic paper by G.F. Still, in the *Medical-Chirurgical Transactions*, London, 1896-97, in which he described arthritis deformans in children. This description represented his M.D. thesis at Cambridge University. He described 22 cases in children, of whom 19 had been seen at Great Ormond Street in London. George Still became the first professor of paediatrics at King's College, London. He also wrote a book of poems for children.

In 1988 A *Collection of Poems Written by Medical Students* was published by the Northeastern Ohio University's College of Medicine in their "Human Values in Medicine Program." The William Carlos Williams poetry competition there attracted many samples of medical undergraduates' writing. This 36-page volume is but a taste of things to come. Medical students may now unlock their dreams and writing abilities, helpfully shielded from the quacking of the various airways. May their tribe increase.

STUDENT SOCIETIES AND STUDENT JOURNALS

Throughout the centuries medical students have been a gregarious lot. William Harvey at Padua was elected head of the English "Nation." In Harvey's time Padua had become a cosmopolitan university with the best medical school in Europe. While there were societies, there were no publications.

The oldest medical society in the English-speaking world is the Royal Medical Society of Edinburgh, founded by students in 1737, and still a sparkling example of a forum in which students can communicate their researches as so many have done historically.

Not to be outdone, the Medical Society of Oxford, launched in 1780 and with 12 student participants, remained in existence for three years. The moving spirit in that little society was William Pargeter, born in 1760, the son of a Hertfordshire rector. In January he entered that Wykhamite bastion, ironically called New College, established in 1379. Pargeter proceeded to St. Bartholomew's Hospital, London, after receiving his Oxford B.A. and took his M.D. degree in Aberdeen in 1786.

Pargeter and his fellow students met on November 1, 1780, as their minute book shows, "having agreed to unite in a body for the Promotion of Medical knowledge within these walls, to hereby incorporate ourselves under the Name of the Medical Society of Oxford. And to the intent that the order of such society be preserved, and the Institution maintain for future Ages, we do upon full deliberation enact" followed by 13 articles. Members in rotation were to read a paper "on some subject intimately connected with medicine" of their own choice. Non-attendance was to be excused only on grounds of illness or absence from the University. There was a penalty for failing to give a paper and members were to meet in each other's rooms until Queen's College could provide suitable space. Disorderly conduct or gross misbehaviour was to lead to expulsion. The subjects discussed in the student papers were diverse: smallpox, gout, rheumatism, hypochondria, disorders of bile, dropsy, chlorosis, the connection of botany with medicine, and "the medicinal virtues of factitious air [nitrous oxide]," a full 18 years before Humphry Davy began his researches.

Unfortunately, the society gave up the ghost when the more active members left Oxford to pursue their clinical studies. A part of the downfall of this little society may have resided in the item in the constitution reading, "when the business has lasted four hours, the President may appoint an extraordinary meeting to be held within three days at which every member shall attend."

At Birmingham under the stimulus of William Bowman, a gifted student contributor to science, a medical society of students was formed. In Paris and later in Boston, Oliver Wendell Holmes and his student contemporaries formed scientific reporting societies which were short-lived but important. The Paris society was named "Société Médicale d'Observation de Paris." Attendance at the weekly meeting was compulsory for the few who had been elected to membership. These included Marshall Hall, Henry Bowditch, James Jackson, Jr., and Oliver Wendell Holmes. These students and others were the pupils of P.C.A. Louis and Gabriel Andral.

In Boston the Society for Medical Improvement filled the void in the intellectual life previously filled by the little society in Paris. At one of the meetings of the Boston Society Holmes learned of the death of a woman from childbed fever whose physician had just assisted at an autopsy. The same physician attended several other women in childbirth and all had come down with puerperal sepsis and fever. Holmes wrote 27 blistering pages for the little-known *New England Quarterly Journal of Medicine and Surgery* and using the methods learned in Paris under Louis, assembled the most damaging case histories that have ever been printed—not a few, but dozens of them—and eventually eliminated childbed fever in America.

As noted in the chapter on anatomy, Ledingham of Aberdeen founded a student paper.

The Clinical Section of the Royal Society of Medicine in London has recently initiated a presentation by undergraduates of papers dealing with their own observations. The papers presented have included a description of squamous cell carcinoma of the right retromolar trigone from a hospital in Glasgow. From St. Mary's Hospital in Paddington a student presented a case of necrotising enterocolitis in a patient with AIDS, the first description of this condition complicating AIDS. A joint description by two medical students from a hospital in Hackney described the successful treatment for a papillary cystic neoplasm of the pancreas. It is to be hoped that other medical societies of high reputation in many countries will follow this excellent example and that medical students will have a chance to make descriptive or research activities better known.

PUBLISHING

For most medical professionals it is impossible to believe that medical students of the past ever became publishers, and yet this is the situation.

John Chapman (1821-1894)

Thanks to Dr. F.N.L. Poynter, the long-time director of the Wellcome Institute of the History of Medicine in London, there is a faithful picture of this "Publisher, Physician and Medical Reformer."

Chapman was born of a father who was both druggist and grocer. At an early age the boy was apprenticed to a watchmaker, but at the same time attended lectures on science and on literature at the Pestalozzian Institution. He ran away to Edinburgh, where he had a brother who was a medical student. The brother was not amused and sent John to Adelaide in South Australia to be a watchmaker and oculist.

Chapman soon declared his independence and arrived at St. Bartholomew's Hospital in London as a student. Then he studied for a time in Paris, where the famous Gay-Lussac was one of his teachers.

In 1844 Chapman returned to Derby and wrote a book, *Human Nature*, which was considered radical. He bought out a retiring publisher and in February 1844 published his own book. He then leased 142 The Strand in London, where his wife ran a hotel in part of it. There they had such guests as Emerson, who stayed for three months, Horace Greely, Noah Porter, W.C. Bryant, and G.P. Putnam from the United States. Mary Ann Evans, later to be known as George Eliot, stayed for two years while she acted as sub-editor in the publishing enterprise. Her first work was her anonymous translation of D.F. Strauss' work, *Das Leben Jesu*. It is said that this two years changed a country girl from Warwick into a knowledgeable friend of Dickens, Thackeray, Carlyle, Froude, John Stuart Mill, Browning, Mrs. Gaskell, Herbert Spencer, Richard Owen, Francis Newman, Leigh Hunt and her future husband, G.H. Lewes.[1]

Chapman published Herbert Spencer's first book, *Social Statistics*. His many associates wrote for his *Westminster Review*, which he acquired in 1851.

At the age of 22 Chapman began thinking about "the survival of the fittest." He was able to applaud Darwin's *Origin of Species*. These were the days in which Herbert Spencer was assistant editor of *The Economist*.

The *Westminster Review* had an interesting history. It was begun in 1824 by James Mill with funds provided by Jeremy Bentham. John Stuart Mill, the son, took over the editing from 1837 to 1840. Chapman bought it in 1851 for £300 sterling. From January 1852 George Eliot became his assistant editor. While they printed only 650 copies, it was an influential journal. Chapman paid £250 sterling in fees to the authors for each quarter. Among his other activities, Chapman had the Booksellers' Association brought into court for price-fixing, a suit which he won. He had some powerful supporters, such as Gladstone, Carlyle, and Dickens, among others.

While all this publishing occured, Barbara Leigh Smith (a cousin of Florence Nightingale) was finally able to persuade Chapman to complete his medical education. She was a determined woman and the founder of Girton College in Cambridge. For the following 19 months, Chapman attended lectures at University College Hospital, King's College in the Strand, and St. George's Hospital Clinics in London. He graduated with the M.D. degree at St. Andrews in Scotland in 1857 at the age of 36.

In 1862 Chapman gave up all business enterprises in order to concentrate on the *Westminster Review* and practice medicine. He wrote on anaesthetics, especially chloroform, and was much interested in the background of Priestley, Lavoisier, Beddoes, Davy, Hickman, Wells, Morton, Bigelow and Snow.

Chapman's interests were eclectic. With mental patients he sought to "track the causes of a large amount of disease into the secret recesses of the soul." He wrote about epilepsy, and even the cooling of the spinal cord. For good measure he patented "Chapman's India rubber bag for hot water," a great boon in Britain's winter weather. He was injured in a cab accident in Paris and died in 1894. He was buried beside George Eliot. Not all medically qualified publishers could claim a life as colourful as Chapman's.

Magnus Gustav Retzius (1842-1919)

Retzius entered the University of Uppsala in Sweden at the age of 18 and then proceeded to the Karolinska in Stockholm for further training. He graduated in medicine at the University of Lund in 1871, having already published his father's contributions to ethnology. In the year of his graduation in medicine he published a volume of sonnets and translated some of the poetry of Robert Burns.

While Retzius was appointed to the department of anatomy at the Karolinska in the same year in which he graduated, publishing was certainly in his blood. For a period of three years, for instance, he became editor-in-chief of the Stockholm newspaper *Aftonbladet*, having married the daughter of its founder. He published biographies of scientists and some of his own poetry. He produced two volumes on brain anatomy and the sense organs of hearing. From 1890 to 1914 he produced 18 volumes of biological researches. Nothing in the nervous system escaped his eye. In 1908 he was invited to give the Croonian Lecture to the Royal Society of London and for that occasion drew his own illustrations. In 1898 he composed a cantata celebrating the chemist Berzelius, and in 1907 another celebrating the birth of Linnaeus. To his great credit Retzius brought to the medical world's attention the undergraduate work of Sandstrom on the parathyroids, which a German anatomical journal had rejected. Retzius reviewed this student effort and helped to establish Sandstrom's priority.

Many early student contributors to science later became founders of medical journals. John Shaw Billings might be considered one of the greatest "publishers" in medical history with his *Index Catalogue* of the Surgeon General's Library (now the National Library of Medicine). Through him it is known that Auguste Théodore Vidal of the Mediterranean village of Cassis, a student at nearby Marseille and at Paris, was instrumental in the founding of the *Gazette des Hopitaux*. As has been already mentioned, John Charles Ledingham (1875-1944), with a fellow student, founded the *Proceedings for the Society of Anatomy and Anthropology* at Aberdeen, short-lived though it was. Sydney Rowland in May 1896, while still a medical student, founded the *Archives of Clinical Skiagraphy*[2]. This journal later became the *Archives of the Roentgen Ray*. Rudolf Virchow, at the age of 26, founded his own journal later known as *Virchow's Archiv*. Both Pierre Marie and Edouard Brissaud founded the *Revue Neurologique*. Henry Head edited the great British journal *Brain* in the formative years 1910 to 1925. Nissl and Alzheimer joined forces in the production of their six-volume work on the histology and histopathology of the cerebral cortex and in the founding of a great journal of neurology and psychiatry in the German language. Alzheimer's thesis for the M.D. degree in 1887 was not as well-known as that of Nissl, but was done in Kölliker's laboratory, on the wax-producing glands of the ear.

In the last year of Sir William Osler's life at Oxford a medical student, **Walter Russell Brain**, studying at New College, put together extracts from the writings of Osler in a publication entitled "Medicine and Nursing," published by the Oxford University Press in *Essays on Vocation*. The title used was *Vocations in Medicine and Nursing*.

Though Brain had entered New College, Oxford, in 1914 he joined the Friends Ambulance Service in 1915 and, while serving with that group and taking evening classes at Birkbeck College in London, was able to reenter New College in 1919 to read medicine. His teachers included the famous John Scott Haldane, Charles Sherrington, Julian Huxley and Cuthbert Bassett. He took his clinical work at the London Hospital, graduating with his Oxford qualification in 1922. His contributions to the study of carpal tunnel syndrome with Dickson Wright and Marcia Wilkinson are well-known. With D.W.C. Northfield and Marcia Wilkinson he went on to describe the symptomatology of cervical disc protrusion with paralysis of the legs. In 1951 he published "Mind, Perception and Science" and in 1959, "The Nature of Experience." His textbook *Diseases of the Nervous System*, published in 1933, went through a sixth edition by 1962.

His poems and verses were notable, beginning with their publication in 1961. He edited the scholarly British journal *Brain* from 1954 until his death in 1966. In total he published 18 books and 150 papers. He was a Fellow of the Royal Society of London, and President of the Royal College of Physicians. He served on the Royal Commission on Marriage and Divorce as well as one on mental certification and detention. He felt that one of his greatest honours was to receive the Osler medal given by Oxford University for distinguished work by a graduate. He died on December 29, 1966, while carrying on his editorial functions.

TRANSLATORS

Martin Lluelyn (1616-1682)

It has long been held that Lluelyn was the translator into English of Harvey's *De Generatione*. As Osler said, "Lluelyn, student of Christ Church, M.A. 1643 and D.M. 1653, was ejected from Oxford in 1648, whereupon he went to London and became a physician, 'prosecuting then his genius as much to physic as before he had to poetry.' (Wood) At the Restoration he was made physician to Charles II and Principal of St. Mary Hall. He retired to High Wycombe in 1664 where he practised until his death. A monument to him is in the parish church." Sir Geoffrey Keynes rather doubts that Lluelyn was Harvey's translator. Keynes admits that Lluelyn "was certainly a friend of Harvey and a genuine admirer of his work," but calls him a "versifier" rather than a poet, as may be seen in his best-known volume, *Men, Miracles and Other Poems*, 1646. Another Cambridge scholar, Dr. Joseph Needham, F.R.S., in his *History of Embryology*, 1959, nevertheless thinks that Lluelyn did the translating.

Thomas Beddoes (1760-1808), as mentioned elsewhere, was a medical student at Oxford when he translated Spallanzani's "Dissertations on Natural History."

Samuel Gross, Sr. (1805-1884), wrote, while still a medical student, that he wished "to spend my leisure to the best advantage. I at once began the translation on a work on General Anatomy, hoping by its publication not only to acquire a little reputation but to obtain means of support which, ere this, had been quite exhausted.... I had determined, long before I had finished my course of studies in Jefferson Medical College to undertake the translation of some French work as soon as I should receive my degree. Doctor Dobson... placed in my hands a book on *General Anatomy* by Bayle and Hollard of Paris just fresh from the press. It was well arranged, concise, and apparently adapted to the wants of the profession in this country. Setting vigorously to work I finished my translation in two months."

One can imagine the consternation on the part of young Gross, when he ran into a brick wall. He wrote in his autobiography:

> An incident happened near the completion of this, my first, literary effort which deserves brief mention. Messrs. Carey and Lea, at that time the principal publishing house in the city, had agreed to publish my translation and to pay me two hundred dollars for it. When the work had sufficiently progressed to be put to press, I placed some of sheets in their hands, and during the conversation which ensued incidentally remarked that I should inscribe the translation to my preceptor Dr. George McClellan. This was enough. In a week the manuscript was returned to me with a note declining the publication. The real cause of its rejection was the fact that the firm was friendly to the University of Pennsylvania, whose faculty were hostile to Dr. McClellan, the founder of Jefferson Medical College. Upon stating the circumstance to him, McClellan consulted Mr. John Grigg... who immediately committed the book to the press.

Ibn Nafis (1210-1288)

Nafis' writing on the pulmonary circuit of the blood to gain oxygenation was translated from the Arabic to German by Dr. M. Tatawi in 1924 as he prepared his doctoral dissertation in medicine at the University of Freiburg: "*Der Lungenkreislauf nach el-Koraschi*." In 1955 a Yale medical student, E.E. Bittar, wrote his thesis at Yale University School of Medicine in New Haven on "Ibn Nafis: A study with translations of two of his works." An essay based on Bittar's thesis won for him the William Osler Medal of 1955.

Maximilien Paul Émile Littré (1801-1881)

This medical student, who never finished his degree, was one of the greatest of medical philologists. Not only did he publish the finest edition of *Hippocrates* with French translation, he also compiled a huge dictionary of the French language, a fresh translation of Pliny's *Natural History*, and wrote historical essays on Celsus, Magendie, Cuvier, Socrates, Pascal and Gil Blas. Osler said of him:

> We owe him an immense debt for his *Hippocrates*, the only complete edition of the Father of Medicine in any modern language. His life is an inspiration. In the touching devotion to his father—see the beautiful dedication in volume I of the *Hippocrates*—he reminds one of Pasteur. A noble man, and a true disciple of Hippocrates. *Bien qu'il n'ait pas prononcé le fameux serment qui lit au sacerdoce médical, il le porte écrit dans son coeur.*

While Littré qualified as an externe and an interne in several hospitals, he never took his final degree in medicine. Nevertheless, he was made a member of the Académie de Médecine. He had serious financial difficulties that probably prevented him graduating. It reminds one of Laennec, whose great success in his studies was unfortunately matched by worsening finances, which were so serious that he wrote to his father stating that for lack of decent clothes he would probably have to postpone his graduation.

MUSIC AND THE ARTS

Finally, in this chapter, a brief word about music and the arts. Two examples must suffice.

Alexander Porphyrievich Borodin (1833-1887) was born in St. Petersburg, Russia, on November 12, 1833. He is said to have been the third of three illegitimate sons of a 61-year-old Georgian prince and a 25-year-old beauty from Narva. Each boy bore the name of a serf belonging to their father, each carrying a different name. Borodin was tutored at home and early in his career began to play the flute. At the same time he dabbled in chemistry, manufactured fireworks and produced pigment with which to paint. At the age of nine he wrote his first musical composition, "A Polka," of which the manuscript has been preserved.

Within a few years he was composing, without formal instruction, a concerto for flute and piano and thereafter a trio for two violins and cello.

At the age of 17 and on the insistence of his mother, Borodin entered the Academy of Medicine and Surgery at St. Petersburg. His many gifts included great ability in chemistry. Two years before completing his medical degree he was appointed assistant to the professor of pathology and therapeutics. In 1858 he graduated with his M.D. degree with honours, presenting a thesis on the analogy between arsenious and phosphoric acids.

In the ensuing three years he travelled in Europe, mixing the writing of scientific papers with the writing of several (unpublished) pieces of chamber music.

Returning to Russia, he collided with the views of the Minister of Education who preached that "Education is harmful to a people born to obey." He and four other composers, optimistically called "the mighty five," pooled their musical interests. Among them were Rimsky-Korsakov and Mussorgsky. Borodin's "Symphony in E Flat Major" was heard publicly in 1867, which brought Russian musicians great international acclaim. Two years later his opera *Prince Igor* was begun. At the same time Borodin worked for the establishment of an Academy of Medicine for Women, the first of its type in Russia, for he believed that women deserved equal professional opportunities. Borodin's musical legacy to the world consisted of two symphonies, several songs and the orchestral tone poem, "In the Steppes of Central Asia," which appeared, in part, as the music for the Broadway production of *Kismet* in 1953, yielding also the popular song "Stranger in Paradise." His opera *Prince Igor* was his masterpiece.

Twenty years after Borodin died, an American phenomenon was born in New York, **Mark David Altschule**. His family lived on the Lower East Side of New York and were highly intelligent Russian immigrants. His parents had in their family many physicians and medical scientists. Mark Altschule was a precocious boy who devoured the works of Plato, Schopenhauer and Nietzsche by the time he was 12 years old. He had already started modelling animals when he was four years of age and while attending the DeWitt Clinton High School, and at the same time studying sculpture at the Educational Alliance. After receiving his bachelor of science degree from the College of the City of New York in 1927, he became a laboratory technician at Montefiore Hospital for two years during which time he applied to six medical schools. Only Harvard accepted him. In order to pay for his education at Harvard he worked part-time in the Beth Israel Hospital laboratory. Thanks to his earlier employment he was able to spend half of his junior year as a pathology house officer at Peter Bent Brigham Hospital.

During his four years at medical school he published his investigation of the embryonic mesonephric tubules and at the same time co-authored five clinical papers. More importantly, perhaps, he studied sculpture at the Copley Society through evening courses. In spite of all this, he achieved his M.D. cum laude in 1933. He developed a research career in several excellent hospitals and was director of internal medicine and clinical physiology research at McLean Hospital for psychiatric patients in Massachusetts. He developed an interest in medical history and had a great love for the Countway Library of Harvard's Medical School, which has few rivals in the world today. Its building, in a comparatively short time, brought together a priceless collection of rare books and prints, portraits and manuscripts.

There is an apocryphal story that is heard whenever the name Countway is mentioned in connection with this wonderful library. The Dean of Harvard Medical School, Dr. George Berry, is said to have parked his car in an apartment garage, immediately next to that owned by Miss Countway. Every morning at 7 a.m., as Dr. Berry was getting into his automobile, the chauffeur was washing Miss Countway's car. One morning the chauffeur remarked sadly that Miss Countway's brother, the head of Lever Brothers in New York, had just died and Miss Countway was wondering how he might best be memorialized. By noon Dean Berry had found the donor for his long-sought new facility that would combine several outstanding Boston collections.

[1] As a memorial to Lewes (1817-1878) she set up a trust, with £5,000 in capital, to provide a fellowship in physiology at Cambridge with the help of Professor Michael Foster. The first fellow was the short-lived C.S. Roy.

[2] In 1965 "An international forum for the advancement of medical science by students," Volume 1, appeared at McGill University in Montreal. Volume 2 appeared in Spring 1996, being edited and written largely by students and covering scholarly clinical and basic science papers, case reports, review articles, epidemiological surveys, clinicopathological reports and medical–legal papers. It has been splendidly produced. The short form of its name is *McGill Journal of Medicine*.

CHAPTER NINETEEN

Unusual Contributors

Medical undergraduates have invented some unusual things. In 1831, Charles Sauria, in France, produced the first phosphorus friction match. Henry Morris in Birmingham "devised the dry photographic plate," according to Oxford medical historical scholar Alastair Robb-Smith.

Henry Woodward, a medical student at Toronto, invented the electric light bulb and later sold the patent to Thomas Edison. James Startin (1806-1874) developed a new and cheap commercial process for stiffening felt hats. He became, logically enough, a successful skin specialist in London. The Russian physiologist Cybolski, to finance his medical education, produced a new mouth wash.

More importantly, a student from Minneapolis, **Elon O. Huntington**, who was studying medicine at Columbia's College of Physicians and Surgeons in New York, made a great if unusual contribution. In walks along the Hudson River on Sundays, he habitually accompanied the Rev. Mr. Gates who was once his pastor in Minnesota. In New York, however, Mr. Gates was the personal adviser to John D. Rockefeller and was searching for a project large enough to usefully absorb his patron's millions. One day Gates asked the student Huntington if he knew of any book on medicine that a layman could understand.

Huntington replied at once that there was one such readable book, William Osler's *Principles and Practice of Medicine*, distilled from the author's vast experience at McGill, Philadelphia, and Johns Hopkins Hospital in Baltimore. Gates bought a copy and, accompanied by a medical dictionary, set off for the Catskill Mountains to read it. On his return he told Mr. Rockefeller that for most diseases the cause was still unknown and that even the methods of prevention or control were in their infancy. The Rockefeller Institute for Medical Research and its successor, Rockefeller University in New York, resulted.

"INDIFFERENT" STUDENTS

It is widely known that Einstein and Röntgen, in mathematics and physics, were considered poor bets by their early teachers, but it is not well-known that some medical students received unfavourable reports from theirs. As a medical student at University College in London, **Henry**

Maudsley received a report from one of his early professors: "Maudsley has great abilities but he has chosen to throw them into the gutter." However, in his five years there he amassed ten gold medals, which he traded for a gold watch. At the age of 24 he was appointed medical superintendent for the Manchester Royal Lunatic Asylum. Six years later he called that "a somewhat rash appointment." Through Sir Frederic M. Mott he gave a large sum of money to build a modern acute psychiatric hospital that he had the pleasure of seeing opened before he died in 1918. Today it is the British Institute of Psychiatry in London.

The Nobelist in Medicine, Joseph Erlanger, has written: "I was not an apt pupil. Indeed my teacher (an excellent one) in the last but one of the grammar grades, advised my mother to let me repeat that year. This I strenuously refused to do. Awakened by that experience, I had no further learning difficulties."

I can't think when I concentrate.
Yogi Berra

William Turner, the anatomist, was labelled an indifferent student by his schoolteacher, but he became the Vice-Chancellor of the University of Edinburgh and was knighted for his contributions. His contemporary Sir James Y. Simpson, who became famous for his induction of chloroform anaesthesia in childbirth, was said to be an indifferent student but for his thesis on peritonitis. Nobelist Niels Finsen was dismissed from his Danish preparatory school for having "small ability and total lack of energy." He was actually suffering from jaundice, measles and kidney disease. Sir Peter Medawar has graphically described the situation in which **P. A. Gorer** (1907-1961) found himself. At age five it was recommended that he be sent to a school for backward children. However, he sped through Charterhouse to Cambridge and Guy's Hospital in London, stopping, en route, to do his classical work on hibernation and in the bacteriological laboratory. He was failed at the oral examination in obstetrics and gynaecology due to a heated altercation over genetics. On his second try he made it. Fortunately he was not put off by this collision with authority and proceeded to unravel the question of blood groups in lower animals, and to investigate the problems of tissue and tumour transplants.

DELAYED GRADUATION

Some medical students had their traditional M.D. programs interrupted by ill health, poverty, war service or by opportunities to engage in teaching or research.

James Lind of anti-scurvy fame did not obtain his M.D. degree at Edinburgh until he left the Royal Navy at age 32. William James went off on an investigation of life forms in the Amazon, and to European universities, not to mention his undiagnosed illnesses, and graduated at Harvard at age 27.

Two important student researchers never actually graduated: William Bayliss, who was so angered by his examiner that he walked out, permanently, in his final year; and Binet in Paris, who became so interested in psychological phenomena at the Salpêtrière that he never had time to complete the M.D. degree. It is said that when Bayliss was summoned to Buckingham Palace to receive his knighthood, he replied that he would be unable to attend because he had an important meeting of the Physiological Society on the same day.

Two of the key people in the insulin story at the University of Toronto had their medical graduations delayed by Banting's discovery. Charles Best had his bachelor of arts degree course interrupted by army volunteer service in the 1914-1918 war. He achieved his B.A. in physiology on one day, and became Fred Banting's invaluable assistant the next. He did not take his M.D. degree until 1925. J.B. Collip, on the other hand, already had his Ph.D. in biochemistry at Toronto when he was pressed into service to purify Banting and Best's insulin but with a heavy teaching load at the University of Alberta did not achieve his M.D. until 1928.

Similarly, C.N.H. Long, Alan Emery, and Arnold Gesell were so occupied with research and publishing their results that they graduated in medicine much later than their colleagues who took a more direct course to the M.D. goal.

The Cambridge physiologists Rushton and Hartridge had research and teaching opportunities that delayed their medical qualification significantly. Lionel Penrose and Russell Brain had service on Red Cross trains for much of World War I, while J.H. Burn began as a motorcycle dispatch rider in that war, completing his M.D. after surviving the worst battles of the Somme and Arras as an infantryman.

Two student researchers became sidetracked for some years through publishing ventures. Gustave Retzius, Jr., married the daughter of the proprietor of the Stockholm newspaper, *Aftonbladet*, and spent three years as its editor-in-chief, before completing his medical degree. John Chapman became immersed in such publications as *The Westminster Review*, where George Eliot worked as his assistant. Only the pointed persuasion of a cousin of Florence Nightingale put Chapman back on track. He eventually took his M.D. degree at St. Andrew's in Scotland.

Service in the Free French Army delayed **François Jacob** in World War II. Having completed his baccalaureate in 1938 he entered the medical school of the University of Paris. With the Nazi triumph over France in 1940 he managed to get to London to join the Gaulist forces. He served as a medical attendant through many of the fierce battles in North Africa. He was wounded in Tunisia and later in Normandy. His M.D. thesis in 1947 was on the tyrothricin of René Dubos. Jacob thereafter joined Monod and Lwoff at the Institut Pasteur in Paris and was awarded the Legion of Honour and the Fellowship of the Royal Society of London.

Not all of the delayed aspirants, or late bloomers, were male. One such student was **Rosemary Biggs,** born in London in 1912. Her research took her to the University of Toronto where she achieved her Ph.D. in 1937. It was not until 1943 that she found time to graduate in medicine from the Royal Free Hospital Medical School in London. Thereafter she was able to concentrate on pathology at the Radcliffe Infirmary at Oxford. From 1967 to 1977 Dr. Biggs was director of the Oxford Haemophiliac Centre where pioneering work was done to permit safe surgery on haemophiliacs.

MEDICAL STUDENT CONTRIBUTORS IN THE ARMED FORCES

For more than a century students have been able to qualify in medicine thanks to a subsidy from the armed forces. Among them were: Emil von Behring, Pavlov, Duchesne the penicillin pioneer, Laennec, Rudolf Virchow, Cornelius Donders, Helmholtz, Ejkman and Laveran.

The conditions varied. Von Behring found that the Military Institute of Medicine in Berlin required one year of service upon graduation for every six months of subsidized study. In his case, he spent seven years in the army, after which he joined Robert Koch's laboratory where he developed vaccination against diphtheria, which disease was killing 70,000 German children each year.

Wars have frequently upset the orderly education of medical candidates. The future Harvard professor of physiology, Henry Pickering Bowditch went off to the American Civil War, delaying his graduation until 1868. In the Spanish Civil War (1936-1939) a future leader of Britain's public health specialists, **Archie Cochrane** (1909-1988) served in a field ambulance supporting the International Brigade. After a year he returned to his medical studies at University College Hospital in London. Upon his re-appearance at ward rounds, the consultant in charge asked: "Had a good weekend?" By the time the Battle of Britain was rending the skies, Cochrane was in the Royal Army Medical Corps, helping to round up German fighter pilots who had been shot down by Spitfire pilots. He had learned German perfectly in Berlin and Vienna after graduating in his premedical courses at Cambridge. This ability was to become a great asset.

Within the year his commando unit had been taken prisoner by German forces invading Crete. He was soon the medical officer to a prisoner of war camp in Salonica, trying to ameliorate "unbelievable levels of infection, malnutrition and Nazi brutality...." It was there that he undertook his "'first, worst and most successful' controlled trial, in search of a cure for famine oedema." In his darkest hours he penned his penetrating war poetry. The scourge of wartime and postwar tuberculosis drove him to a "scientific study of diagnostic and prognostic error," to quote his great friend, Sir Richard Doll. Cochrane's overarching concern as a medical student, both undergraduate and postgraduate, was to cut through the fog of clinical therapeutic claims and to launch randomized clinical trials whose outcome could be trusted. Today, when such undertakings are legion, it is necessary to think of a medical student, personally dogged by porphyria but brave in war and peace. Following is a sample of Cochrane's doggerel: "But death was near and hunger, and prisoners' dreams were rare. The doctor at Salonica sat down and tore his hair."

I am all for the Public Schools but I do not want to go there again.
Winston Spencer Churchill (1874-1965), F.R.S. 1941

Another German-speaking medical student was **Michael H. McPharlin** who, despite great hardships, managed to take his premedical requirements at Bowdoin College in Maine, and at Heidelberg in Germany. He was admitted to Duke University Medical School in 1936, where he became a great favourite, who because of his short stature was christened "wee Michael." He ran out of money and went to sea on freighters and tankers. Eventually he entered the Royal Canadian Air Force where he was soon given a commission and sent to Camp Borden in Ontario to receive basic training. Thereafter he and his American friends received advanced training in their Eagle Squadron (RAF Squadron 71). From Hawker Hurricanes they advanced to the famous Spitfires, and it was while being attacked on the way home from the Canadian raids on Dieppe that McPharlain was set upon by the Luftwaffe and ended up in the sea. He was well-known to the German pilots because he could harangue them in their own tongue. Infuriated, they "went for him." He was sighted in his minute dinghy by a lighthouse keeper who rescued him in a hypothermic state. He returned to his station to find a "wake" for him in progress. After transferring to Mustangs with an American Squadron, he engaged in the bombing of railways during the Normandy landings on D-Day. There he and his flight were killed when a group of 15 Nazi fighter planes dove on them.

RHODES SCHOLARS

Duke University comes into the picture from another era through the activities of its first dean of medicine, Wilburt Davison, and his fellow Rhodes Scholars in World War I, Wilder Penfield and Emil Holman. All were students of Sir William Osler and Professor Charles Sherrington at Oxford. The American triumvirate consisted of two Princeton graduates of 1913 and Emil Holman, a Stanford premedical graduate of 1911, who had spent two years thereafter as secretary to David Starr Jordan, Stanford's president.

Davison was an early volunteer for service at the Red Cross hospital in France, where he became both wound dresser and anaesthetist. Holman was recruited by Herbert Hoover to help with the supervision of foodstuffs sent to the starving Belgians through neutral Holland. Sherrington at Oxford arranged a leave of absence for his star student, Davison (about twice Sherrington's height), to join a voluntary medical group going to war-torn Serbia. Typhus killed there, in 1915, 150,000 people, including 30 per cent of all Serb physicians.

Davison returned to Oxford, at least part way, in the luxury of the yacht *The Erin* with its owner Sir Thomas Lipton of tea fame, who had carried on it volunteers to Salonica. One of the guests on board was the editor of London's *Daily Mail*, who promised Davison, a citizen of a neutral nation, the large sum, for a student, of £15 sterling to proceed from Naples overland to Britain, and to write of his experiences in the news-hungry British press.

En route Davison learned from a convalescing but alcoholic German officer that poison gas was about to be used. British officialdom ignored his report, which was proven true 10 days later as chlorine gas was used against the Allies at Ypres. Penfield had tried to visit the ancient Italian universities but was harassed by border guards, so he returned to Britain and took courses in anatomy at Edinburgh during the summer vacation. Holman became an ambulance driver in a French field hospital.

In the six-week vacation at the end of Oxford's fall term, Penfield crossed to France to the same Red Cross hospital, and was soon carrying on medical responsibilities never given to a second-year medical student in peacetime. In the spring vacation he arranged to return to the hospital at Ris Orangis, travelling from Folkestone across the Channel on the steamer *Sussex*. Unfortunately it was torpedoed with loss of many passengers including Enrique Granados, the Spanish pianist. Penfield was thrown into the air by the explosion and landed on the deck with a badly fractured leg—an injury that dogged him the rest of his life, especially after long brain surgeries in the operating room at

McGill. Sir William Osler sprang into action and had "his" Rhodes scholar brought to his home at Oxford, known for good reasons as "The Open Arms." There Lady Osler—great-granddaughter of Paul Revere—looked after the wounded in style.

These three Americans and a South African Rhodes Scholar, Krige, were all pressed into service as guinea pigs by Osler, so that the new vaccine against typhoid and paratyphoid could be speedily tested. There was no sense in waiting, during a war, for a Home Office licence needed to test the vaccine on rabbits. Thus these students were propelled into the medical literature of 1917.

Davison and Penfield, with letters of recommendation from their pater familias, Sir William Osler, left Oxford for Johns Hopkins Hospital Medical School in Baltimore to complete their M.D. degrees. Davison so astounded Halsted, the famous professor of surgery there, with his knowledge of the care of infected war wounds that Halsted immediately offered him a surgical internship. Penfield carried on, with Professor Howell in physiology, the replacement of blood in wounded soldiers, with fluid substitutes. Holman's record amazed the Hopkins surgeons who surveyed his record as a medical student at Oxford: performed 33 autopsies; anaesthetized more than 100 patients; removed tonsils and adenoids in 24 cases; one hernia repair; several amputations; delivered 31 babies at The Rotunda in Dublin. Cecil Rhodes smiled.

> **[Constant interruptions] deafen with little bells the spirit that would think.**
> Pierre Curie

One cannot view the human losses suffered by the world's youth in recurrent wars—some of that youth being medical students—without remembering the words of medical student contributor Sir Victor Horsley, the many-sided genius, who in 1916, before he died in Mesopotamia, where he was serving as senior surgeon to the British Army, described "the drunken misdirection of our military affairs" and the "apathy and indifference of the whisky drinkers." He said his toughest job was "trying to make the aged and incompetent realize that the British soldier is a human being." He was echoing the words of Florence Nightingale, whom Lytton Strachey describes as an "eagle and no swan": "The three things which all but destroyed the army in the Crimea were ignorance, incapacity and useless rules, and the same thing will happen again unless future regulations are framed more intelligently and administered by better informed and more capable officers."

UPHILL STRUGGLES

Poverty has imposed a barrier and a hurdle to be overcome in the lives of many medical student contributors. Ambroise Paré, destined to be France's greatest surgeon, had to wait from 1536 to 1541 to accumulate enough money to pay the fee required for certification in Paris as a "barber-surgeon." (Paré was specifically spared by Charles IX in the St. Bartholomew's Day massacre of French Protestants in 1572.)

Prejudice has been another barrier to be surmounted. In 1855 Augusta Klumpke, who was born in San Francisco, described an important neurological paralysis when she was a medical student in Paris. She was the first woman in France to be named "interne des hôpitaux" and the furious controversy that ensued was settled only when Paul Bert, the Minister of Public Instruction, confirmed the appointment.

Maude Abbot (1869-1898)

When the future world's expert on congenital heart disease, Maude Seymour Abbott, was a student at Bishop's University Medical School, she was about to be expelled because her case reports on ward patients at the Montreal General Hospital were never completed. The mystery was solved when the professor of surgery, Francis Shepherd caught the hospital's superintendent "red-handed" destroying them. Osler stood by "Maudie" throughout his life, as did Paul Dudley White.

David Gruby (1810-1898)

Another student contributor in the cardiovascular field, and for decades thereafter, was David Gruby. As an undergraduate, he was not allowed to sit in the classrooms of the Piarist Gymnasium in Pesth because of his race. Instead, he heard the lectures while listening quietly outside the lecture hall door, until his teacher, impressed by his ability, broke all rules and admitted him.

Prejudice against women scientists has not been the monopoly of medical institutions alone. Emil Fischer required Lise Meitner to work with Otto Hahn in the carpenter shop, since his institute's laboratories were to remain male preserves. (The same view has held at London's Athenaeum since 1823, to the distress of the Royal Society of London, next door.)

John Beresford Leathes (1864-1956), a son of the Rev. Stanley Leathes, D.D., attended Winchester School and its Wykhamist "cousin" New College, Oxford, in preparation for life in the church. However, Leathes came to the conclusion that he could do more for the world as a medical doctor, and entered Guy's Hospital Medical School, London. As a result his father cut him off with all but one shilling per week. This medical student managed to live with an aunt at Highgate, who gave him breakfast and supper. He walked six miles into London and six miles home again in all sorts of weather. In 1890-91 he worked as a student research assistant to Professor Starling on veratrine and demonstrated in anatomy.

After graduation Leathes never practised medicine, but had a brilliant career studying body metabolism. He was invited to give the Croonian Lectures at the Royal Society of London on "The Role of Fats in Vital Phenomena" and the Harveian Oration at the Royal College of Physicians on "The Birth of Chemical Biology." He taught at the University of Toronto from 1909 to 1914. His last paper (1939) was with another student researcher, Professor John Mellanby at Oxford on thrombokinase.

Harold Scheie was born into a homesteading family in North Dakota, and grew up in a sod house on the Berthold Indian Reservation. He worked his way through the University of Minnesota, where he graduated with honours in 1935, and took up ophthalmology at the University of Pennsylvania. In World War II he served in the U.S. Army in China, India, and Burma, retiring as a brigadier-general. Pennsylvania made him professor of ophthalmology and chairman of his department, from which he retired in 1975.

J. Bruce Beckwith, of the Beckwith-Wiedemann Syndrome, was born in the Flathead Indian Reservation at St. Ignatius, Montana, in 1933.

In 1816, I was consulted by a young woman labouring under general symptoms of diseased heart, and in whose case percussion and the application of the hand were of little avail on account of the great degree of fatness. The other method just mentioned (ear to chest method of Hippocrates) being rendered inadmissible by the age and sex of the patient, I happened to recollect a simple and well-known fact in acoustics, and fancied at the same time, that is might be turned to some use on the present occasion. The fact I allude to is the augmented impression of sound when conveyed through certain solid bodies, as when we hear the scratch of a pin at one end of a piece of wood, in applying our ear to the other. Immediately, on this suggestion, I rolled a quire of paper into a sort of cylinder and applied one end of it to the region of the heart and the other to my ear, and was not a little surprised and pleased, to find that I could thereby perceive the action of the heart in a manner much more clear and distinct than I had ever been able to do by the immediate application of the ear. From this moment I imagined that the circumstance might furnish means of enabling us to ascertain the character, not only of the action of the heart, but of every species of sound produced by motion of all the thoracic viscera.

R.T.H. Laennec,
Auscultation Médiate (1819),
Forbes translation

As a medical student at the University of Washington in Seattle, he developed an early interest in embryology and histology. In 1964 he became the director of pathology at the Children's Orthopaedic Hospital in Seattle and in 1980 was named the distinguished medical alumnus of the school of medicine of the University of Washington. He later filled the directorship of pathology at the Children's Hospital in Denver. His syndrome, described with Professor Wiedemann, the paediatrician and geneticist at Kiel in Germany, was characterized by exophthalmos, macroglossia and gigantism.

Dr. Grey Dimond was another ingenious student. Not only did he finance his medical education from an almost hopeless start, but he later developed a new kind of medical school known today as the University of Missouri-Kansas City School of Medicine.

Dimond entered Purdue University in the state of Indiana on a football scholarship, of which he wrote years later: "Without exaggeration I can say that the two years at Purdue were so stressful, so physically demanding, and such a painful load, lack of money, deterioration of Dad from drink and Mother from cancer... that the rest of my life has been relaxing." Transferring to the University of Indiana for pre-medical studies, he lived in a "funeral home" where he took night calls in exchange for a free room. After a summer spent in tutoring students and swotting embryology and comparative anatomy, and standing up to "a little Caesar" of a medical school dean, he entered upon his four-year medical course.

"I did nothing but study, figure out how to buy a meal, and get enough ahead for rent, tuition and books." He "cut corners" on textbooks, bought an aged microscope for $10, and used up his meagre savings from his janitorial job at Eli Lilly's main factory where he washed windows, mopped floors and emptied wastebaskets. Dimond's mother was able to send him $10 per week. From 5 p.m. to 7 a.m. he worked as an oxygen dispenser, on call at University Medical Centre, at $50 per month, with free room, board and laundry. He took on an additional job as cashier from 5 p.m. to 7 p.m. for another badly needed $50 per month. Understandably, his weight dropped.

Then came, as he said, "the break of breaks." "A notice appeared on the elevators that the Medical Centre's cardiologist needed someone to read medical journals to him for two hours an evening, two evenings a week, and the pay would be two hundred dollars a month." The cardiologist had lost his central vision. A compensatory ability to hear heart sounds through his stethoscope made him the most admired cardiologist in the university. Simultaneously, all medical students were inducted into an army program that supplied free tuition and free uniforms and an income of $600 per month. "By the end of my senior year I had to ask myself when ever again would I be so prosperous! Graduation was a financial blow."

Dimond for all his travail became, with his blind tutor, an outstanding cardiologist. He not only read the entire periodical literature that then existed, but also learned to describe in minute detail the electrocardiographic tracings, and to use the ophthalmoscope on his tutor's patients. For two and a half years as a medical student and for 18 months of house officer training, Dimond studied the patients and their cardiograms with a great teacher.

CHAPTER TWENTY

Serendipity

Lord Cohen of Birkenhead was a great clinician and medical historian. In his Nuffield Lecture to the Royal Society of Medicine on "The Fruits of Error and False Assumption," he quotes Bacon: "Men are rather beholden generally to chance, or anything else, than to logic, for the invention of arts and sciences." Cohen, a member of the Wellcome Trust panel on the history of medicine continued: "The role of the chance observation in scientific discovery... has attracted to itself the word 'serendipity,' first coined in 1754 by Horace Walpole after he had read a fairy tale entitled 'The Three Princes of Serendip' (the ancient name for Ceylon). Writing to his friend, Horace Mann, Walpole suggested that 'serendipity' might be added to our language because 'as their highnesses travelled they were always making discoveries, by accident or sagacity, of things they were not in quest of.'" Osler gave the example of Hearn, the Oxford bibliophile, who thanked Providence "in a particular manner" for "one act when I unexpectedly met with three old manuscripts yesterday."

Serendipity is often the backbone of after-dinner chit-chat by scholars in front of a wood fire—as at New College, Oxford, where a little trolley warms the port before it is repeatedly passed around the circle of Fellows. There one learns of the "lab boy" fed up with the tiresome job of distilling water for the chemical or physiological experiments. One hears of the University College Hospital physician in London, Sidney Ringer, who was able to keep a frog heart beating for a short time only. When, however, the bored laboratory assistant decided to take a shortcut, and to surreptitiously substitute tap water for distilled water, the heart kept on beating for hours. This happy result was then traced to the calcium content of the city's water supply. Ringer added potassium as well, thus producing his solution used universally today.

Paul Ehrlich, working long into the night, left some microscope slides of tubercle bacilli on his laboratory stove. When the *diener* lit the stove next morning the bacteria became exquisitely stained, thus inaugurating, serendipitiously, a new method for demonstrating "acid fast" bacteria. A puzzled Professor Murray Barr at the University of Western Ontario asked his histological technician in 1945 why the nerve cells of some rats showed a particular "dot" in the nucleus while those of other rats failed to show it. Recourse to the records showed that this represented the first cellular difference seen to that date between males and females--the "Barr body"—opening a new chapter in genetics.

Sir Henry Dale, who wrote the wise and subtle foreword to *Young Endeavour* was researching the question of allergic reactions when he found a dead guinea pig whose muscle tissue reacted violently and uncharacteristically, to the slightest trace of horse serum. Dale later wrote: "It occurred to me that many guinea-pigs in that laboratory were used for testing the strength of anti-toxic horse serum and that an economically minded colleague might have provided me with a survivor from such a test. The verification of that suspicion gave us a new idea about the meaning of the anaphylactic or allergic condition." In 1914 Marshall and Davies set out to study the distribution of urea in body tissues. Instead of "wasting" 50 cents on two normal dogs, they used a pair in which Crowe and Wislocki had removed the adrenal glands. They found such an amazing increase in the tissue urea that they discovered the totally unexpected influence of the adrenals on the kidney.

Osler noted in his great *Bibliotheca*, when referring to that apprentice medical student Humphry Davy that Thomas Beddoes had written a paper: "Proposal for the Preservation of Accidental Observations in Medicine." It might well have applied to Davy's observation that nitrous oxide relieved his headaches, and to his prophetic if neglected statement in his "Researches" of 1800: "As nitrous oxide...appears capable of destroying physical pain, it may probably be used with advantage during surgical operations in which no great effusion of blood takes place."

The work of the third-year medical student Alfred Vogel in Vienna on the diuretic effect of mercurial compounds, as opposed to their effect in syphilitic infections, was detailed in the chapter on chemistry. Willius and Dry in their *History of the Heart and the Circulation* considered that Vogel's discovery "has completely revolutionized the treatment of congestive heart failure."

Dr. Michael Smith, recently awarded the Nobel Prize in Chemistry, has told his students at the University of British Columbia that many discoveries are achieved "by people looking at something they're interested in, and making an observation which may not have been directly connected to what they are looking for." While on a sabbatical year at Cambridge University on an entirely different project, he indulged in the traditional laboratory coffee break, and there was suddenly struck by the idea of working with a re-programmed synthetic gene. He, with his colleagues in Vancouver, pursued this idea with great success. He has described the process: "No one sat down and said 'Design a specific mutagenesis method.' We wouldn't have done it. We were doing other things and realized it was something we could apply elsewhere."

And so the journey of the three princes of Serendip goes on.

CHAPTER TWENTY-ONE

Great Teachers of Student Contributors

Throughout this volume it has been evident that the medical undergraduates whose research was noteworthy enjoyed the support, not to say the inspiration, of some great teachers. All these teachers deserve praise. However, a happy load was carried willingly by some notable scholars, such as Purkinje, the great Czech patriot and Ramón y Cajal, in his isolation beyond the Pyrenees. Not all were great lecturers in the narrow classroom sense. Sherrington and Banting shared a halting delivery but energized whole generations of student researchers. Sherrington may have overcompensated by producing at Oxford three other Nobel laureates, Eccles, Florey and Granit. Banting, from personal experience, believed more in students than in professors and set up a foundation to aid young researchers.

William Osler "embodied within himself a whole medical centre. [He was] the gentle sage... The whole world of medicine lays its tribute at his feet."
Brigadier General Francis Winter,
U.S. Army Medical School

He was a very parfit practisour.
Chaucer's Doctor of Physick

The personal factor in the student contributors was clearly one of the propelling forces. When a visitor to Cambridge University asked what Sir Michael Foster, the bearded professor of physiology, had discovered, he was answered in one word, "Men." As already mentioned, Sir William Osler recruited men and women as researchers at Johns Hopkins Medical School in Baltimore, and at Oxford he dragooned three male American Rhodes scholars, Davison, Penfield, and Holman, and one from South Africa, Krige, into being guinea pigs for trials of vaccines against typhoid and paratyphoid, made urgent by the horrific casualties in World War I.

Some of these great teachers influenced whole generations by their lectures and their writings. Osler also qualified for membership in this celebrated group, by writing the most widely read textbook in clinical medicine, which incidentally led to the development the two great research-minded foundations—the Rockefeller and the Nuffield.

From clinical teachers such as Boerhaave in Holland, John Hunter and Joseph Lister in Britain, Louis, Andral, Laennec, Charcot and Pierre Marie in France, Kocher in Switzerland, Paul Dudley White and Harvey Cushing in America, Penfield in Canada, and Billroth in the Germanic world, came an impetus to focus on basic research and its eventual application.

Others served to recruit several generations to the cause of research, such as Thomas Huxley, Peter Medawar, Johannes Müller, Walter Cannon, Rudolf Virchow, and Paul Ehrlich. Through their felicitous pens William

Boyd the Canadian pathologist and Lewis Thomas at Sloan-Kettering in New York awakened a wider interest in research by young hands and minds. John Fulton turned his physiological laboratory at Yale into an international powerhouse in every branch of physiology from synapses to the frontal lobes of the brain, to aviation medicine, and to the history of medical discoveries.

Two statesmen of science, Sir Henry Dale and Dr. Alan Gregg opened the floodgates of research support for young minds. Though Dale was a Nobelist in Medicine, he never held a university professorship. Instead, he became chairman of Britain's Medical Research Council and later of the Wellcome Trust. Gregg, as Director of the Medical Sciences Division of the Rockefeller Foundation, helped to establish medical research facilities around the world. He was keener on brains than on bricks, but he helped on both fronts, through catalytic matching funds.

One medical school dean in Britain described his problem this way: "Our students come to us ignorant but curious. They leave us, ignorant but no longer curious." Times are changing, however, and enlightened foundations are seeking out hospitable medical schools where student research is welcomed and promoted. The future is bright for those who follow in the footsteps of the early pioneering students whose lives are chronicled here.

Another great teacher was **Florence Rena Sabin** (1871-1953), who was born near Denver, Colorado, and graduated from Smith College in zoology and mathematics in the year 1893. In 1896 she entered Johns Hopkins Medical School after three years of teaching experience in Denver and at Woods Hole Laboratories. Her first publication (1897), "On the Anatomical Relations of the Nuclei of Reception of the Cochlear and Vestibular Nerves," has become a classic. In 1900 she published her student research on "A Model of the Medulla Oblongta, Pons and Midbrain of a New-born Babe." This was based on serial microscopic sections—a method used ever since in constructing models in plasticine of the human brain.

In 1917 Dr. Sabin became the first woman to achieve a full professor's rank at Johns Hopkins Hospital Medical School as professor of histology. That was only the beginning. She then took up the study of the lymphatics and, as well, the technique known as supravital staining. By 1924 she was the first woman to become president of the American Association of Anatomists, and a year later the first woman member of the Rockefeller Institute. She was the first woman to be elected to the National Academy of Sciences. In 1934 she published the biography of her mentor and research guide, *Franklin Paine Mall; The story of a Mind*. By then she had accumulated 15 honourary degrees. In 1951 she received the prestigious Lasker Award of the American Public Health Association, and had a building named after her at the University of Colorado School of Medicine, a centre for the study of cellular biology. Dr. Sabin died in 1953 and there is a school in Denver named the Sabin Public School. In the National Statuary Hall in Washington, D.C., there is a statue of Dr. Sabin by Mrs. Joy Buba. In addition to this recognition, Dr. Sabin was awarded the Trudeau and the Jane Addams medals. She was a great teacher.

Dedicatory letter To William Osler, a Master in Medicine.

We, the graduates of the Johns Hopkins Medical School, present to you this collection of our published papers on the occasion of your withdrawal from the Professorship of the Principles and Practice of Medicine in the Johns Hopkins University to accept the Regius Professorship of Medicine at Oxford.

We wish at this time to record our debt of gratitude to you for the influence you exerted on us while we were your students.

We consider it a rare privilege early in our medical work to have had the inspiration of your presence, your precept and your example.

We have learned to esteem you as a teacher and to love you as a man.

You have been an exponent to us of the highest ideals in the science and practice of medicine.

You taught us the importance of careful observation, the necessity for the application of exact methods, and the advantage of the closest relationship between the laboratory and the clinic.

You have inspired us with the desire to contribute, in so far as we are able, to the advancement of medical knowledge.

It is with the deepest regret that we see you leave the Johns Hopkins University, but we are certain that the influence exerted by you during your sojourn there will continue as a great force in the upbuilding of American Medicine.

We give you Godspeed, rejoicing that we could have been your pupils.

May 1st, 1905.

Letter of transmission accompanied by 500 contributions in 12 volumes

Osler wrote:

My chief treasure... A splendid record.

Conclusions

And some seed fell on the good ground and grew and brought forth fruit a hundred fold.

The foregoing chapters have shown the kaleidoscopic nature of life as it has been lived by students and contriibutors over the past 400 years. And yet it is basically a study in growth of men and women and of their ideas, with much depending on the seed, the soil, the nourishment provided, the losses and wastage, and the weather at harvest time.

The seed was the obvious critical factor throughout. Without it there would be nothing to discuss. These students obviously had gray matter. Some critics feel that some of the gray matter in the population is not getting within hailing distance of today's universities.

Some may ask: "If we had the brightest high school graduates within our universities would we have any more student discoverers? Do we not, in some institutions, tend to have a rigid set of rewards and blessings heavily inclined towards the spectacular performer in the classroom?" As James Kendall remarked in his delightful book, *Young Chemists and Great Discoveries*, the Leipzig chemist, Wilhelm Ostwald, used to say that his pupils who later became famous contributors were not those at the head of their classes, but those who had not been satisfied with what had been routinely given out in the classroom. The student contributors in the present volume could be said to have had a constructive curiosity. It is of the type exhibited by the youthful Michael Faraday—son of a blacksmith and apprenticed to a bookbinder—whose early education consisted in the surreptitious reading of the volumes he was binding. This constructive curiosity may be seen in the lives of such physician botanists as Valerius Cordus, Haller, Linnaeus, Garden, Schleiden and Withering, such physician geologists as Bright, Stensen and Jenner, or such ornithologists as T.S. Roberts, the Minnesota paediatrician, and Max Peet, the Michigan neurosurgeon. Some educators feel that with the hubbub of modern university campuses some of the best seed never even falls to the ground, so diverse are the currents of air which sweep over the students and so powerful are the tribal organizations that mold them socially. The passive role of the student is taken for granted in so many colleges that the student who seeks new answers may be a cause for official alarm. Just as college athletics have become spectator sports instead of participant sports, so medical education may have become

Nobody knows how the kindling flame of life and power leaps from one life to another. What is the magic quality in a person which instantly awakens faith? You listen to a hundred persons unmoved and unchanged; you hear a few quiet words from the man with the kindling torch and you suddenly discover what life means for you forever more, and you become forthwith another man, carrying perhaps, your own torch.
Rufus Jones

He who ceases to try to do better ceases to do well.
Oliver Cromwell

Medicine is a science which hath been more professed than laboured, and yet more laboured than advanced, the labour having been more in a circle than in progression.
Lord Bacon

Youth, however eclipsed for a season, is undoubtedly the proper, permanent and genuine condition of man.
Nathaniel Hawthorne

Greater even than the greatest discovery is to keep open the way to future discoveries.
J.J. Abel (1915)

spectator-centred, with real participation by students glossed over.

Whether some of the seed is unusual in appearance or behaviour is patently irrelevant to the main matter of the scientific contribution to be made. Semmelweis, Horsley, Holmes and Carrion were no ordinary men, to mention only a few in this student group, but they advanced humane science.

Another question may be asked: "Was fame the spur in the students discussed in this volume?" It is inconceivable that Semmelweis lived only for the day when his researches on tartar emetic in experimental pneumonia would make him famous, though it was the beginning of his interest in infection. Lister, gazing through his microscope at the muscles of the iris, was not consciously launching his crusade against sepsis, though the talents that he later developed at the microscope led him there. William Harvey, assisting in the researches of his teacher Fabricius, in Padua, little dreamed that he would gather fame in the field of the circulation of the blood, or that he would, as a result, lose half his practice in England.

Then there is the question of the soil, as seen in the laboratory of William Sharpey at University College, London, where Lister, Huxley and James Blake made their early contributions. In Johannes Müller's laboratory, in Berlin, Remak, Helmholtz and Gruby first put their hands to research. Carl Ludwig taught the techniques of investigation to Henry Bowditch, who, in turn, encouraged the student Walter Cannon to apply x-rays to the movements of the gut in animals in his Boston laboratory. In more modern times the laboratories of Sir Henry Dale and Sir Charles Sherrington became nurseries in which hundreds of researchers received their initial stimulus. Sympathetic teachers have done much to encourage discovery.

Sir Geoffrey Jefferson, in his review of some British pioneers in neurology, comments on students who have been, reciprocally, great fertilizers of their teachers' imaginations. He tells of James Ross (1837-1892) holding a bedside clinic at the Manchester Royal Infirmary, on the subject of pleurisy in that part of the lung which touches the diaphragm, sometimes causing a sharp pain in the tip of the shoulder. Ross recorded: "In observing a case of pleurisy a few days ago and casting about for an explanation, one of the students suggested that, considering the connections of the phrenic, the pain might be caused by that nerve." This student, without knowing it, opened up one of the most interesting fields in medicine, that of "referred pain." Purkinje was famous for allowing students to announce, in papers they wrote, discoveries he had made.

Students' medical societies and students' medical libraries have had a great catalytic effect in this field. Sir William Bowman, whose name remains attached to structures in the eye and the kidney, read papers at his student society on haemorrhage, influenza and paraplegia. William Withering as an undergraduate at Edinburgh read two papers to his student society on dropsy, little realizing that as a practitioner in Shropshire he would soon learn from "Old Mother Hutton" of the value of foxglove in the treatment of this disease. A good library and a sympathetic librarian are essential to the development of student contributors. Thanks to the goal set by John Shaw Billings as an undergraduate, all students today have access to the world's medical literature through indices and current lists of the contents of journals, and through microfilms, computer networks and photostats from the National Library of Medicine in Washington, D.C. He started an information revolution.

The choice of a target has helped some to contribute where there was no hospitable soil for the germination of ideas. John Hunter set himself to study inflammation when he was an almost illiterate student; his great work on this subject was published in the last year of his life. (It is related that Abraham Lincoln, floating down the Mississippi on a river barge, at the age of 19, picked out his target—and held to it until the slaves were freed.) Semmelweis marked out his own target as he took special work in obstetrics a few months before he graduated. On seeing the crude barbers doing the dissecting in Paris, Vesalius decided to wrest the scalpel from them, and later to describe in his book the true structure of the human body. Carrion, like an arrow, went straight to the heart of Oroya fever and died in the process. These students lacked the guidance of teachers, and indeed made their contributions despite deep-rooted opposition.

Historically, the nourishment of the seed in the soil has taken some strange forms; the means of support were sometimes pitiful in the extreme. Cotugno lived on radishes and bread and the charity of a hospital for incurables in Italy. Billings lived on a diet consisting, according to Weir Mitchell, of nothing but eggs and milk and the charity of a pioneer hospital in Ohio. Others served in assistantships or as demonstrators, such as Christopher Wren, who, after serving Harvey's pupil Sir Charles Scarborough as a dissector sought to make his way through Oxford University by assisting Thomas Willis, whose arterial circle in the base of the brain he was to illustrate in this capacity. Jean Fernel, and the rejected playwrights Claude Bernard and Brown-Séquard in Paris, lived on their earnings as tutors while pursuing medicine.

The time lost to study, in some of these pursuits, is discussed by Sir Weldon Dalrymple-Champneys in his paper, "The Medical Student Through the Ages," read before the Royal Society of Medicine in London in 1955. He quotes the complaint of a poor student at Bologna in the 15th century: "The time I should spend at lectures and in study I am driven to waste in begging from door to door, crying scores and scores of times, 'Charity, charity, dear masters,' and getting the answer 'Begone, and God be with you.' I appeal both to ecclesiastics and laymen, and am mostly driven from the door, or perchance one may say 'Wait a bit,' when I get a dirty scrap of bread which a dog would reject, or I may get fusty beans, bits of skin or gristle, or sour wine."

Tribute should be paid to the military agencies that subsidized such medical students as Helmholtz, Donders and Pavlov, to name only a few. At a later stage in his career Billings was to have the blessing and financial support of General Barnes in the development of the Surgeon General's Library. To what better use were residual canteen funds ever put after a bitter war?

Wastage may result from poor methods of tilling the soil, and against this evil the best seed is not proof. Charles Robert Darwin (1809-82) was lost to medicine because of the teaching he encountered. His interest in variation in species dates from his early childhood when he told an unsuspecting eight-year-old playmate that he could develop any colour in primroses by merely watering them with coloured solutions. The truth proved to be stranger than even this fiction. He went to study medicine

From my point of view there is only one intellectual infection of any permanent value to the medical student—the scientific spirit and outlook and attitude of mind, which he gets, often unconsciously from his teachers and fellows. If good, it leavens his life work. That he may be steeped in it and be at the same time thoroughly practical is the experience of scores of teachers and scores of pupils, of men of the type of Bowman and Paget. The practical man (whom Mr. C-G. has lauded) was well defined by a general practitioner in my company a few moments ago as one who never learns anything after leaving his hospital. I should be grievous sorry to have any student in whom I was interested come under the influence of a man who in these days could say that 'scientific education may be excellent as an ideal but I doubt if it materially assists the average practitioner in the treatment of disease.' Mr. G. represents a type —the men who jeered at Harvey, scoffed at Pasteur and scorned Lister — the carpenters in surgery and the pill-mongers in medicine, without vision beyond the bench or the counter. The tragedy is that the type persists.
William Osler (1913)

It is not within the power of the properly constructed human mind to be satisfied.
Sir Frederick Banting

"The greatest liberation of thought achieved by the scientific revolution was to have given human beings a sense of a future in this world."
Sir Peter Medawar

"One of the hard things to learn in medicine, even harder to teach, is what it feels like to be a patient."
Lewis Thomas, M.D.

at the University of Edinburgh where his brother was completing his training. Of his own experiences there, Darwin wrote:

> The instruction at Edinburgh was altogether by lectures, and these were intolerably dull, with the exception of those on chemistry by Hope. Dr. Monro (tertius) made his lectures as dull as he was himself, and the subject disgusted me.

The harvest weather has varied considerably for this group of contributors. Einthoven's work was accepted from the first and he lived to see demonstrations of affectionate homage. But the unorthodoxy implied in searching for new truths, and in replacing old ideas with new, has usually collided with orthodoxy in some guise or other. Wilfred Trotter used to say that the mind welcomes a new idea about as graciously as the body welcomes a foreign protein. As mentioned, Harvey lost a large part of his practice. George Sarton has remarked on the tactics of his critics; at first they said his "facts" were not true; then, in retreat, they argued that they were already well-known. Vesalius was pilloried by the "practical men," whom he reviled as being fit only to prescribe for the bowels. His contemporary, Servetus, was burned at the stake by John Calvin who fancied himself divinely guided and who would brook no rival views on theology even when mixed with the discovery of the circulation of the blood through the lungs. Similarly, Morton's ether anaesthesia was attacked by some clerics whose unctuous rectitude was exceeded only by their ignorance. Semmelweis was turned out of the General Hospital in Vienna, as was Freud 40 years later. Stensen was attacked by his teacher Blasius, and Galileo was eventually imprisoned.

What a pity there were no volcanos in the Holy Land. They would have suited the old Hebrew prophets perfectly. Mr. Gates, shaking his fist at a sedate but respectfully attentive board shouted,... `And when you die and come to approach the Judgement of Almighty God, what do you think he will demand of you—yes, each of you? Do you for an instant presume to think He will inquire into your petty failures, your trivial sins, your paltry virtues? No! He will ask you just one question. What did you do as a Trustee of the Rockefeller Foundation?'
Alan Gregg, M.D., 1923

I have come to the conclusion that the stimulation of research is possible when salaried academic personnel can in addition to their teaching duties, do research work. But if that free time is so small that they have to employ additional academically trained assistants...then it becomes a case of creating research—not encouraging it.
Alan Gregg to William C. Gibson, 1954

What does the future hold for the young minds passing through medical schools today? Educators are conscious of the need for prescribed courses for men and women who will one day care for the sick. There is no substitute for that central core of factual knowledge, but, as Alan Gregg has remarked, the mistakes in medicine are not made by those who don't know, but by those who don't care. By overloading undergraduates with a huge amount of detail in some subjects, the sick person is obscured and students become de-sensitized. Over and above the legal minimum of instruction, however, there is the question of how best to develop the enquiring mind. Surely this mind is the patient's greatest guarantee of good diagnosis and rational treatment. The intellect is also the critical factor in discovery and progress in medical science.

Educators can encourage enquiring minds in medicine. Harvey Cushing's criticism of medical education was that it proceeded in convoy fashion, the speed of the fleet being measured by the speed of the slowest ship. He would agree with Fuller's sentiments expressed in 1639 in his *Holy Warre*: "Good is not good when proceeding from them from whom farre better is expected." Is enough expected from the brighter students? Are they challenged to educate themselves, or are they forced to become cynical young onlookers?

What sort of opportunity should be given to "dangerous young infidels" on their way through medical school? It is to be hoped that a new generation of medical comets will be further encouraged in their endeavours after reading these accounts of the pioneers who came before them.

Index

mn=marginal notes